WHEAT
BELLY
COOKBOOK

WHEAT BELLY
COOKBOOK

150 Recipes to Lose the Wheat, Lose the Weight, and Find Your Path Back to Health

WILLIAM DAVIS, MD

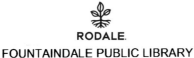

RODALE.

FOUNTAINDALE PUBLIC LIBRARY

300 West Briarcliff Road
Bolingbrook, IL 60440-2894
(630)   759-2102

Exclusive direct mail edition published by Rodale Inc. in October 2012 as *Lose the Wheat, Lose the Weight! Cookbook.*

© 2013 by William Davis, MD

Photographs © 2013 by Rodale Inc.

Rodale books may be purchased for business or promotional use or for special sales.
For information, please write to:
Special Markets Department, Rodale Inc., 733 Third Avenue, New York, NY 10017

Printed in the United States of America

Rodale Inc. makes every effort to use acid-free ♾, recycled paper ♻.

Photographs by Mitch Mandel/Rodale

Before/After photos courtesy of the test panelists

Book design by Carol Angstadt

Library of Congress Cataloging-in-Publication Data

Davis, William
Wheat belly cookbook : 150 recipes to lose the wheat, lose the weight, and find your path back to health /
William Davis, MD.
pages cm
Includes bibliographical references and index.
ISBN 978–1–60961–936–7 hardcover
1. Gluten-free diet—Recipes.   2. Reducing diets—Recipes.   I. Title.
RM237.87.D378 2013
641.5'63—dc23   2012031662

Distributed to the trade by Macmillan

4   6   8   10   9   7   5   3   hardcover

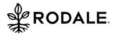

We inspire and enable people to improve their lives and the world around them.
rodalebooks.com

To everyone who has come
to understand the liberation that
emerges with wheatlessness.

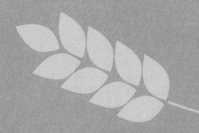

CONTENTS

INTRODUCTION

The truth will set you free, but first it will piss you off.
GLORIA STEINEM

WHEAT IS NOT the "healthy whole grain" it was pretending to be. Like a faithful spouse exposed as a philanderer and polygamist, wheat is not to be trusted. Held up as an icon of health, it is in reality a major contributor to the world's worst epidemic of obesity and an astounding list of health problems, from simple annoyances like dandruff to incapacitating conditions like dementia.

This is a cataclysmic revelation for most people: It's unsettling, it's upsetting, it's downright inconvenient. The condemnation of wheat is as paradigm shifting, earth shattering, and life changing as the emergence of the Internet, the packaging of collateralized debt obligations and the collapse of mortgage markets, the upheavals of the Arab Spring . . . events that shook core beliefs, upended comforting habits, and changed worldviews.

Wheat is the Enron of the food world, the tobacco industry all over again—frauds, both intentional and inadvertent, conducted on an international scale. Charming and engaging on the outside, sociopathic and destructive on the inside, it works its way into your life, wreaking havoc in every conceivable health-destroying way.

These are, for those of you unfamiliar with the arguments set forth in *Wheat Belly: Lose the Wheat, Lose the Weight, and Find Your Path Back to Health* (Rodale, 2011), undoubtedly bold assertions that fly in the face of nutritional wisdom. The Dietary Guidelines for Americans issued by the USDA and the US Department of Health and Human Services, as well as the American Heart Association, the American Diabetes Association, and the Academy of Nutrition and Dietetics all agree: Healthy whole grains should make up a substantial portion of your diet.

This is colossally bad advice. "Eat more healthy whole grains" is among the biggest health blunders ever made in the history of nutritional advice. Modern health care, treating millions of people at the cost of hundreds of billions of dollars every year for hypertension, high cholesterol, obesity, arthritis, acid reflux, irritable bowel syndrome, fibromyalgia, migraine headaches, depression, diabetes, various forms of neurological impairment, and on and on, is really treating . . . wheat consumption. And the endlessly repeated advice to eat more "healthy whole grains" fuels this fire, much to the appreciative applause of the pharmaceutical industry. After all, the pharmaceutical industry funds a good part of the wheat lobby promoting and propagating this message. Oh, you didn't know that? Yes, a long list of drug manufacturers have close financial ties to the organizations that lobby Congress, help establish school lunch policy, and get cozy with the USDA to maintain the lofty nutritional role of "healthy whole grains."

And, yes, the clinical studies documenting these arguments have already been performed, but rarely do they make the light of day in media supported by Big Food, who count wheat products among the handful of commoditized ingredients, subsidized by the US government, that serve as the basis for most processed foods.

In health, as in software, we are living examples of the principle of *garbage in, garbage out*. Put this stuff, the creation of geneticists from the 1960s and 1970s, into your body, and you get all manner of unanticipated health effects.

Since the release of *Wheat Belly*, I have become convinced that not only is this an incredibly big issue for health, the situation is *worse* than it first appeared. It has affected far more people than I originally anticipated and to such an extraordinary degree that it is difficult to overestimate the severity of this problem. This is no fad that will flare and then burn out, much as the misguided low-fat notion has. This is *not* a dietary precept like "get more fiber." It is an exposure of the genetic and biochemical changes introduced into this common foodstuff, all in the name of increased yield-per-acre, but with no questions asked about its suitability for human consumption.

We are, in effect, experiencing the consequences of a grand agricultural experiment gone sour.

Hey, Marlboro Man: Have a Bagel!

Remember this? "According to a nationwide survey: More doctors smoke Camels than any other cigarette"? In the mid- and latter 20th century, the national discussion went from gushing about the pleasures and health benefits of smoking, to studies documenting the health damage caused by smoking, to executives denying any wrongdoing to Congress, to uncovering concealed documents demonstrating the industry's knowledge of the adverse health effects of smoking *decades* earlier.

We are reliving the tobacco experience with wheat in its place. I believe that smart food scientists stumbled on the *appetite-stimulating effect* of the gliadin protein in wheat *25 years ago*. How else do we explain why wheat is in virtually all processed foods, from tomato soup to licorice? In 1960, you would have found wheat in bread, rolls, and cakes—obvious places that make sense. Go up and down the food aisles in your local supermarket in the 21st century, and you will find that nearly *all* canned, packaged, and frozen foods contain wheat in some form. Is wheat that necessary for taste, or for texture? I don't think so. I think it's put there for one reason: to stimulate your appetite and increase sales.

The transformation of the gliadin protein in newly created strains of wheat was accompanied by an increase in calorie consumption of 440 calories per day. By putting wheat in everything, the food industry, especially Big Food, ensured that you come back for more. Just as tobacco manufacturers increased nicotine content of cigarettes to ensure addiction, so adding wheat to every processed food created addictive behavior in response to all things wheat. Eating 440 more calories per day, 365 days per year—not only does that add up to a lot of calories and a lot more food consumed, it adds up to a lot more weight. (Using a simple calories-in calculation, this yields 160,000 calories, or *45.8 pounds* gained in a year. This is an oversimplification, since calories-in, calories-out is a flawed concept, but it nonetheless illustrates how substantial this effect can be.) The introduction of the new form of gliadin was followed shortly thereafter by a nationwide increase in weight. After people gained 30, 50, 60, or more pounds, an explosive surge in diabetes followed. We are now in the midst of the worst epidemic of diabetes ever experienced by humans, such that the curve showing the number of people with diabetes is in a vertical climb straight upward, a trajectory that is likely to engulf your children and grandchildren.

The gliadin protein of wheat ensures that wheat products, such as whole grain or white breads, bagels, and muffins, are *addictive:* They generate a need for more . . . and more, and more. Gliadin is an *opiate*, you will discover, with its own form of euphoria and its very own *opiate withdrawal syndrome* when wheat consumption stops that can also be provoked with opiate-blocking drugs.

So the inadvertent transformation of wheat gliadin into a much more potent appetite stimulant, recognized quickly by observant food scientists, brought us here, to this overweight, diabetic situation that now plagues Americans and much of the rest of the developed world . . . while we are advised to eat more "healthy whole grains." No doubt, many people profited handsomely—and continue to do so—from this message, but the public has paid the price, both with their pocketbooks and their health.

There's Power in Them Tweets

Since the release of the first *Wheat Belly*, social media has served the role of a worldwide stage for these arguments to play out.

Some things, when enacted in real life in real people, are so consistent and powerful that, despite their anecdotal nature, they serve to reinforce what we learn through scientific observation. If I hit my head with a hammer and it hurts, and my head stops hurting when I stop hitting it, do I need a double-blind, randomized clinical trial to prove that hitting my head with a hammer causes head pain? The association is so consistent and obvious that you can safely accept the premise that the hammer is the cause. Likewise, eliminating wheat has been demonstrated, through the thousands of people who have embraced these ideas, to produce life-changing transformations of health and weight that most thought were impossible, allowing them to throw away multiple medications and leave behind years of pain, wheezing, diarrhea, cramps, swelling, fatigue—within *days* of saying goodbye to their bran muffins or breakfast cereal.

In the Middle East, social media allowed the masses to organize, communicate, and overthrow despotic dictators. In no other time in history could dissent disseminate so rapidly, revolt be organized within hours. Likewise, social media is now showing us, on an unprecedented scale and abbreviated timeline, that rejecting all things wheat is among the most powerful and liberating health strategies imaginable. We purge this Muammar Gaddafi of diet using the facility and speed of Twitter, Facebook, and other electronic media, spreading the word of dietary revolution using the very same tools.

This is not a popular message at the USDA, or in the halls of Big Food and Big Agribusiness. It's not uncommon, for instance, for agribusiness giant Monsanto to spend more than $2 billion *per quarter* to lobby the federal government to influence policymakers—and that's just one company.

Dollar for dollar, we cannot even begin to compete with such forces. Ah, but we can talk to each other and share our experiences, something that these dominating corporate forces are unlikely to do with us.

Lose the Wheat, Lose the Weight . . . and the Acid Reflux, and the Edema, and the Mental "Fog" . . .

Much like when you stop hitting your head with a hammer and the headache miraculously goes away, so eliminating all wheat from the diet is followed by the majority of people experiencing abrupt and substantial weight loss along with relief from a long list of health conditions.

In other words, the proof of this concept is in your own hands, a simple rearrangement of food priorities in your own pantry. You don't have to wait for a large-scale clinical trial to know whether this is relevant to your health situation. If you decide to wait for national advice to embrace this concept, you are going to wait a very, very long time. How do official agencies undo the disastrous advice of the last 40 years without losing credibility, without incurring legal liability for the unimaginable economic damages—and without losing the revenue stream that this corrupt message has generated? You don't have to wait. You can start the process and know within *days* whether this thing called wheat has been to blame for your health and weight.

The total effect experienced in eliminating wheat is greater than the sum of its parts: It's a 2 + 2 = 11 phenomenon. That's no typo. Getting rid of wheat is *that* big. Despite our knowing about many of the undesirable changes introduced by geneticists into modern wheat, the health changes—health *transformations*—experienced by most people who say good-bye to wheat are often *far greater than we'd predict*. It makes for some of the most compelling success stories in weight and health you could imagine.

Gluten-Free . . . and Other Blunders

A growing number of people are declaring themselves gluten free, thereby buying and consuming gluten-free foods.

Big mistake. Yes, it's a very good thing to avoid the gluten from wheat. But this can take you down the path of gluten-free processed foods. Oddly, the majority of manufacturers of gluten-free foods have chosen to base their products—with rare exceptions—on rice starch, cornstarch, potato starch, and tapioca starch. While they may provide a reasonable facsimile of gluten-containing wheat flour–based products in taste and texture, they are among the few foods that raise blood sugar *even higher* than the high levels generated by wheat products. In other words, gluten-free multigrain bread or gluten-free pasta, from the perspective of high levels of blood sugar and its consequences, are

poor choices as replacements for wheat.

So we should be *wheat* free and *gluten* free, but also *free of gluten-free foods* made with junk carbohydrates.

A bit confusing, yes. This was part of my motivation for adding the *Wheat Belly Cookbook* to the discussion, to help you re-create delicious foods without wheat and without the rice starch, cornstarch, potato starch, and tapioca starch of commercial gluten-free foods. The recipes presented herein are tasty, don't screw with blood sugar, don't trigger appetite, and are truly healthy—a novel concept!

Lettuce and Cardboard?

For many people, the prospect of giving up wheat is daunting, even downright terrifying, especially since wheat comes with its very own withdrawal syndrome. Not only might you be deprived of something that yields an addictive relationship, but what foods will remain? Will you starve? Will you have to live on lettuce, cardboard, and tasteless replacement foods?

Not at all. As many wheat-free people will attest, foods minus wheat are actually *more* enjoyable. A fundamental change occurs when you remove this addictive food: You enjoy food for its own sake, not because there is an appetite stimulant present making you eat anything you can get your hands on. Taste is heightened: You are better able to discern the nuances of foods, but also more sensitive to sweetness, with formerly tasty treats now sickeningly sweet. You are less hungry to the tune of 440 fewer calories per day; what you eat, you enjoy *more* since you are having *less*.

Foods can be wonderfully varied without wheat. In addition to beef burgundy and pizza, you can have muffins, cookies, pies, scones, and other former wheat-containing foods, made using truly healthy ingredients. These are among the 150 recipes in the *Wheat Belly Cookbook.*

What this is *not* is a gluten-free cookbook. No food manufacturer or author of a gluten-free cookbook I know of yet understands the principles of healthy wheat-free, gluten-free eating sufficiently to craft truly healthy gluten-free food. If you want to get fat and diabetic, develop cataracts and arthritis, and grow a belly full of inflammatory visceral fat, eat gluten-free substitutes sold in stores or follow the recipes in the newest gluten-free cookbook. So the recipes I've developed here are indeed free of wheat and gluten, limited in carbohydrate exposure—and truly healthy.

Quit Your Bellyaching!

"Don't you miss it?" and "Aren't you tempted to eat a doughnut?" are among the common questions from those contemplating a life sans wheat.

If, by the end of these opening chapters, you aren't eyeing your beloved multigrain bread or onion ciabatta with suspicion or outright horror, then I haven't done my job. I see my role as exposing these arguments to the light of day for all to see, not just the tarted-up, hunky-dory version presented to us by those who profit from influencing the message. My hope is that, by the time you have finished reading the first few chapters, you will understand that not only is this creation of genetics research awful for weight and health, it is downright deadly. Removing it is . . . liberating. It's the rainbow after the storm, remission after cancer treatment, viewing bright colors after a lifetime of blindness.

Be sure to read the success stories that I've peppered throughout the recipe section detailing many of the compelling tales of health and weight turnarounds that have come my way ever since this message has gained an international audience. Read real stories of dramatic weight loss, relief from crippling health conditions, transformations of children's behaviors—all from people denying themselves the effects of this creation of modern genetics research called wheat.

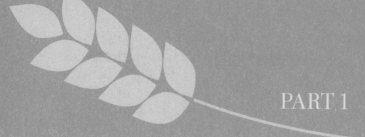

PART 1

HEALTH, WEIGHT, AND LIFE THE WHEAT BELLY WAY

Let's begin by surveying the wheat landscape. We find that it is no longer a field of beautiful "amber waves of grain," but a field of something different. It is also a battleground of obesity, diabetes, and legions of people who have succumbed to its effects.

We begin the discussion on modern wheat in three parts.

FRANKENGRAIN

Agricultural scientists have stitched the genetics of this thing together, concocted from extensive, sometimes bizarre experiments to increase yield-per-acre of wheat.

How has it changed? Just as the Frankenstein monster, the creature created with body parts woven together in a laboratory, terrorized the countryside, so this Frankengrain has worked its way onto your kitchen table, doing its dirty deeds on your health. This gets a bit complicated, but you will discover that the deeper we dig, the worse it gets. You will gain an understanding of just how far off course this thing has been taken from its natural state.

WHY DOES MY STOMACH HURT? AND WHY DO MY JOINTS ACHE, AND MY BOWELS RUMBLE, AND MY FEET SWELL, AND MY . . .

It's not wheat. At least it's not the wheat of 1950, and certainly not the wheat of centuries past. It's no more wheat than rapper Snoop Dogg is Wolfgang Amadeus Mozart.

This creation of the genetics laboratory is different, altered in fundamental ways that increase appetite, ignite inflammation, grow visceral fat, skyrocket blood sugar, destroy intestinal and joint health, and wreak a long list of other havoc on health and metabolism.

WELCOME TO THE WONDERFUL STATE OF WHEATLESSNESS

If consuming modern wheat makes us fat and destroys our health, then removing it should undo the entire mess . . . and it does!

Remove sugar and you lose a few pounds and blood sugar trends down. Remove wheat and joints feel better, acid reflux goes away, rashes disappear, mental "fog" disappears, energy increases, sleep is deeper, food obsessions are gone, asthma improves or disappears, leg swelling shrinks—oh, and you lose a few pounds and blood sugar trends down. Nothing—*nothing*—matches the health impact of losing the wheat, the "healthy whole grains," in your diet.

We go one step further: If you eliminate wheat, health and weight are not necessarily ideal if you continue to consume soft drinks, gumdrops, and their dietary equivalents. So we also discuss why limiting nonwheat carbohydrates is important, too, especially if you are trying to lose weight.

We then tackle the day-to-day particulars in . . .

ASSEMBLING YOUR WHEAT BELLY KITCHEN

Here we discuss everything from what to banish from your kitchen to what wheat-free flours to choose to re-create cupcakes, cookies, and cheesecake. Life is good after saying goodbye to wheat! You are healthier, more energetic, and more slender—while indulging in delicious brownies and pizza.

Okay, let's get started and kiss your sorry wheat-consuming butt goodbye!

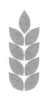

FRANKENGRAIN

WHEAT ENCAPSULATES a fundamental dilemma of our technological age: How much should we permit modern agriculture to modify our food, change its genetics, alter its biochemistry—but not tell us *what* they did, *how* they did it, *why* they did it, and that there are potentially uncertain effects on us unwitting humans who consume it with our breakfast burrito?

If your hairdresser one day decided to give you a new hairdo and dye your curls red, surely she would discuss this with you first. If your spouse decided that life would be better in Anchorage, Alaska, wouldn't it first come with a bit of discussion?

The production of our food does not seem to adhere to such common courtesies. Food crops and livestock are changed, you

buy them, you eat them—no questions asked. The changes introduced are not just that of a new color, or an adaptation to grow under some unique condition. The food is, in many cases, fundamentally changed.

More than any other common foodstuff, wheat stands apart as the most changed. Selling bread, pretzels, or ciabattas to you under the guise of wheat is a deception that you would not tolerate in other areas of your life, certainly not from your hairdresser or spouse.

Modern wheat represents the technological capabilities of agricultural geneticists that predate the age of genetic engineering and genetic modification, the use of gene-splicing technology to insert or delete a gene. Wheat represents the brain-child of genetics manipulations that were employed before such technologies were developed. Wheat represents the product of genetic methods that were crude, often stumbling, less controllable, less predict-able—*far worse* than genetic modification. Yes, believe it or not, modern genetic modification using gene-splicing technology to insert or delete single genes, as frightening as it may be in its implications to mess with nature's design, represents a substantial *improvement* over what geneticists were doing previously.

Using breeding methods that predate genetic modification, geneticists were unable to precisely control which genes were changed, which genes were turned on or turned off, and whether entirely new and unique genetic traits were created by accident. They simply looked for the characteristics relevant to their own interests, such as shorter height or greater yield, but had no real interest in nor insight into what the total package did to humans. Why would they, since none of us ever asked?

And yet the products of these stumbling early efforts at creating "improved" genetic variations of your food are already on your store shelves. And you've been consuming them for something like 35 years.

Healthy Whole . . . What?

"Healthy whole grains." It is the mantra you hear and see repeated dozens of times each day in TV commercials, on cereal boxes and bread wrappers, and by well-meaning people offering nutritional advice. The message is delivered by happy moms, sports figures, superheroes and well-dressed leprechauns, well-intended nutritionists and concerned physicians. Whole grains are good for everybody, they say: every man, woman, and child, from infancy on up to our retirement years. Whole grains reduce weight gain, colon cancer, diabetes, and heart disease. Whole grains make you regular. Whole grains should represent the biggest part of your diet every day.

Just what are "healthy whole grains"? By "grains," we nearly always mean wheat. After all, how many times a day do you sit down to a sandwich with bread made of sorghum flour, breakfast cereal made of quinoa, or pancakes made with millet and buckwheat? If you are like most people, it is rare to never. It's wheat that constitutes nearly all of what most people consider "whole grains" and thereby dominates consumption. Whole wheat, along with white flour products in their many and varied forms, dominates the diets of most people, adding up to 20 percent of all human calories. It's wheat that's in your pizza crust, bagels, pretzels, bread, pasta, muffins, breakfast cereals, doughnuts, hamburger and hot dog rolls, dinner rolls, bread crumbs and breading, pitas, wraps, subs, and sandwiches. And those are just the obvious sources.

Grains occupy the widest part of the former Food Pyramid, and now the largest segment of the Food Plate, the graphic renditions of the Dietary Guidelines for Americans. School lunch programs aim to include more "healthy whole grains," and educators teach children that "healthy whole grains" should be a part of every child's daily eating habits. Grains, we are told, are good for us, and without them our health will suffer.

So, just what is this thing called "wheat" that occupies a huge chunk of the modern diet?

It's not what you thought it was. I would argue that it's not wheat, or at least it is far removed from the wheat of 1950 that predates the extensive genetics transformations introduced during the 1960s and 1970s. But these crude genetics efforts were successful in delivering what geneticists were striving for: increased yield. To a lesser degree, efforts in wheat breeding were aimed at cultivating characteristics like resistance to drought or high temperature, or the ability to fight infestations like molds. But most of the genetic changes introduced into modern wheat were performed to increase yield-per-acre. And, from the perspective of yield, the new genetic strains of wheat were successful—on a grand scale. From the perspective of Third World countries, for instance, that adopted high-yield wheat strains in the 1970s, famine was converted to surplus within a year of their introduction. High-yield strains of wheat became cause for celebration.

But the day after the big party brings the . . . hangover. Sure, it yielded previously unimaginable riches in yield and fed the hungry. But at what price?

This modern product of genetics research looks different. Nearly all the wheat grown today in all parts of the world stands 18 inches to 2 feet tall, a semi-dwarf strain (full dwarf strains stand 12 to 18 inches tall) with a thick shaft that resists buckling in the wind and rain, a large seed head, and larger-than-normal seeds. (Seeds are harvested to make flour.) With heavy nitrogen fertilizer application, modern semi-dwarf wheat yields tenfold more per acre than its traditional 4½-foot-tall predecessor.

But changes in height and yield are only the start. Outward changes in appearance are unavoidably accompanied by changes in biochemical makeup. Just one hybridization, for instance, of two parent wheat plants can yield 5 percent unique proteins not found in either parent. Modern high-yield, semi-dwarf wheat is not the result of a few hybridizations, but the result of thousands of hybridization events conducted by geneticists, repeated breeding to select for qualities like height and seed size, resulting in the creation of many unique proteins and other compounds. And breeding efforts ventured much further than just crossing two plants, often employing techniques we'd consider extreme or bizarre. It means that this new breed of wheat introduces hundreds of unique compounds to consuming humans never before encountered in nature. More on that later.

Problem: Geneticists assumed that, regardless of the degree of genetic changes introduced into the plant, no matter how severe the change in appearance, no matter how bizarre some of the methods used to generate those changes, it remains suitable for human consumption.

Tinkering with the Dinkel

Modern wheat is not wheat, any more than a human is a hairless chimpanzee.

As primates, we keep company with chimpanzees, orangutans, gorillas, and baboons. While apes have 48 chromosomes and humans have 46 (due to the fusion of two ape chromosomes), I'm certain you would object if I brought an orangutan to your home for dinner. Despite the extensive overlap in genetics, the outward differences are obvious. And there are internal biochemical and physiologic differences hidden beneath the obvious.

I have 46 chromosomes. You have 46 chromosomes. A Yanomamo tribesman from the Amazon rain forest has 46 chromosomes. A 4-foot-10-inch, dark-skinned Tasmanian Aboriginal woman has 46 chromosomes, as does a Nunavut Inuit hunter from northern Canada. There are marked outward differences among us humans, yet we all share an identical number of chromosomes.

Not so with wheat. Einkorn wheat, ancestor of all modern wheat, harvested by hunter-gatherers in the Fertile Crescent 10,000 years ago, is a 14-chromosome wild grain. The wheat of the Bible, emmer wheat, also grew wild in the Middle East and bears 28 chromosomes. Strains of wheat that predate human genetic intervention, the crop cultivated by humans during the Middle Ages through the 19th and early 20th centuries in North America and Europe, were 42-chromosome plants. Modern wheat of the 21st century is also a 42-chromosome plant. But our modern strains, thanks to genetic changes introduced by humans for our own purposes, contain new and unique characteristics, among them an inability to survive in the wild. Modern wheat is many thousands of years and many genes apart from 14-chromosome einkorn, 28-chromosome emmer, and even the 42-chromosome wheat of the 19th century.

The genetic story behind the evolution of wheat has only come to be appreciated over the last 100 years. In 1913, a German scientist named Schultz developed the first genetic classification of wheat. He divided wheat into three categories: einkorn, emmer, and dinkel. Five years later, a Japanese scientist performed a chromosomal analysis, making the determination that einkorn contained 14 chromosomes, emmer 28 chromosomes, and dinkel 42 chromosomes. The dinkel of that day was pretty much untouched by genetic changes, representing only the crude year-over-year efforts by farmers to select for qualities such as hardiness and ability to survive a cold spell. (Since then, kamut has been identified as another 28-chromosome form of wheat and spelt another variation on 42-chromosome wheat.)

It's dinkel that now dominates the world's wheat and has been the recipient of all the attentions of geneticists. With 42 chromosomes, dinkel proved to be better suited to the tinkering of geneticists. Now called *Triticum aestivum*, dinkel wheat is a hardy "hexaploid" version, meaning it comes with three complete pairs of chromosomes ("hex" means six), unlike einkorn's single and emmer's two paired sets. The greater genetic potential of hexaploid *Triticum aestivum* means more adaptability and hardiness—and greater potential for genetic changes to be introduced by clever human geneticists.

So dinkel, 42-chromosome hexaploid *Triticum aestivum*, is the form of wheat that geneticists fiddled with, striving to increase yield-per-acre during the 1960s and 1970s. While the Cold War was smack in the center of consciousness at that time, the full realization of the power of science to do both good and bad had not yet focused on agriculture. Agricultural science was still young and full of promise, not yet having acquired the tarnished reputation that was to come in the future with herbicides like 2,4-D and 2,4,5-T (the two main components of Agent Orange, used to defoliate the jungles of Vietnam, Laos, and Cambodia, resulting in the maiming of hundreds of thousands of natives and American soldiers) and pesticides like DDT that were linked to infertility and birth defects.

During those years, agricultural geneticists worked free from concerns about toxicity and the implications for humans consuming the products of their genetic redesigns. It was still the age of science for the sake of science, with little to no thought devoted to potential consequences for exposed humans.

The techniques used to transform dinkel wheat involved plenty more than just mating two plants. The current strains of wheat—high-yield, semi-dwarf strains—were generated using repetitive hybridization (crossing two strains), wide crossing (crossing two very dissimilar plants, even distantly related wild grasses, to generate unique genetic combinations), repetitive backcrossing (repeatedly crossing to winnow out a specific genetic characteristic), embryo "rescue" (artificially sustaining an embryo of a hybrid that would have died naturally due to mutations), and chemical, gamma ray, and x-ray mutagenesis (the purposeful provocation of mutations, followed by cultivation of desired mutants). Most modern strains are the result of many, if not all, of these techniques.

Semi-dwarf wheat started with the 42-chromosome mutant spawn of the Norin 10 dwarf strain from Japan and the Brevor 14 strain from Washington. Progress in developing an especially high-yield strain of wheat was accelerated with the dedication and ingenuity of Dr. Norman Borlaug and colleagues working in Mexico City at the International Maize and Wheat Improvement Center (IMWIC). Thousands of hybridization experiments, crossing strains repeatedly, shuttling seeds back and forth between two very different climates (the high-temperature, low-altitude plains of the Yaquí Valley and the lower-temperature, high-altitude mountains of the Sierra Madre Oriental), helped create a unique, never-before-seen strain of wheat: exceptionally high-yield (tenfold greater yield-per-acre), short (18 to 24 inches tall), with a thick stem and large seeds.

Mexican farmers quickly recognized the production advantages of this super-yielding strain. It was exported to other countries, including the United States, Canada, India, China, and elsewhere. Adopted reluctantly at first in the United States and Canada in the late 1970s because farmers thought it looked peculiar, word spread quickly about this new odd-looking semi-dwarf strain once the remarkable yield-per-acre became evident, and it was embraced widely by the early 1980s. By 1985, virtually all wheat grown in the United States and Canada was the high-yielding semi-dwarf strain. Today, nearly all wheat grown worldwide is the semi-dwarf strain, with only small odd pockets of older strains still under cultivation in southern France, parts of Italy, and the Middle East.

This brings us to the present. Today, the wheat products you are sold in the form of whole grain or white bread, bagels, cookies, cakes, pretzels, pizza, and breakfast cereals, as well as the myriad other clever ways food manufacturers have managed to transform this grain, originate with the semi-dwarf brainchild of genetics research.

It's not wild einkorn, it's not biblical emmer, it's not spelt or kamut of the Middle Ages, it's not the dinkel of the 19th century. Modern wheat with its newly introduced genetic changes is uniquely and genetically suited to accommodate our demands for increased yield, more desirable baking characteristics, and more pliable dough.

It's just not perfectly suited for human consumption.

What Changed?

While wheat has been a problematic food for as long as humans have consumed it (with records suggesting celiac disease, or intestinal damage from wheat gluten, for instance, as long ago as AD 100), modern changes introduced by geneticists made it much worse.

Now, if you take me at my word that wheat has been changed extensively at the hands of geneticists but don't care to know all the details, then skim the heavy stuff over the next several pages. But if you desire a deeper understanding of what exactly changed, then pour yourself another cup of coffee and read on. Warning: The discussion unavoidably gets a bit complicated for the next several pages. But there are truly important details here for those of you who want to know just what happened.

So what exactly changed?

First, there are obvious outward changes visible to the naked eye. The knee-high semi-dwarf plant has a shorter stalk that diverts less fertilizer and nutrients from the seeds. This change in height is due to changes in Rht (reduced height) genes that code for the protein gibberellin, controlling stalk length (discussed later). The seed head is larger, with seeds that are also bigger and different in shape. While there is variation among the 25,000 modern strains, semi-dwarf wheat also tends to have reduced protein content and higher carbohydrate content, and it yields different baking and texture characteristics.

The differences in outward appearance are accompanied by internal genetic and biochemical differences.

Gliadin

Gliadin is among the most interesting—and most destructive—of all the many components of modern wheat.

Gliadin is one of the proteins in the gluten family of proteins. Gluten is actually a combination of smaller gliadin proteins and lengthier glutenin molecules. While gluten is often fingered as the source of wheat's problems, it's really gliadin that is the culprit behind many health issues.

Gliadin can assume many forms, with more than 200 gene variants coding for as many variations of gliadin protein. The past 50 years of genetics research has introduced extensive changes into gliadin structure, but the full implications of these changes have not been fully mapped out, as they were assumed to be benign. And, after all, this research was performed by agricultural scientists, not physicians or people with insights into human health. Changes in gliadin have therefore been dismissed as

harmless, despite the fact that gliadin is capable of increasing intestinal "leakiness" to foreign proteins and triggering cross-reactions with human structures (i.e., triggering an abnormal immune response to similar, though not identical, proteins in the body, a process called molecular mimicry), such as nervous system proteins like synaptin, cells of the intestinal lining (enterocytes), or the ubiquitous calcium-modulating protein calreticulin, potentially triggering inflammatory and immune responses to these proteins.

The changes introduced over the past 50 years in particular have increased the expression of the Glia-α9 amino acid sequence within gliadin that has been most closely linked to triggering celiac disease. While the genetic sequence coding for Glia-α9 was absent from most strains of wheat from the 19th and early 20th centuries, it is now present in nearly all modern varieties. Glia-α9 is a perfect fit for the transglutaminase enzyme that activates it into the form that strongly binds immune-activating ("HLA DQ") molecules lining the intestinal wall, activating the characteristic T-cell immune response that sets celiac disease in motion. The dramatically increased presence of Glia-α9 likely explains why there has been a fourfold increase in celiac disease since 1948. (Interestingly, the Glia-α9 sequence, coded for on the sixth chromosome of the "D" collection of genes in modern wheat, is also absent from primitive strains of wheat that lack "D" genes, such as einkorn, which contains only the "A" set of genes, and emmer, which contains the "A" and "B" sets of genes.)

Opiates, such as heroin, have been shown to activate appetite in addition to pain relief and euphoria. Likewise, the new forms of wheat gliadin have been shown to have effects on the human brain via binding to opiate receptors—yes, opiate receptors, the very same receptors that are activated by heroin, morphine, and Oxycontin. The opiate-like effects of wheat gliadin, however, are less of a "high" and more that of increased appetite and increased calorie consumption, with studies demonstrating a very consistent increased calorie intake of 400 or more calories per day (see "Wheat Gliadin and Exorphins: The Ultimate Obesogens" on page 10). Blocking gliadin with opiate-blocking drugs like naloxone and naltrexone has been shown to reduce calorie consumption by 400 calories per day and induce weight loss of 25 pounds over 6 to 12 months.

Glia-α9 represents just one change introduced into so-called α-gliadins. Changes have also been introduced into the three other fractions of gliadin, including the Ω-gliadin responsible for some forms of wheat allergy and anaphylaxis, and γ-gliadin that, along with the α form, bind HLA DQ. The full effect of these changes, given the widely held assumption that wheat is good for health, has not been fully explored.

Gluten

Gluten is the stuff that confers the viscoelastic properties that are unique to wheat dough, the stretchability and moldability that allow it to be so accommodating to bakers and shapeable into so many varied configurations, from pretzels to pizza. Gluten is also popular as an additive to processed foods like sauces, instant soups, and frozen foods, causing the average person to ingest from 15 to 20 grams per day.

Gluten is a diverse collection of proteins that vary from wheat strain to wheat strain. Gluten is the recipient of much genetic manipulation, as the long chain and branching structure of the glutenin proteins within gluten determine baking characteristics (firmness, sturdiness, bendability, stretchability, crust formation). Geneticists therefore bred and crossbred wheat strains repeatedly to achieve desired baking characteristics, bred wheat with nonwheat grasses to introduce new genes, and used chemicals and radiation to induce mutations that included new and unique changes in glutenin characteristics.

In addition to adding lightness to doughnuts and chewiness to wraps, gluten is also among the most destructive of proteins in the human diet, thanks to its ability to bind to what are called HLA DQ proteins (via gliadin) along the insides of the human intestinal tract. People with specific genetically determined forms of the HLA DQ proteins, such as DQ2 and DQ8, are especially prone to this effect, yielding inflammatory responses that result in celiac disease or sensitivity to gluten. Up to 30 percent of the population has either the DQ2 or DQ8 genes—by no means rare, though only around 1 percent of people with either DQ gene will develop the full-blown celiac disease syndrome, while another 10 percent develop gluten sensitivity. (It's not entirely clear why some people develop gluten sensitivity with symptoms of abdominal cramps, gas, diarrhea, etc., while others develop more severe celiac disease.)

Other important changes have been introduced into gliadin proteins of gluten (see page 9), including enrichment of the

Wheat Gliadin and Exorphins: The Ultimate Obesogens

Obesity research has raised an intriguing question: Are we being exposed to industrial chemicals that cause weight gain and contribute to the obesity epidemic? Bisphenol A (BPA), which is found in polycarbonate plastics and the resin lining of cans, and the pesticide atrazine, for instance, are two compounds suspected to provoke weight gain by blocking or distorting various glandular responses. These chemicals have been dubbed *obesogens*—compounds that cause obesity.

Could something new in wheat also be an obesogen?

The gliadin proteins of wheat are degraded in the gastrointestinal tract to a group of polypeptides named *exorphins*, or exogenously derived morphine-like compounds. Several different exorphin compounds, called gluteomorphin or gliadorphins by researchers studying these curious compounds over the last 30 years, have been identified. Not only do wheat-derived exorphins bind to the brain's opiate receptors, but they are blocked from interacting with brain opiate receptors by the opiate-blocking drugs naloxone and naltrexone, the very same drugs used as antidotes, for example, for heroin or narcotic overdose.

So what is the evidence that the opiate-binding compounds that derive from wheat gliadin, in particular the newest forms of gliadin in modern wheat, via wheat exorphins, stimulate appetite? Here's a sampling of the research.

- Celiac disease, intestinal destruction from wheat gluten/gliadin, is traditionally regarded as a condition yielding emaciated, malnourished people, but has, over the last 40 years, become a disease of the overweight and obese.

- Overweight people with celiac disease who eliminate all wheat and gluten *lose 26 to 27.5 pounds of weight in the first 6 months*. Growing, overweight children with celiac disease lose fat mass and return to normal body mass index (BMI) with elimination of wheat and gluten. (These effects, by the way, tend to be short-lived because of the common mistake of resorting to weight-increasing gluten-free foods.) Note that in all of these studies, weight was lost without restricting calories, grams of fat, or anything else except eliminating wheat and gluten (and thereby gliadin).

more harmful Glia-α9 sequences that likely underlies the quadrupling of celiac disease over the past 50 years.

The breeding methods used prior to modern techniques of genetic modification to alter gluten quality did not always result in predictable, controllable changes. For example, just one hybridization event between two different wheat plants can yield as many as 14 new glutenin protein

---

- People who eliminate wheat consume, on average, *418 fewer calories per day*, or 14 percent fewer daily calories compared to wheat-consuming people in another study.
- Normal volunteers injected with the opiate-blocking drug naloxone consumed *400 fewer calories* in 1 day's time compared with those administered a placebo.
- People who suffer with binge-eating disorder (who often experience binge and "purge" cycles and are usually obese) consume 28 percent fewer calories during a binge after administration of naloxone.
- Multiple studies have recently demonstrated the efficacy of the oral opiate-blocking drug naltrexone (in combination with the antidepressant bupropion) for weight loss. Participants receiving the combination drug lost 25 pounds over the first year and experienced substantial reduction in food cravings. (These studies served as the basis for a pharmaceutical company's 2010 application to the FDA for a weight-loss indication for this drug.)

This is perfectly in sync with what I witness in my office every day, what I've witnessed over the past 5 years in people who have eliminated all wheat from their diet, and what I have seen unfold many thousands of times in the people who have read and followed the advice provided in *Wheat Belly*: Lose the wheat, lose the weight.

Wheat, in effect, is a powerful obesogen. Exorphins from the wheat protein gliadin increase appetite and increase calorie consumption by 400 or more calories per day; blocking the morphine-like effects of wheat exorphins with opiate-blocking drugs reduces calorie consumption and results in weight loss. The introduction of modern high-yield, semi-dwarf wheat in the late 1970s, with widespread adoption by 1985, was accompanied by a surge in weight gain, an explosive increase in the number of Americans classified as obese, and, after a lag of a few years, the greatest epidemic of diabetes ever seen.

Say goodbye to wheat, say goodbye to wheat gliadin and exorphins, say goodbye to excessive appetite, and say goodbye to weight—a lot of it.

sequences within gluten, the great majority of which have never before been consumed by humans. New genes for glutenin proteins within gluten have been described in modern forms of wheat that have never been found in older forms, such as the unique glutenin genes GluD3-3 and GluD3-12.

Usually as part of efforts to change the genetics of wheat to increase yield or enhance baking characteristics, new and unique gliadin, glutenin, and other proteins have resulted, none of which were tested for suitability for human consumption prior to their introduction into your food—they are just produced and sold, no questions asked.

Lectins

Lectins are a class of protective molecules found in plants. Lacking such things as cellular immunity and antibodies like we higher mammals have, plants instead rely on proteins called lectins to protect themselves from molds, insects, and other would-be predators. Because it is an effective defense against pests, geneticists have genetically engineered the gene for wheat lectin, wheat germ agglutinin, into other plants, such as corn, as an insecticide, given its lethal effects on the larvae of a pest known as the European corn borer.

The lectin of wheat, wheat germ agglutinin, is toxic. Found at highest concentration in wheat germ that many people regard as especially healthy, it has peculiar effects at many levels in wheat predators such as humans. Unlike gluten and gliadin, whose toxic potential is amplified in the genetically susceptible through HLA DQ genes, wheat germ agglutinin can do its damage directly, no genetic assistance required. It binds to the lining of the intestinal tract, disrupting cellular structure and microvilli, the short absorptive "hairs" on intestinal cells, and causing "hyperplasia," i.e., abnormal cell growth, of the small intestinal lining. These phenomena increase intestinal permeability, suspected to explain why foreign substances are able to gain entry into the bloodstream in the presence of wheat germ agglutinin. Wheat germ agglutinin is unique in that it is resistant to digestion in the human gastrointestinal tract, as well as to cooking, baking, sprouting the seeds, or sourdough fermentation. Because of its relatively small size, in addition to allowing other intruding compounds into the bloodstream, it is itself readily able to penetrate the intestinal lining and gain access to the bloodstream, with many people expressing antibodies against wheat germ agglutinin.

Once it gains entry into the bloodstream, wheat germ agglutinin has the capacity to exert an entire range of peculiar and unhealthy effects, including amplifying the effects of insulin on fat cells (increasing fat storage) and stimulation of abnormal immune responses such as that underlying rheumatoid arthritis. Wheat germ agglutinin is believed to worsen celiac disease; studies suggest that wheat germ agglutinin alone is sufficient to generate celiac disease–like intestinal damage.

Oddly, wheat germ agglutinin resembles

the protein hevein, the lectin from rubber plants responsible for latex allergy. The three variants of wheat germ agglutinin in modern wheat, isolectins A, B, and D, all contain eight copies of the hevein sequence. The full implications of this peculiar juxtaposition have not been explored in humans, though it has potential for allergic and immune consequences, given the frequency and severity of latex allergy.

The genetic changes inflicted on wheat have potential for expressing altered forms of wheat germ agglutinin. The structure of this protein in modern wheat is different by several amino acids from that of the ancient wheat strains emmer and einkorn. Unfortunately, what is not clear, given the general lack of interest among agricultural scientists and the recent development of technology able to make such distinctions among molecules, is whether new forms of lectins created over the last 50 years are more harmful than older forms. (It might turn out, for instance, that wheat lectins are bad for humans no matter what form they take.)

Rht Genes

Nearly all of the world's wheat is the semi-dwarf variety, a high-yield 18- to 24-inch-tall plant. Dwarfism is controlled by reduced height, or Rht, genes that reduce the production of the protein gibberellin, which stimulates growth of the stalk. Genes for dwarfism were originally obtained during the flurry of genetics research conducted in the 1960s and 1970s through repeated crossings with the mutant Norin 10 strain from Japan.

As with many mutations, one "defective" (or, in this case, desirable) gene is often accompanied by other genetic changes. Changes in Rht genes are accompanied by other changes in the genetic code of the wheat plant. Reduced height is also associated with thicker shafts, greater nutrient uptake in the seed heads (which are ground to produce flour), yielding larger and an increased number of seeds, and variations in other proteins expressed, such as alpha amylase inhibitors. As with much of the research of this age, some of the characteristics created were desirable to agricultural scientists, some not, but most were not even identified nor outwardly expressed or visible to the eye since the nature of the methods used did not seek to identify each and every change, just the obvious ones. (Imagine, for instance, I provoke a mutation for height in a chimpanzee. A 12-inch-tall chimpanzee dwarf might also have mental impairment, odd hair texture and color, endocrine abnormalities, etc., some of which are apparent to the eye, many of which are not.)

What consequences do these unique genes and proteins have for humans consuming various Rht mutants with their accompanying changes? Nobody knows, since the question was never asked.

Alpha Amylase Inhibitors and Other Allergens

Allergy to wheat is on the increase (along with allergies to peanuts, dairy, and other foods). This means that more people generate an IgE (immunoglobulin E) antibody response to various protein triggers, or "allergens," in wheat. Eighteen percent more children today have various dietary allergies, including wheat, than children did as recently as 1997.

Numerous allergens have been identified in modern wheat that were not present in ancient forms like einkorn. Wheat contains alpha amylase inhibitors, probably the most common among proteins responsible for wheat allergy in children (usually resulting in hives and/or asthma, cramps and diarrhea, and eczema). The structure of alpha amylase inhibitors of modern wheat overlaps with that of alpha amylase inhibitors of ancient strains by 90 percent, meaning that 10 percent of the genetic code and alpha amylase inhibitor structure are different. As any allergist will tell you, just a few different amino acids can spell the difference between no allergic reaction and a severe allergic reaction, even anaphylaxis (shock). When it comes to allergy, little changes can have big consequences.

Unfortunately, with the numerous protean changes introduced into the 25,000

Clearfield wheat was created through a process called *chemical mutagenesis*. Developers exposed wheat seeds to the chemical sodium azide, NaN_3. Sodium azide is highly toxic to animals, bacteria, and humans, with human ingestion of small quantities yielding effects similar to those of cyanide. With accidental ingestion, for instance, the CDC recommends not performing CPR on the victim (in effect, just letting the victim die), since the CPR provider could be fatally exposed along with the victim. The CDC also advises not to dispose of any vomit into a sink, since it can explode (and this has actually happened).

In addition to methods of chemical mutagenesis, gamma and x-ray radiation are also used on seeds and plant embryos to induce mutations. These methods of inducing purposeful, though unpredictable, mutations all fall under the umbrella of "traditional breeding methods."

So plants subjected to all manner of chemical- and radiation-based hybridization techniques are unleashed on the unwitting public, all presumed to be safe for human consumption, without safety testing in animals, just . . . used to create your foods.

There are some efforts made to analyze carbohydrate content, fiber content, and other crude measures of compositional change. Oh, you'll be happy to know that they also did test for its ability to yield cohesive cookies and light sponge cake.

strains of modern wheat, it is a virtual impossibility to track which strain contains which form of alpha amylase inhibitor. The loaf of bread you bought at the grocery store, the Cinnabon from the mall, the bagel from the bagel store—none are labeled, of course, with the strain of wheat they are sourced from. You can begin to appreciate the difficulty in tracking which strain of wheat might be associated with a specific individual's allergic reaction. But one thing is certain: Modern forms of wheat, thanks to busy geneticists, are associated with increased potential for allergy, some of which are due to changes introduced into alpha amylase inhibitor genes.

There are other forms of wheat allergy as well, with people in the baking industry who develop a condition called Baker's asthma. There is also the peculiar condition called wheat-derived exercise-induced anaphylaxis (WDEIA). a severe and life-threatening allergy induced by exercise after eating wheat. Both conditions are likely due to allergy to a gliadin protein fraction.

In addition, many other proteins—such as lipid transfer proteins, Ω-gliadins, α-gliadins, serpins, and low-molecular-weight

(continued on page 18)

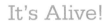

It's Alive!

"Come on! Wheat can't be that bad! If it's so bad, how come my mom ate bread every day and lived until she was 85 years old in perfect health?"

What we are being sold today is so far removed from the wheat of even 50 years ago that I challenge that it should even be called wheat any longer.

Let me weave you a scary tale that helps illustrate what has been done to this thing called wheat. This story might freak you out. So put the kids to bed, close the door, and make sure no nosy neighbors are watching.

Okay. Imagine you and I are evil scientists. We want to know what happens when we mate a 4-foot-7 Mbenga Pygmy tribeswoman from the Congo with a 6-foot-4 blond Swedish male. We obtain the offspring, a child somewhere in between the Pygmy mom and Swedish dad. Once it reaches sexual maturity, we mate this Swede-Pygmy with yet another Pygmy, but this time chosen for the shortest stature among this short race. We repeat this process several more times over several generations. We also introduce mates that have other characteristics, such as hairlessness or resistance to malaria. We also ignore some of the unexpected genetic characteristics that emerge, such as peculiar facial features, missing limbs or other body parts, or unique metabolic derangements.

Then the really creepy part starts. We mate our Swede-Pygmy descendant with some nonhuman primates, such as an orangutan, because we'd like to see whether our creature can be made to ably climb trees. The offspring are not always viable, but that's not our concern. We just keep our creations alive with whatever artificial means are required. It might require surgical correction, antibiotics, or artificial nutrition. We also take pregnant mothers and expose them to chemicals that induce mutations in the developing fetus *in utero,* and use gamma radiation and high doses of x-rays, also to induce mutations. Most of the mutations are grotesque and nonviable. But every so often, we're lucky and the mutant survives. It may be really weird looking, with odd facial features, deranged teeth, and deformed bones, as well as peculiar health problems, but that's also not our concern.

At the end of this process, repeated over and over again over many years, what do we call the creatures we've created? We can't call them Swedish humans. We can't call them Pygmies. They are artificially created things that bear no name, no resemblance to anything that occurs in nature because we used unnatural methods to create them. Maybe they're 3-foot-tall creatures that, permitted some mix of synthetic food for sustenance, provide a unique service that we've sought, e.g., climbing trees to harvest coconuts.

Thankfully, nobody outside of Nazi Germany conducts such horrific practices in humans and our close primate relatives. But such practices are commonplace in plant genetics.

Apply something similar to wheat of the early 20th century: repeated crossings to select for specific characteristics such as short stature, ease of release of the seeds, extreme oil production to discourage birds, resistance to mold and fungi; occasionally mate with non-wheat grains to introduce entirely unique genetic characteristics; salvage otherwise fatal mutants by embryo "rescue"; and expose the seed or embryo to the process of chemical or radiation mutagenesis to induce random mutations that occasionally are useful—well, those are the techniques that agribusiness and geneticists like to call traditional breeding methods. These are the methods that lobbyists for the wheat industry don't talk about, choosing instead to say things like "modern wheat is not genetically modified," meaning gene-splicing techniques have not been used to insert or delete a gene.

So the truth of it is that "traditional breeding methods" used to create modern semi-dwarf, high-yield strains of wheat were cruder, less controllable, much less predictable, and prone to produce consequences outside of the intended characteristic. In short, they were far *worse* than genetic engineering, yet these products made it to your supermarket shelf, dinner table, and gastrointestinal tract . . . no questions asked.

The result: what I call a *Frankengrain*, the result of extensive genetic changes, unable to survive without artificial chemical support, genetically stitched together with parts from various sources, like the creature created using the pieces from cadavers and charnel houses by Dr. Victor Frankenstein.

Except this Frankengrain isn't terrifying the countryside–we willingly invite it onto our dinner tables, package it in clever eye-catching ways, and feed it to our children.

This raises a fundamental question that has not yet been answered in agriculture or agricultural genetics: How much genetic and biochemical change can a plant like wheat undergo, after being subjected to extensive efforts to change its genetics, yet still be called wheat?

At the very least, we should be informed of the degree of change introduced into our foods, but even that modest concession is vigorously opposed. For instance, witness the intense lobbying agribusiness has waged to block the Truth in Labeling Act that would require food companies to declare whether a genetically modified ingredient is contained in a product. Nobody is asking them to *stop* generating genetically modified crops, but just to *tell us* if they did it. But even this modest disclosure is vigorously opposed.

No, the extreme changes introduced into the genetics of food crops like wheat are a well-kept secret, not divulged on labels, certainly not discussed in advice to "eat more healthy whole grains."

glutenins—have also been shown to trigger IgE-mediated allergic reactions to wheat. It is unclear whether the changes introduced in modern wheat have been associated with increased allergy to any of these wheat proteins, but clearly the potential is there.

So we have increasing allergy to modern strains of wheat, occurring most commonly among children. Surely, such a substantial increase in allergic reactions in children would sound the alarm among geneticists and prompt some serious questions, perhaps even a moratorium on any additional changes? Nope. Changes introduced into wheat continue unabated, allergy or no.

Products made from wheat flour are delicious, smell great, and make for all sorts of clever variations, from pita bread to wedding cake. But wheat flour is a delivery vehicle for all manner of compounds that exert undesirable effects on the human body, including new forms of gliadin, new and unexplored glutenin sequences, new forms of lectins, new alpha amylase inhibitor sequences, and many other new forms of proteins never before consumed by humans.

Surely, regulatory agencies like the USDA or FDA scrutinize each new change, study the biochemical changes introduced, examine the evidence of safety for every genetic alteration, look at animal safety testing, and then ask for human safety data when necessary? Nope. No such thing.

Geneticists create new strains of wheat with its collection of genetic changes, agribusiness sells it, farmers grow it, bakers put it to use, and then you and your family eat it.

Imagine one day the FDA announces that pharmaceutical manufacturers no longer need to file an FDA application to introduce new drugs; they can just develop and sell them, should they see fit. Pandemonium would result, of course, a scramble to introduce new drugs with uncertain side effects in the hopes of accelerating profits. Such a laissez-faire attitude, of course, would never be acceptable to the public—but that is precisely what has been going on in agricultural genetics.

When you examine the health effects of the various pieces within modern wheat, you can't help but conclude: It is a perfect poison.

Why Pick On Wheat?

Why am I so intent on bullying poor wheat? Surely there are other problems in the modern diet and lifestyle besides wheat.

The proliferation of high-fructose corn syrup as a sweetener, causing fructose consumption from corn sweeteners to skyrocket from an annual average per capita exposure of almost none in 1960 to 39 pounds in 2005, has undoubtedly contributed to obesity and other distortions of metabolism. Fructose in high-fructose corn syrup, as well as that in sucrose, is a uniquely metabolized sugar that does not generate satiety and is converted to triglycerides, introducing unique distortions that contribute to heart disease, insulin resistance, diabetes, and weight gain.

Corn, soy, beets, and potatoes have been genetically modified, i.e., gene-splicing technology has been used to insert or delete single genes, while wheat has not. Roundup Ready corn and soy, genetically modified organisms (GMOs) engineered to be resistant to the herbicide glyphosate (Roundup), dominate corn and soy fields on most farms today, meaning much of the processed food now sold contains these GMOs (as well as glyphosate residues). Preliminary observations of undesirable health effects in experimental animals suggest that they contribute to health problems, including weight gain, too.

Of course, the favorite explanation from "official" sources for the widespread weight gain, obesity, and diabetes epidemic is laziness and gluttony: You watch too much TV, spend too much time behind the computer or desk, don't exercise enough, eat too much fat, and drink too many soft drinks. In this worldview, we are a bunch of indulgent, slothful, chip- and soda-consuming people, no different from many 14-year-olds.

So why is wheat different? Why is wheat so bad, especially if the wheat sold today is not genetically modified?

First of all, the gliadin protein, the opiate-like compound that stimulates appetite, is unique to wheat. No other food or additive—high-fructose corn syrup, GMO corn, sucrose, fat, food colorings, preservatives, etc.—stimulates calorie consumption like wheat. Eat wheat, increase calorie consumption by 440 calories per day; remove wheat, reduce calorie consumption by 440 calories per day. The phenomenon is consistent and predictable. No other food is capable of such a phenomenon.

Second, due to the unique properties of the amylopectin A of wheat, few foods increase blood sugar and thereby insulin as much as wheat. Ice cream, Snickers bars, and Milky Way bars do not increase blood sugar and insulin as much as two slices of whole wheat bread. Recall that foods that increase blood sugar and insulin the highest are the most likely to stimulate growth of visceral fat, the deep abdominal fat that is uniquely inflammatory. Grow visceral fat, increase inflammation, which in turn further blocks insulin and causes worsening resistance to insulin—around and around, until you have a big swollen collection of visceral fat, a "wheat belly," that underlies even more health conditions, such as diabetes, hypertension, heart disease, and cancer.

Third, the intestinal "leakiness" (the increased entry of foreign substances into the bloodstream from the intestinal tract) encouraged by the lectin in wheat, wheat germ agglutinin, is unique to wheat. No other lectin in any other plant is capable of disrupting intestinal health in such a way—not the lectin in lentils, nor the lectin in elderberries, nor the lectin in peanuts. This likely explains why eating lentils does not cause or worsen rheumatoid arthritis, lupus, or polymyalgia rheumatica, but consuming

(continued on page 22)

Can We Go Back?

Can a return to the old ways teach us some useful lessons about wheat?

If the product of 1960s and 1970s genetics research, high-yield, semi-dwarf wheat, is the source of so many modern problems, what happens if we reject this genetic mutant and bring back some of the older, even ancient, forms? Are the predecessors of modern wheat free of all its problems? Should we ask farmers, for instance, to resurrect wheat strains ("landraces") popular during the 19th century, such as Russian and Red Fife, or the wheat that Moses and the Israelites carried with them in their flight from Egypt, emmer wheat?

Recall that modern wheat is a 2-foot-tall strain bred primarily for exceptional yield. It is the combination of three unique genetic codes, designated the *A, B,* and *D* sets of genes (genomes), the most recently added *D* genome being the recipient of most of the genetic manipulations and the source of unique glutens, glutenins, and gliadins that make modern wheat such a nasty creature.

In other words, say you, me, and Sherman accompany Mr. Peabody in the WayBack Machine, and we sample the wheat of bygone ages. If we go back in time, we'll encounter:

Wheat of the early 20th century—i.e., *Triticum aestivum,* or 42-chromosome wheat that predates the extreme breeding and mutation-generating interventions of the latter 20th century, with its genetics relatively untouched. These strains of *Triticum aestivum* share the *A, B,* and *D* genomes, but this *D* genome lacks all the extreme changes introduced by 20th-century geneticists. This includes strains such as Sonora, a strain that flourished in rural late-19th- and early-20th-century California, and Ladoga, which was transplanted from Russia to Canada in the late 19th century and spawned several successful 20th-century varieties.

19th-century and previous landraces—These are the strains of *Triticum aestivum* wheat that developed unique to specific climates and terrains, similar to wine grapes' *terroir.* Strains adapt to a location's humidity, temperatures, soil, day-night cycles, and seasonal changes. This includes several thousand varieties, all of which also share the *A, B,* and *D* genomes.

Spelt—Spelt is a 42-chromosome *A,B,D* wheat dating from prebiblical times and cultivated widely until the Middle Ages.

Emmer—Emmer is the 28-chromosome *A,B* offspring of an ancient natural cross between einkorn wheat and a wild grass. Emmer is likely the wheat of the Bible. It lacks the *D* genome that contains most of the genes coding for the most disease-causing forms of gliadin.

Kamut—Kamut shares genetics similar to that of emmer, i.e., 28 chromosomes, and the combined genes of einkorn wheat and a wild grass. Like emmer, kamut contains the *A* and *B* genomes, but not the *D*.

Einkorn—The great-granddaddy of all wheat, the grain first harvested wild, and the source of the original 14 chromosomes, the *A* genome, of wheat.

Obviously, experience with the various forms of wheat, particularly the varieties of ancient wheat, is extremely limited. But we do know a few things.

Hunter-gatherer humans who first began to incorporate wild einkorn into their diets experienced a downturn in health, including more dental disease, bone diseases, and possibly atherosclerosis and cancer. Likewise, modern hunter-gatherer cultures who do not consume wheat are spared these conditions.

We also know that celiac disease is *not unique to modern wheat* but was described as early as AD 100 by ancient Greek physician Aretaeus and by others many times over the centuries, meaning it likely occurred with consumption of emmer, spelt, kamut, and *Triticum aestivum* landraces, though the relative frequencies were likely much lower.

If we go back step-by-step from modern semi-dwarf wheat, back to the wheat of 1950 that predates human genetic intervention, back to the wheat of the early 20th and 19th centuries, back to the wheat of the Middle Ages and the first millennium, back farther to the wheat of the Bible, then the wheat of prebiblical civilizations, and finally to the einkorn wheat harvested wild, wheat becomes less and less destructive each step of the way, less likely to trigger human illness.

But does wheat ever become entirely benign, perhaps healthy, the farther back we go?

Here's a tough question: How much *better* does a wheat strain have to be in order to be acceptable to most people—50 percent, 70 percent, 80 percent, 100 percent better than our modern choice? What level of risk would you be willing to accept in order to consume foods made of this grain? If I had a cigarette, for instance, that posed 80 percent less risk of lung cancer than conventional cigarettes, is that safe enough for you to consider?

There are no right or wrong answers. It will be something to ponder in the coming years as information and experience with the older forms of wheat grow. In the meantime, given what we know (and don't know) about these older forms of wheat, my commonsense advice is to steer clear of all forms of wheat, new and old, and be *certain* you have great health and nutrition.

wheat does. Wheat lectins therefore heighten inflammation that, in turn, worsens insulin resistance, causing visceral fat to accumulate.

Fourth, and very importantly, wheat is about so much more than weight. Consumption of modern wheat is about acid reflux and irritable bowel syndrome. It's about neurological impairment and celiac disease. It's about water retention and leg edema. It's about allergies, asthma, and chronic sinus congestion and infections. It's about inattention and behavioral outbursts in children with ADHD and autism. It's about worsening symptoms of bipolar illness and schizophrenia. It's about mental "fog" and depression. It's about acne, dandruff, seborrhea, psoriasis, and a whole host of other skin conditions. It's about triggering the number one cause of heart disease, small LDL cholesterol particles.

Fifth, what other food contains the gluten protein that causes celiac disease, neurological impairment (gluten ataxia, peripheral neuropathy, and dementia), dermatitis herpetiformis, and non-celiac gluten sensitivity? Yes, barley, triticale, rye, bulgur, and perhaps oats overlap with the immune properties of wheat, but the gluten of wheat remains the Emperor of Gluten. Corn syrup, sucrose, candy, "trans" fats—none of these foods can cause the range of diseases caused by wheat.

In other words, even if you struggle to come to grips with the appetite-stimulating and blood sugar–provoking effects of wheat, there is so much more to wheat's effects on health that you've got to conclude that weight is among the least important of wheat's effects. Yes, it's an important effect, but the many components of modern wheat impair human health in so many other varied ways.

Put all these pieces together in the form of modern wheat, and you've got a heck of a health-distorting foodstuff. In short, wheat is the dietary perfect storm capable of generating in humans undesirable health effects that no other plant or food can match. And it enjoys the endorsements of "official" agencies, all urging us to eat more "healthy whole grains."

So, yes, wheat is the worst.

What's in the Future?

While no current commercially produced wheat products on the market today are, in the language of geneticists, genetically modified, i.e., the product of gene splicing techniques to insert or delete a gene, they are coming. Their appearance on your grocery store shelf is inevitable.

Genetically modified wheat has been around since the mid-1980s, when gene splicing techniques, such as exposure of wheat embryos to polyethylene glycol (the same as in antifreeze), electrical current, and particle bombardment that force insertion of new genes, made their appearance in genetics laboratories. Monsanto has been sitting on several strains of GM wheat but has not yet marketed the seed to farmers due to public resistance—but it's coming, public resistance or no.

Semi-dwarf wheat strains with new genes for high-molecular-weight glutenins (a component of gluten) to improve viscoelasticity are in the works, as well as efforts to reduce the blood sugar–raising potential of wheat amylopectin A. Extensive work is also ongoing to generate new strains resistant to various pests, fungi, and molds by inserting genes encoding viral coat proteins, antifungal proteins, and proteinase inhibitors.

Characteristic of the naive thinking of plant geneticists when considering the effects on humans who consume their products, much genetic research with wheat has focused on ways to disable the adverse health effects of gluten. In their way of thinking, breeding new strains of wheat that lack the 33 amino acid sequences most likely to stimulate the immune response of celiac disease would yield a more benign form of wheat. The problem: All the other problem components of wheat remain, including wheat germ agglutinin, amylopectin A, and alpha amylase inhibitors, not to mention the unanticipated effects of altered forms of gliadin, glutenin, and gluten created by these genetics efforts never before consumed by humans.

With all that uncertainty, surely there will be extensive biochemical analyses, experimental animal assessments, and human volunteer studies testing these products of genetic modification prior to introduction of such genetically and biochemically unique products . . . but probably not. Genetically modified wheat can be produced, marketed, and sold in the supermarket, but there does not have to be any record of safe consumption in humans. After all, there hasn't been any such effort for any genetically modified food before. And agribusiness has been spending tens of billions of dollars to lobby the federal government every year to oppose legislation that would only require that genetically modified food say so on the label.

Eat It . . . and Weep

Now that I've scared you silly with the science behind this crazy genetic monster called modern wheat, let's now turn to understanding how this thing fiddles with your health.

What happens to us humans who, unadvised of the genetic changes introduced, consume this stuff every day?

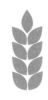

WHY DOES MY STOMACH HURT?

AND WHY DO MY JOINTS ACHE, AND MY BOWELS RUMBLE, AND MY FEET SWELL, AND MY . . .

EAT SOME JELLY BEANS, and you get a blood sugar rise, grow some tummy fat, and rot your teeth. Drink a carbonated soft drink, and you get a blood sugar rise, grow some tummy fat, and rot your teeth. End of story.

But eat wheat, and you get a blood sugar rise, grow some tummy fat, rot your teeth—and experience increased appetite, addiction, acid reflux, bowel urgency, joint pain, leg swelling, migraine headaches, skin rashes, dandruff, moodiness, sleeplessness, depression, seizures, dementia, and on and on. No other food is capable of such head-to-toe destruction of health—not jelly beans, not bag after bag of M&M's, not soft drinks by the liter bottle, not high-fructose corn syrup. (I know of a few poisons that can do the same, however.)

We consume this genetically altered (notice that I did not say genetically modi-

fied, the imprecise and elusive terminology of those wily geneticists) form of wheat. You've been eating it, sharing it with friends and family, feeding it to your kids. You've been choosing multigrain over white because you were told it was a healthier choice. You've been loading up with bran cereal at breakfast to keep your colon working smoothly. And pasta? A low-fat staple at the dinner table.

The problem: Modern wheat is not the wheat of your mother's day, nor is it the wheat of the 19th century. It is far removed from the wheat of the Bible and vastly different from the wheat that grew wild and was first consumed by hunter-gatherer humans.

So what happens to us modern humans who've been consuming this stuff, told by all "official" sources of dietary advice to eat more "healthy whole grains" that come from high-yield, semi-dwarf strains of wheat?

I'm afraid it's not a short list. The list of effects—no, the catalog of effects—that derive from consuming quantities of this modern creation of genetics research reads like a description of all the ills of modern life, hauntingly familiar in that it likely describes the people around you, perhaps even you.

Every wheat-consuming individual will not experience all of the effects discussed. You might experience, for instance, "only" acid reflux and disrupted intestinal health, or "only" appetite stimulation and addictive behavior. But no individual is entirely immune to the effects. Let me say that again: No individual is entirely immune to the effects of consuming modern wheat. In other words, no matter who you are, no matter how good you look and feel, whether you are a winner on *Dancing with the Stars* or a champion at horseshoes, wheat works its magic on you. Nobody escapes the effects of modern wheat, whether you perceive them or not. And, given its ubiquity and incredible potential to exert so many effects on health, it is wise always to consider wheat as the culprit in just about any health condition you develop.

While most people perceive symptoms that can be blamed on consumption of wheat, some people have no symptoms at all but just have distortions of multiple metabolic phenomena beneath the surface. It might be high blood sugar or hidden inflammation from amylopectin A and gliadin; it might be increased flow of abnormal foreign substances into the bloodstream from wheat germ agglutinin—but it's all there, smoldering away, taking its toll on long-term health.

This is why I do not advocate gluten elimination only for the gluten sensitive; I am advocating wheat elimination for everybody because we all experience undesirable effects from consuming this thing, not just the relative few with celiac disease or blood-test-proven gluten intolerance.

So what does the unwitting wheat-eating individual experience by eating more wheat-containing "healthy whole grains"? Let's pick the effects apart, one by one.

Blood Sugar Disasters

Consult any table of glycemic index (GI) values that describes how high blood sugar ranges over the 90 to 120 minutes after consuming any food. You will see that two slices of whole wheat bread have a higher glycemic index than nearly all other foods—higher than 6 teaspoons of table sugar, higher than a Snickers bar, higher than ice cream.

GI of whole wheat bread = 72

GI of sucrose (table sugar) = 59 to 65

(The GI of sucrose varies in different studies.)

GI of a Snickers bar: 41. Ice cream: 36.

Whole grains, such as 12-grain or multigrain breads that contain more fiber, do indeed have a somewhat lower GI, typically in the 50 to 55 range, around the same as a Milky Way bar.

Being told to "eat more healthy whole grains" thereby provides advice to consume foods that send blood sugar through the roof for breakfast, lunch, dinner, and snacks. And note that the GI of foods is nearly always obtained by examining blood sugar behavior in young, slender volunteers. The blood sugar rise is often far higher in older and overweight people. GI therefore describes the best-case scenario.

High blood sugar is unavoidably accompanied by high blood insulin, since insulin is required to clear the bloodstream of sugar and move it into muscles and organs for energy, and fat cells for storage. Just as wheat products, especially whole wheat products, increase blood sugar levels higher than nearly all other foods, wheat products also increase blood insulin levels higher than nearly all other foods, too.

Repetitive high levels of insulin set the stage for creating resistance to insulin, i.e., reduced responsiveness in muscle, the liver, and other organs to the body's own insulin. Insulin resistance is the fundamental process that leads to prediabetes and diabetes, situations in which the body can no longer cope with the carbohydrates driving repetitive high blood sugar, allowing blood sugars eventually to increase. Insulin resistance also causes the growth of deep abdominal fat, visceral fat, a form of fat that is highly inflammatory. Filled with white blood cells (like that in pus), visceral fat emits inflam-

matory proteins into the bloodstream, thereby increasing inflammation everywhere in the body, from your knees to your heart to your brain.

By the way, this metabolically messy situation of insulin resistance, prediabetic or diabetic blood sugar levels, and the visceral fat of a wheat belly is nearly always accompanied by having an abundant quantity of small, dense LDL particles, by far the most common cause of coronary heart disease and heart attack today.

So high blood sugar leads to high blood insulin that, in turn, generates insulin resistance. Insulin resistance generates visceral fat that amplifies inflammation, which worsens insulin resistance and increases blood sugar and small LDL particles, starting the whole cycle over again, worse and worse and worse.

And it all started with your morning bagel.

Opiate of the Masses: Addiction and Withdrawal

The gliadins in wheat, particularly the new forms crafted by geneticists, are opiates. Wheat is therefore an opiate. Yes, wheat keeps company with Oxycontin, heroin, and morphine.

It has been known for a century that opiates, when administered to laboratory animals or to humans, increase appetite. It was discovered around 30 years ago that the gliadin protein of wheat is, in effect, an opiate, as it yields digestive breakdown products that bind to the opiate receptors of the brain.

Gliadin is degraded in the gastrointestinal tract to smaller polypeptides called exorphins (exogenous morphine-like compounds), such as gluteomorphin and gliadorphin, that, once absorbed into the bloodstream, penetrate into the brain and bind to the opiate receptors, exerting effects similar to those of opiates such as morphine. Wheat opiates, however, stimulate less of a "high" but are more potent stimulants of appetite.

The appetite-stimulating effect of wheat gliadin explains why people who eat more "healthy whole grains" typically experience constant hunger: a 7:00 a.m. breakfast of "high-fiber" cereal followed by a growling stomach at 9:00 a.m. with the need for a snack such as low-fat pretzels or crackers, hungry again at 11:00 a.m., hungry just a couple of hours after lunch, dinner at 6:00 p.m. followed by a need to snack at 8:00 p.m. Many people "graze" all through the day or eat many small meals every 2 hours, a strategy endorsed by dietitians but representing nothing more than a pointless and counterproductive means of dealing with the constant cravings of the wheat-consumer.

Stop consuming wheat and appetite plummets. People report going through the day barely hungry at all. A common experience is having breakfast at 7:00 a.m. followed by noticing that "It's 1:00 p.m. Perhaps I might eat something, but I'm not really that hungry." The after-dinner munchies that many people struggle with disappear. Total calorie intake drops by 400 or so calories per day, documented in both clinical studies and in real life. And that's the average experience: Some people reduce calorie intake less than 400 calories per day, while others experience far greater reduction. Four hundred fewer calories per day, multiplied by 365 days per year—that's a lot of food, 146,000 cumulative calories, and a lot of weight that can be lost effortlessly.

You can see why the failure to eliminate wheat explains why so many people struggle with weight-loss diets: because they failed to remove this appetite stimulant. Reducing calories becomes torture, like waving a syringe full of heroin at a helpless addict.

Where there's spaghetti, there are meatballs. And where there's addiction, there's withdrawal. Yes, indeed: withdrawal from the opiate in wheat. Don't believe it? Try this little experiment: Stop feeding your husband or kids wheat during a 72-hour period when you can control their diet (e.g., a long weekend), then sit back and watch the emotional fireworks. You're likely to observe crying, yelling, nausea, incapacitating fatigue, begging for a roll or pretzel, sneaking off to the nearest convenience store for a "hit." (Wheat withdrawal is such an important phenomenon that I discuss it in more detail in the next chapter.) You'll quickly realize that you've been living with a family of opiate addicts, consuming their drug of choice cleverly disguised as a bran muffin, breakfast cereal, or pizza.

Another caution: The longer you are wheat free, the more likely you will develop undesirable reactions when re-exposed, inadvertently or intentionally. I call these awful experiences wheat "re-exposure reactions." (Readers and social media followers of Wheat Belly say they've been "wheated.") Say you've been wheat free for 4 weeks, lost 15 pounds, been freed from irritable bowel syndrome symptoms and the funny rash that wouldn't go away for 5 years. You eat a few of the crackers you let sit in your cupboard—what the heck, you've been so good!—and you've got yourself a case of diarrhea and cramps, bloating, pain in your elbows and shoulders, and a recurrence of the rash, very common re-exposure reactions. Other common re-exposure reactions include headache, asthma and sinus congestion (in those prone), and emotional effects, especially sadness, hopelessness, anxiety, and anger. Re-exposure reactions last from hours to days. Gastrointestinal reactions like diarrhea tend to dissipate over a day or two, while joint pains can persist for days to weeks. You will survive, but for many of us, the experience is so unpleasant that no indulgence makes it worth the pain and hassle.

Weight Gain: Grow Your Very Own Wheat Belly

If the gliadin protein of wheat, changed by geneticists in their efforts to increase yield, stimulates appetite and increases calorie consumption by 400 or more calories per day, 365 days per year, what happens to us

unsuspecting participants in this national experiment? We get fat. Given the unique properties of wheat's amylopectin A to raise blood sugar and insulin levels, we gain the weight mostly around our middles, evidenced on the surface by what I call a wheat belly, and evidenced on CT scans and MRIs as deep visceral fat encircling the intestines and other abdominal organs.

And we don't just get a little bit fat. Many of us get really fat, sufficient to send our body mass indexes (see "What Is Your Body Mass Index [BMI]?") to 30 and above, falling into the range classified as obese, or even morbidly or super-obese with BMIs of 40 and over, the group growing the fastest. Such classifications have only become a matter of necessity in the last 25 years, since these extreme ranges of overweight were previously uncommon, rarely seen outside of circus tents and peep shows.

Recall that modern semi-dwarf strains of wheat were introduced in the mid- to late 1970s, with only a few percent of farmers adopting this crop viewed as peculiar in 1979. As more and more farmers began to observe the startling surges in yield-per-acre of high-yield, semi-dwarf strains, this wheat was rapidly embraced in the early 1980s. By 1985, virtually every wheat product you bought—white, whole grain, organic, sprouted—came from high-yield, semi-dwarf wheat.

Oddly, data collected by the USDA and Centers for Disease Control and Prevention (CDC) show that 1985 also marks the year when calorie intake began to climb,

What Is Your Body Mass Index (BMI)?

To calculate your BMI, plug your weight and height into the following equation:

BMI = [weight in pounds ÷ (height in inches)²] x 703

Alternatively, go to the National Heart, Lung, and Blood Institute's BMI calculator at www.nhlbisupport.com/bmi.

BMI is often used as an assessment of the appropriateness of weight for height, or as an index of health. It is not perfect, as it does not factor in such differences as body shape, muscle mass, and other variations among us humans. Nonetheless, it is often used to compare differences in weight in populations and is often cited in clinical studies.

Classifications of BMI:

Underweight = <18.5

Normal weight = 18.5–24.9

Overweight = 25–29.9

Obese = 30 or greater

Super-obese = 40 or greater

---

increasing 440 calories per day, every day, 365 days a year. Increased calorie intake leads to weight gain, year after wheat-consuming year. It means we have obese adults, obese elderly, obese teenagers, obese children—more overweight, obese, and super-obese people than ever before in the history of man.

Recent findings in experimental models also suggest that the lectin in wheat, wheat germ agglutinin, may block the hormone leptin, meaning the body becomes unresponsive to the satiating effects of this hormone. Obese people have inappropriately high levels of this hormone when it should be low, given their overnourished state. If this holds true in future studies and wheat lectins prove to block the satiating effect of leptin, it will become clear that wheat consumption essentially equals weight gain. "Eat more healthy whole grains": a perfect formula for obesity.

Diabetes: You Get What You Ask For

The "official" explanation for the 30-year climb in collective weight and the diabetes that results from it? We are all lazy and gluttonous. We drink too many soft drinks and watch too much TV. If we would just exercise more and cut our calories, we would return to the age of slender Jimmy Stewarts and Donna Reeds.

Let's consider an alternative explanation. If the amylopectin A of wheat, what dietitians call a complex carbohydrate, increases blood sugar more than simple sugars such as table sugar and many candy bars, then surely it must increase the likelihood of diabetes. Wheat products increase blood sugar every time you eat them. Eating more "healthy whole grains" ensures high blood sugar levels, along with all the phenomena that follow, including insulin resistance that results in diabetes.

It is well-established fact that foods with a high glycemic index promote diabetes, while foods with a low glycemic index—or, even better, no glycemic index—make diabetes less likely. What food has among the highest glycemic indexes of all foods out there? Yup: Foods made of wheat. Ironically, whole wheat is worse than white (though both are bad, of course). Whole grain and multigrain products improve the situation a bit, but remain triggers of high blood sugar despite the extra fiber and B vitamins. After all, whole grain, whole wheat, white—it all comes from the same semi-dwarf wheat plant bearing the same amylopectin A.

Gain 30, 40, 60, or more pounds, especially in the visceral fat of the abdomen, and most people become prediabetic or diabetic. And, indeed, during the mid- to late 1980s, as products made with semi-dwarf wheat flour proliferated, expanding from only breads and rolls to licorice, instant soups, frozen dinners, and nearly all other processed foods, a surge in the incidence of these conditions began, accelerating through the 1990s. The numbers reflecting the incidence of diabetes are now a vertical climb, straight upward since 2008.

Conventional wisdom, of course, argues the opposite: Consuming more healthy whole grains is associated with reduced likelihood of diabetes. And that is true—if you compare whole grain consumption to consumption of processed white flour products. Study after study conducted over the past 30 years, including such ambitious studies as the Nurses' Health Study of 80,000 women, or the Physicians' Health Study of 30,000 professionals, all demonstrated the significant health benefits of consuming healthy whole grains . . . over white flour. Okay, so let's follow the logic of these studies.

If you replace something bad with something less bad and there is an apparent health benefit, then a whole bunch of the less bad thing must be good.

If there are health benefits to consuming something less bad, what are the effects of complete removal? In other words, what happens when wheat products, white and whole grains, are completely eliminated from the diet? That, too, has indeed been studied, but the dramatic weight loss and reductions of blood sugar and HbA1c (a measure that reflects blood sugar fluctuations over the prior 2 to 3 months) are often dismissed as due to malnutrition (discussed further in the next chapter). As with many things wheat, the answers have been there all along—just not recognized for what they were.

Recall that wheat is also an opiate, due to the gliadin protein that converts to exorphins upon digestion, and that this opiate acts as an appetite stimulant. It means that consumption of modern wheat sends blood sugar higher than nearly all other foods while stimulating appetite to consume more calories. Eat more calories, desire more food, send blood sugar higher again and again, and you've got yourself a perfect situation to cultivate diabetes.

But you, your friends, and your family are all accused of being gluttonous and lazy. You've gained weight, developed insulin resistance, and become prediabetic or diabetic because of your love affair with chips, Mountain Dew, and your sofa. I believe all that is true—for many 10- to 14-year-olds. But what about all the health-conscious adults who exercise, avoid junk foods, and eat more "healthy whole grains"?

Unwinding this metabolic disaster is powerfully accomplished by eliminating all things wheat. Additional benefit is obtained, however, by restricting other carbohydrates as well, from candy bars to fruit. More on that in the next chapter.

The Gastrointestinal Battleground

You deliver wheat products directly into your gastrointestinal tract, starting at the mouth and on down for another 30 or more feet. It therefore serves as the front line for the wheat battle.

We know that many people experience gastrointestinal distress from gluten in wheat (actually the gliadin within gluten, as well as glutenin). Of course, gluten is primarily responsible for celiac disease, a condition marked by destructive changes in the intestinal lining that result in abdominal pain, cramps, diarrhea, impaired absorption of nutrients, hemorrhage, and occasionally death; it affects approximately 1 percent of the population. Of the approximately 2.4 million Americans who have celiac disease, 90 percent don't know it, making it among the most underdiagnosed of chronic diseases. And it's gotten worse: Over the last 50 years, we've witnessed a quadrupling of the incidence of celiac disease, a doubling over the past 20 years.

Gluten also disrupts the gastrointestinal tracts of people without celiac disease, resulting in common complaints such as acid reflux, heartburn, excessive gas, abdominal cramping, diarrhea, and constipation. (See "Gluten Sensitivity: Is There Such a Thing?" on page 32.) Gluten sensitivity can develop in people with abnormal antibodies to gliadin; it can develop in people without abnormal antibodies to gliadin. Celiac disease and gluten sensitivity combined affect up to 10 percent of the American population, but the intestinal disruptive effects of wheat add up to far more than 10 percent of the population, with more people experiencing the heartburn of acid reflux, the bowel urgency and crampiness of irritable bowel syndrome, and the worsening of symptoms (diarrhea, cramps, gas, pain) of ulcerative colitis and Crohn's disease.

The lectin in wheat, wheat germ agglutinin, because it has a direct toxic effect on the intestinal tract, adds to the intestinal disruption of gluten. After all, lectins are potentially poisonous proteins in plants meant to protect them from insects, molds, and other predators. Wheat germ agglutinin is the stuff that permits abnormal intestinal permeability to develop, allowing foreign substances—including wheat germ agglutinin itself—to gain access to the bloodstream in small quantities. (In larger quantities, direct injection of wheat germ agglutinin into the bloodstream of laboratory animals is rapidly fatal.) Once in the bloodstream, wheat germ agglutinin and its

Gluten Sensitivity: Is There Such a Thing?

For years, many physicians denied that there was such a thing as celiac disease, the intestinal destruction that develops from wheat gliadin/gluten consumption in genetically predisposed individuals. But only the most intransigent (read: "crazy") among my colleagues can continue to deny that celiac disease is a genuine—and potentially devastating—disease.

Physicians are now struggling with the notion of *gluten sensitivity,* a reaction to the gluten in wheat but not achieving the severity of celiac disease. While not everybody agrees on how to define gluten sensitivity, the most common definition is that of showing symptoms of sensitivity to wheat gluten, such as acid reflux, abdominal pain, cramps, and diarrhea, that disappear with elimination of wheat. Despite the apparent response to wheat/gluten removal, intestinal biopsy (which usually reveals extensive damage in celiac patients) shows either *no* evidence of damage in those with gluten sensitivity, or inflammatory changes without damage.

One recent and important Italian study demonstrated that 56.4 percent of people identified with gluten sensitivity, but lacking the intestinal damage associated with celiac disease, are positive for the IgG antigliadin antibody (i.e., an antibody to the gliadin protein in wheat), but not for other markers. In other words, many people demonstrate evidence of an abnormal antibody response to the gliadin protein in gluten but don't have celiac disease.

Other studies have demonstrated that gluten consumption, even when subjects are blinded to what they are consuming, generates symptoms in people without celiac disease.

Gluten sensitivity can extend beyond the gastrointestinal tract, with new descriptions of neurological impairment, especially cerebellar ataxia (loss of coordination and bladder control due to destruction of the cerebellum at the base of the brain) and peripheral neuropathy (destruction of the nerves of the legs, arms, and organs). In one study, 57 percent of people with unexplained neurological impairment were positive for antibodies against gliadin, while only 5 percent of people with neurological impairment from known diseases (e.g., stroke) showed positive gliadin antibodies. Typically, people with these forms of neurological impairment do *not* have celiac disease.

hordes of unwanted foreign compounds then migrate to your liver, joints, brain, and just about everywhere else in the body, leading to inflammation and abnormal conditions in these organs. It means that people who consume wheat, and thereby wheat germ agglutinin, are more likely to experience inflammatory diseases or experience worsened symptoms of existing conditions, such as lupus, rheumatoid arthritis, Sjögren's syndrome, polymyalgia rheumatica, polymyositis, Hashimoto's thyroiditis, seborrhea, psoriasis, and a long list of other inflammatory and autoimmune conditions.

In short, the human intestinal tract is poorly equipped to endure the onslaught of

This is not just an academic debate. Observations suggest that gluten sensitivity not only can result in intestinal inflammation and neurological symptoms, but also *increases mortality.*

Because it required about 40 years for the concept of celiac disease to even *begin* to gain wide acceptance in the medical community, it is another leap for most physicians to believe that there is another form of intolerance to wheat gluten that extends beyond celiac disease.

Problem: If 56.4 percent of participants in the Italian study experienced relief from abdominal symptoms with wheat removal, it means that the remaining 43.6 percent experienced relief by saying goodbye to all foods containing wheat—but had no evidence of abnormal immune response to gliadin. Researchers from the world of gastroenterology don't know what to do with this bothersome 43.6 percent, dismissing it as an uncertain group, a group prone to placebo effects, or just plain nuts.

Now that you have a better appreciation that wheat is about more than just gluten and gliadin, you can readily surmise that at least *some* of those 43.6 percent in the Italian study who had symptoms associated with wheat consumption and experienced relief with wheat elimination included people who likely reacted to wheat germ agglutinin, or experienced reactions to glutenin, alpha amylase inhibitors, or any one or more of the many other relatively uncharted and unique compounds in modern wheat. *It's not all about gluten.*

One lesson is clear: If modern medicine cannot identify the blood marker or the biopsy evidence that active destruction of some organ is actively occurring, then *there's nothing wrong.* (You know how many people I've seen placed on antidepressants, pain-relieving drugs and narcotics, and antiseizure drugs, all to treat wheat consumption? I lost count long ago.)

In the march of scientific progress in charting the adverse consequences of consumption of modern wheat, along each step of the way we learn that many of the people who complained of a variety of health problems, but were dismissed as cranks, nuts, or undiagnosable, prove to have some form of unhealthy reaction to one or another component of wheat.

the dual toxic effects of wheat gluten and lectin, resulting in a battleground strewn with casualties, experienced as an astounding range of gastrointestinal and inflammatory illnesses, and managed with all manner of drugs and procedures.

Neurological Impairment: Wheat Brain

Among the most disturbing associations between wheat and ill health are the associations being made between consumption of this man-made grain and the deterioration of the brain and nervous system.

Anecdotally, mind "fog" is exceptionally common with consumption of wheat. It is likely due to the mind effects of gliadin that are also responsible for addictive behavior, worsened by the hypoglycemia that typically develops after amylopectin A's extravagant blood sugar high. But the effects of wheat on the human brain go far deeper than that.

While celiac disease is usually regarded as a disease confined to the intestinal tract, over the last few years celiac disease has become less a disease of diarrhea and cramps, and more a disease of nervous system impairment and psychiatric problems. Rather than developing diarrhea, people with celiac disease more recently tend to demonstrate impaired coordination, difficulty controlling their bladders, and a wide variety of other nervous system derangements.

Most nervous system involvement has been confined to people with abnormal immune markers (such as increased levels of transglutaminase, endomysial, or gliadin antibodies) to wheat typical of celiac disease or gluten sensitivity, though many do not experience intestinal symptoms. Nervous system involvement is especially worrisome, as it is difficult to diagnose, since it yields symptoms that most physicians would not associate with wheat consumption, and is not fully reversible. Cerebellar ataxia, for instance, involving loss of balance and bladder control and destructive changes in the cerebellum (the region of the brain responsible for coordination) seen as atrophy (shrinkage) on MRI, with a typical age of onset of 48 to 53 years, has been linked to wheat consumption. Peripheral neuropathy, the loss of sensation in the legs or the loss of bladder and bowel control, may be due to wheat consumption in as many as 50 percent of those afflicted when no other cause can be identified. Even dementia from wheat has been identified, recently documented by a study from the Mayo Clinic and identified at autopsy—yes, fatal dementia from wheat.

The effects of wheat consumption on the human brain can also involve seizures, typically of the temporal lobe variety but also grand mal, and migraine headaches.

You don't have to have celiac disease or gluten sensitivity for wheat to exert effects on your brain. We know that gliadin gains access to the brain, yielding the appetite-stimulating opiate effect that increases calorie consumption. Gliadin is also the probable cause of behavioral effects (reduced attention span and behavioral outbursts) in children with autism and attention-deficit hyperactivity disorder (ADHD). Gliadin is likely to blame for the worsening of auditory hallucinations, social detachment, and paranoia of paranoid schizophrenia and the manic phase of bipolar illness. Gliadin effects in these conditions are reversible: They occur with wheat consumption; they dissipate with wheat avoidance.

In most of us, wheat does not generate auditory hallucinations or destruction of the cerebellum. But it does induce appetite to the tune of 400 or more calories per day, every day. Think about this: What if Big Food and Big Agribusiness got hold of such information? Would they warn us—or just put wheat in everything?

Inflammation: Going Down in Flames

Signs of inflammatory processes gone awry in the wheat-consuming individual are common. Typical signs include painful wrists and hands, painful elbows and shoulders, worsening of arthritis in knees and hips, and tender ankles and shins when touched. If any form of inflammatory disease is present, such as rheumatoid arthritis or lupus, wheat is the gasoline on the fire, typically worsening inflammation and resulting in greater pain, swelling, rash, etc.

Inflammation is a fundamental process that underlies an astoundingly wide range of conditions, such as lupus, rheumatoid arthritis, ulcerative colitis, Crohn's disease, diabetes, Sjögren's syndrome, scleroderma, polymyositis, polymyalgia rheumatica, coronary disease and heart attack, even cancer—to name just a few in a long, long list. The elaborate processes of inflammation can be initiated by a variety of triggers, including nutritional deficiencies (e.g., vitamin D, omega-3 fatty acids), chronic infections (e.g., gingivitis, intestinal bacterial overgrowth), ingestion of oxidized compounds (e.g., polyunsaturated fatty acids, foods cooked at high temperature), autoimmune processes in which the body's immune defenses mistakenly attack normal tissue (e.g., Hashimoto's thyroiditis, autoimmune hepatitis), and ingestion of toxic substances. The last two paths are especially relevant to our wheat conversation.

Wheat is an especially prominent player in the complex web of inflammation: The direct toxic effects of wheat germ agglutinin and the indirect toxic effects of gliadin get the fires of inflammation started; autoimmune processes are set in motion by the abnormal entry of foreign substances into the bloodstream allowed by wheat germ agglutinin; and the inflammation-stoking effects of visceral fat further fan the flames.

The process starts with the direct toxic effects and intestinal leakiness created by wheat germ agglutinin. Foreign compounds gain access to the bloodstream, some of which intensify ongoing inflammatory responses, while others mistakenly generate autoimmune responses, immune responses errantly waged against the body's own proteins, which is the signature process underlying conditions such as autoimmune hepatitis and Hashimoto's thyroiditis.

Gliadin, the wheat protein responsible for celiac disease, indirectly provokes inflammation in the lining of the intestinal tract. Gliadin triggers the entry of inflammatory T-cell lymphocytes, damaging the fine hairlike villi lining the intestinal tract, and invites a barrage of inflammatory proteins such as interferons and interleukins. People with non-celiac gluten sensitivity show inflammation from gliadin. Although it doesn't wreak the same degree of destruction of the delicate villous lining, inflammatory changes, such as infiltration of inflammatory lymphocytes, are seen.

The visceral fat of the wheat belly that lines the intestinal tract or encircles the liver, pancreas, and kidneys, thanks to repeated bouts of high blood sugar and insulin, amplifies inflammation. Visceral fat is itself inflamed. If biopsied, it appears to be riddled with white blood cells, not unlike the pus that oozes from an inflamed wound. Visceral fat, often reflected on the surface as "love handles" or a "muffin top," also pours inflammatory proteins into the bloodstream, proteins like tumor necrosis factor and leptin that export inflammation out from visceral fat and into all other areas of the body.

All the pieces in wheat add up to an incredibly effective vehicle for generating inflammation in multiple organs, head to toe. How'd those cookies taste?

Make Your Skin Crawl

The skin is the largest organ of the human body, serving functions such as temperature regulation, insulation against water loss, and protection from bacteria and other potential invaders.

Think of the skin as the outward reflection of internal health. Rashes, acne, itchiness, pain—all can reflect something going on inside. Skin health may especially reveal gastrointestinal health. So a rash may not simply be a rash; it may provide insight into some process gone awry in, say, the small intestine, pancreas, and liver.

Dermatologists typically biopsy rashes, then treat them with steroid creams and toxic drugs like dapsone, sulphamethoxypridazine, and isotretinoin (Accutane). It is not uncommon for dermatologists to have no idea why you have a rash and have no choice of treatments except to shotgun it with drugs, wear long-sleeved shirts and long pants, and grin and bear it.

Skin problems are rampant in wheat-consuming individuals. The most frequent problem is a dry red rash along the edges of the nose and on the cheeks. Dermatologists call this seborrhea. However, it is so common and so typical of wheat consumption that I recognize this as a wheat rash.

Dandruff, itchy rashes of eczema, and seborrhea-like rashes on the elbows are also common expressions of wheat consumption. The thick, silvery, scaly rash of psoriasis is another very common expression of wheat consumption.

Dermatitis herpetiformis, a herpeslike rash (but not caused by the herpes virus), is the signature rash of people with a celiac disease tendency (characterized by having abnormal immune markers to wheat, such as increased levels of transglutaminase antibodies). It is an angry-looking, itchy rash that occurs symmetrically on the body. Although it occurs in people with a genetic susceptibility to celiac disease, intestinal symptoms of celiac disease are not usually present.

In truth, the list of skin conditions that can develop from consumption of wheat is easily four pages long. It includes such peculiar conditions as acanthosis nigricans, black velvety patches on the back of the neck, armpits, and elbows; dermatomyositis, a rash that occurs along with muscle weakness and inflammation, resulting in difficulty walking and climbing stairs, and blood vessel inflammation; and alopecia, or hair loss from the head or other areas. Wheat causes so many skin conditions that I believe it makes sense to always consider wheat consumption as the underlying cause of all rashes until proven otherwise.

Death, Taxes, and Wheat

Nobody escapes the effects of wheat. They might be visible on the surface, they might be hidden deep within your stomach, intestinal tract, bloodstream, or brain, but they're there, working their effects.

If I told you that eating green peppers triggered increased appetite, wreaked havoc on your gastrointestinal tract, exerted neurological destruction in susceptible people, screwed with insulin and blood sugar, damaged joints, etc., then I'm sure you would say, "Well, I'll never have a green pepper again!" (Innocent green peppers do not do any of this, of course.) So why is it so hard to persuade people that these things happen with consumption of their beloved bagels, croissants, and pancakes? Most people say convenience: Wheat products are portable and available. But I think it's more than that. I say it's because this thing has a hold on you, an opiate-like comfort that you crave, and distinctly unpleasant feelings when you lack it. And this effect is not lost on the food industry, which happily accommodates your addiction, making sure it includes a bit of wheat in everything.

We then take medications for acid reflux and irritable bowel syndrome, drugs for joint pain, diuretics for leg swelling and water retention, cholesterol drugs for high cholesterol, anti-inflammatory drugs for inflammation and pain. . . . We are, in effect, treating the effects of wheat consumption.

You cannot avoid taxes. You certainly cannot sidestep death. But you can sure say goodbye to wheat.

WELCOME TO THE WONDERFUL STATE OF WHEATLESSNESS

IF MODERN WHEAT is associated with addictive behaviors, appetite stimulation, and so many abnormal health conditions, then removing it completely from the diet should result in reversal of the whole kit and kaboodle.

And indeed it does. The contrast is so dramatic that I give the wheat-free lifestyle a name: I call it wheatlessness.

Say goodbye to wheat and you say goodbye to the appetite-stimulating protein, gliadin, that acts as an opiate on your brain. You say sayonara to the altered forms of gliadin that cause celiac disease, such as the Glia-α9 sequence, now found in nearly all modern forms of wheat. Say adios to the lectin, wheat germ agglutinin, that directly damages the intestinal lining and acts like a Trojan horse for foreign substances to gain access to your bloodstream and organs. Say arrivederci to amylopectin A in wheat that provokes a roller-coaster ride of high blood sugar, followed by plummeting blood sugar

and the mental "fog" of hypoglycemia and insatiable hunger. Say au revoir to unique alpha amylase inhibitors in wheat and lose many wheat allergies.

Remove onions and . . . you remove onions—nothing more, nothing less. There is no withdrawal process, no weight loss, no relief from any pain, no religious epiphany, nothing except no onions with your fried liver or bratwurst.

But remove wheat . . . and it's like removing a poison from your body. After withdrawal subsides, health transformations result.

Critics of *Wheat Belly* have argued that these ideas represent nothing more than a low-carbohydrate diet for weight loss in disguise. But they've missed the essential point: Eliminating modern wheat, this product of genetics research, is about so much more than weight loss. Sure, you lose weight—often a lot of weight—but it's all the other stuff that results from wheatlessness that makes this approach such a powerful and life-changing concept. (For those of you interested in maximizing weight loss in as short a time as possible, or trying to undo severe carbohydrate intolerance, as in diabetes or prediabetes, we will discuss how going beyond elimination of wheat and restricting all carbohydrates provides additional benefits.)

It's part of what I call wheat's "whole is greater than the sum of the parts effect." Despite all we know about this destructive high-yield, 24-inch mutant, the benefits of removing it from diet exceed expectations. Although we already know plenty about the destructive health effects of gliadin, lectin, amylopectin A, and other components of wheat, get rid of the whole package and health benefits enjoyed by the majority are greater than you'd ever anticipate.

Let's be clear: This is not about gluten elimination for gluten-sensitive people. Given wheat's effects that spare no one, I am advocating wheat elimination for everybody.

Downside: Tell this to the average wheat-eater and they find it a bit difficult to swallow, to say the least. You may be on the receiving end of yelling, swearing, sobbing, and physical confrontation. No other food elicits such forceful reactions because no other food has such a hold over the consumer's mind. Imagine taking a trip into the inner city and swiping the stash from a heroin addict—it wouldn't be pretty. Remember: You are, in effect, trying to persuade a wheat-eating opiate addict that their source of comfort in times of good and bad is really

undoing health, making them the unwitting victim of a "food" that gains access to the brain to influence behavior.

So what can modern wheat-consuming individuals expect when they rid themselves of this thing? Let's discuss that next.

Happier Joints, Happier Bowels, Happier Minds

Your body is healthier and happier when all things wheat are removed.

But before we get to the "hard" observations, the effects on various diseases and conditions that we can expect with elimination of wheat, let's talk about the many "soft"—but not to say insignificant—effects that develop, the subjective experiences many or most people report on saying goodbye to modern high-yield, semi-dwarf wheat. Subjective effects are tougher to measure but are nonetheless consistent and reproducible. I've personally witnessed these subjective effects unfold many thousands of times.

Typical subjective observations that emerge with elimination of wheat include:

Thinking is clearer. Most people describe a lifting of mental "fog." (I personally experienced this effect to a dramatic degree.) The constant struggle to maintain concentration is replaced by the ability to focus for prolonged periods.

Mood is improved, dark moods lessened. People are happier and less depressed. I've witnessed many people with lifelong struggles with depression who were able to reduce or stop antidepressant drugs.

Energy increases. Not only is energy increased throughout the day, but the cycles of ups and downs diminish or disappear.

Sleep is deeper. It becomes closer to the profound, restful sleep that children experience.

Appetite is reduced. The predictable 2-hour cycle of hunger is replaced by eating followed by many hours of no interest in food. When you redevelop hunger, it seems to match physiologic need, providing interest in just obtaining what you need to live and function—not the bizarre excess of calories typical of modern habits and exemplified by such phenomena as all-you-can-eat buffets and food bars. The effects are especially fascinating in people who've been labeled with eating disorders such as bulimia, anorexia, and binge eating disorder, many of whom experience normalization of appetite and food perceptions.

People feel younger. Twenty years younger is the most common observation. (I truly don't fully understand why this happens—reduced inflammation, shifts in hormones—but it is incredibly consistent.) At the very least, the perceived sense of youthfulness seems to be the combined result of increased energy, deeper sleep, and reduced stiffness and pain.

Menstrual cycles are milder. Women experience reduced cramping and moodiness.

The "heartburn" of acid reflux improves or disappears in the majority of people. Those labeled with irritable bowel syndrome typically experience less bloating, less gas, and less unpredictability in bowel habits.

Less joint pain and swelling. Most characteristically, this involves reduced pain and swelling in the joints of the fingers, hands, and wrists, but also in the elbows and shoulders. Tenderness and swelling of the shins and ankles also recede, as do leg and ankle swelling.

Naysayers, of course, jump on unquantifiable subjective benefits as mass hysteria, a group placebo effect that develops because I have such incredible powers of persuasion. But the experience that counts is yours and that of your family and friends. The wonderful thing about this is that you can decide for yourself: Just eliminate all things wheat. There are no prescription drugs, no nutritional supplements, no meetings to attend—just no wheat.

But there is a complicating factor, because when you deny your body all things wheat, there is . . .

Wheat Withdrawal

Removing wheat, for many people, is downright terrifying.

If the gliadin protein of modern wheat acts as a morphine-like opiate, then halting the flow of wheat can generate withdrawal. Aside from alcohol, I know of no other food that has a genuine addiction—and I mean actual physical addiction, not just intense desire—and withdrawal associated with it, certainly no food that you share with friends and serve your children.

The addictive property of wheat is a very real phenomenon. Most people intuitively know that when deprived of their opiate of choice, they will begin to experience unpleasant effects within hours. They experience overpowering hunger that leaves them foggy and shaky. They feel the unpleasant low mood of lacking wheat, the desperation that causes you to seek relief, leading you to eat stale crackers from a year-old box, eat your children's food, or snap at the waitress because you've been waiting more than 5 minutes for your food. Like all addictions, it recedes with a sigh of relief when the next "hit" of wheat arrives, at least for the next few hours.

But what if that next hit never comes? What happens when you commit yourself to doing away with all things wheat and trigger wheat withdrawal on purpose?

It means that many of the short-term phenomena of withdrawal—fatigue, shakiness, low mood, cravings for wheat and sugar—will be sustained and worsen over time. Wheat withdrawal closely resembles withdrawal from other opiates like morphine, Oxycontin, and heroin, just less severe. The effect generally lasts from 24 hours to several days, occasionally weeks. But it does not last forever. I've witnessed it in men, women (who seem to get wheat withdrawal worse than men), Republicans, Democrats, young, old, even children. When it recedes, it can do so quite dramatically, with many describing a palpable surge in energy and mood and the disappearance of cravings. The drop in energy with wheat elimination is also partly due to the delayed conversion of metabolism from a constant flow of easily burned carbohydrates, like the amylopectin A of wheat, to that of fat oxidation, or the mobilization of fat stores. This conversion is necessary to lose weight, which generally proceeds rapidly and is mostly lost from the abdomen.

Some disruption of bowel habits is also typical, with some people experiencing loose stools, others constipation. This is most likely the result of the change in bowel flora that results from depriving the bacteria in the intestinal tract of the components of wheat, amylopectin A, gliadin, and lectins. (More on this later.)

Not everyone is subject to wheat withdrawal. The wheat withdrawal syndrome affects around 35 to 40 percent of people who stop consuming wheat products. Thankfully, while I won't minimize its severity in some people, it is not as traumatic as withdrawal from, say, heroin. The process of wheat withdrawal, aside from the emotional turmoil and aches, is harmless. Everyone has survived.

Despite the low mood and emotional turmoil, most people choose simply to grin and bear the process, allowing their bodies to adjust to the loss of this opiate on brain function and the slow activation of fat oxidation. Because the withdrawal process can be disruptive and unpleasant, it is worth not triggering again with a return to wheat and repeated withdrawal, thus my motto: Once wheat free, always wheat free.

The Wonderful State of Wheatlessness

Life without wheat is, for so many of us, so utterly different from our former wheat-consuming lives. It's America after the

Revolution, race relations after Martin Luther King, Kirstie Alley after *Dancing with the Stars*. The transfiguration is that dramatic.

Wheatlessness means eating to meet your body's needs, not submitting to the perverse appetite-stimulating effects of wheat gliadin. It means enjoying mental clarity and the capacity for sustained concentration unclouded by the opiate of wheat. It means being slender, happier, with fewer body aches, better bowel health, and fewer rashes. It means ridding yourself of the grotesque metabolic distortions that develop in wheat-consuming people and instead enjoying marked improvements in metabolic health reflected by lower blood sugar, reduced measures of inflammation, reduced triglycerides, and improvement of an entire host of other health parameters.

In short, life is transformed when you say goodbye to wheat and join in the Wonderful State of Wheatlessness. Let's consider each of these effects in greater detail.

Weight Loss and the Magical Shrinking Wheat Belly

What happens when you reduce calorie intake—and hunger—by 400 or more calories per day?

You lose weight. Multiple studies have demonstrated weight loss of 26 pounds, on average, in the first 6 months of being wheat free. And that is what I have witnessed over and over again (some people less, others more, but an average of 26 pounds during the first 6 months) in people who say goodbye to the appetite-stimulating effects of wheat gliadin. The weight lost exceeds the quantity of wheat calories lost.

The weight is lost primarily from the abdomen, with typical reductions of 2 to 3 inches in waist circumference within the first 4 weeks of wheatlessness. Although the reasons for such a selective, specific process around the waist are not entirely clear, it is at least partly due to the absence of amylopectin A that had previously been responsible for extravagantly high jumps in blood sugar and insulin that stimulate visceral fat accumulation. I also have to believe that receding inflammatory responses—removal of wheat germ agglutinin, restoration of leptin sensitivity—in visceral fat cells have to play a central role in the exaggerated loss of waist size.

So, no, you are not overweight because you failed to eat a sufficient quantity of "healthy whole grains." Chances are that you are also not overweight because you are lazy and gluttonous, as many official sources claim. If I were to peek in your family room some day, I doubt I'd catch you lying flat on your back watching *Survivor* reruns, snacking on a bag of chips, and drinking Coca-Cola by the liter bottle. In fact, I wouldn't be surprised if instead I caught you walking on your treadmill or riding your stationary bike, frantically trying to work off the excess pounds.

You and many others are overweight because you were given bad advice—advice that actually causes weight gain. Reject that advice, remove the appetite-stimulating effects of wheat gliadin and amylopectin A, and weight loss can finally proceed without effort.

But, as powerful as wheat elimination is, I can't say that you will lose all the weight you want if you eliminate all wheat but then eat all the candy and drink all the soda you want, or consume "healthier" equivalents of these insulin-provoking foods. Add to this the fact that the majority of adults are now diabetic or prediabetic (you may not even know it), meaning they have abnormal resistance to insulin, have disordered leptin signaling, and are unable to properly metabolize carbohydrates. If weight loss and reversal of diabetes/prediabetes are on your agenda, then restricting total carbohydrates will accelerate your success (see "Can I Eat Quinoa? Carb-Counting Basics" on page 44).

Diabetes: Kiss "Healthy Whole Grainitis" Goodbye

Type 2 diabetes and "healthy whole grains" are so tightly tied to one another that they are nearly one and the same: Eat "healthy whole grains," become diabetic or prediabetic. Reject "healthy whole grains," and diabetes and prediabetes improve or disappear in the majority. But that, of course, is not what you are told by "official" sources of nutritional advice.

Type 1 diabetes, incidentally, is also increasingly looking like a disease of wheat consumption. This is not to say that all type 1 diabetes is caused by wheat exposure, but an important minority of children who develop this lifelong condition do so because of wheat exposure if genetically susceptible. Note that children with type 1 diabetes have ten- to twentyfold greater likelihood of developing celiac disease, and children with celiac disease have tenfold greater likelihood of type 1 diabetes.

You've likely heard the argument that if whole grains replace white flour products, the likelihood of diabetes is reduced. That is indeed (a little bit) true. The next step—elimination of all things wheat, especially modern wheat—is not talked about. But that is when the real magic happens and appetite drops, visceral fat recedes and waist circumference shrinks, inflammation that drives insulin resistance drops, blood sugar drops, and hemoglobin A1c (a common measure that reflects the prior 60 to 90 days of blood sugars) plummets.

Credit the absence of gliadin that stimulates appetite and the amylopectin A that drives blood sugar higher for improvements in diabetic blood sugars. Over time, improvements are compounded by dropping body weight and shrinkage of inflammatory visceral fat. That's when most prediabetics become nonprediabetic and many, if not most, diabetics become nondiabetic, or at least experience marked improvements in blood sugar and reduced reliance on diabetes medication.

Wheat elimination represents the exact opposite of the advice offered by the American Diabetes Association and other purveyors

(continued on page 46)

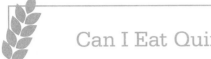

Can I Eat Quinoa? Carb-Counting Basics

It's a frequent question: Can I eat quinoa, beans, brown rice, or sweet potatoes? Or how about amaranth, sorghum, and buckwheat? Surely corn on the cob is okay!

These are, of course, nonwheat carbohydrates. They lack several undesirable ingredients found in wheat, including:

Gliadin—The protein that degrades to exorphins, the compound from wheat digestion that exerts mind effects and stimulates appetite.

Gluten—The family of proteins that trigger immune diseases and neurological impairment.

Amylopectin A—The highly digestible carbohydrate that is no better—*worse,* in fact—than table sugar.

Wheat germ agglutinin—The protein that is directly disruptive in the intestines and can generate celiac-like destructive changes, as well as piggyback foreign substances into the bloodstream.

So why not eat all the nonwheat grains you want? If they don't cause appetite stimulation, behavioral outbursts in children, addictive consumption of foods, skin rashes, dementia, etc., why not just eat them willy-nilly?

Because they still increase blood sugar and insulin.

Conventional wisdom is that these foods have a lower glycemic index than, say, table sugar, meaning they raise blood glucose less. That's true, but misleading. Oats, for instance, with a glycemic index of 55 compared with table sugar's 59 to 65, will still send blood sugar through the roof. Likewise, quinoa, with a glycemic index of 53, will send blood sugar to, say, 150 milligrams/deciliter compared with 158 milligrams/deciliter for table sugar—yeah, sure, it's better, but it still stinks. And that's the result in people who don't have diabetes. It's *worse* in people with diabetes and prediabetes. You can be wheat free and lose the appetite-stimulating effects of gliadin, but consuming larger servings of oatmeal, quinoa, and rice will serve to stall or reverse your weight loss. Because it is gluten free, quinoa in particular has acquired a reputation for being problem free. Not true. Consume a cup of cooked quinoa containing 34 grams of "net" carbs, for instance, and you will trigger insulin and stall weight loss.

Of course, John Q. Internist will tell you that, provided your blood sugars after eating don't exceed 200 milligrams/deciliter, you'll be okay. What he's really saying is "There's no need for diabetes medication right now. You will still be exposed to the many adverse health consequences of high blood sugar similar to, though less quickly than, a full diabetic, but that's not an urgent problem. You're probably lazy and gluttonous, anyway, and can't follow a diet program. We'll just keep an eye on you until you need medication."

In reality, most people can get away with consuming *some* of these nonwheat grains, provided portion size is limited. Limit portion size and you better manage carbohydrates to ensure that metabolic distortions, such as high blood sugar, glycation (glucose modification of proteins associated with conditions like cataracts, hypertension, heart disease, and arthritis), and small LDL particles (the worst LDL particles of all, the bad of the bad), are not triggered.

These nonwheat carbohydrates, or what I call intermediate carbohydrates (for lack of a better term; low glycemic index is falsely reassuring), still trigger all the carbohydrate phenomena of table sugar. Is it possible to obtain the fiber, B vitamins, and antioxidant benefits of these intermediate carbohydrates without triggering the undesirable carbohydrate consequences?

Yes, by using small portions. Small portions are tolerated by most people without triggering all these phenomena. Problem: Individual sensitivity varies widely. One person's perfectly safe portion size is another person's deadly dose. For instance, I've witnessed extreme differences, such as blood sugar 1 hour after eating 6 ounces of unsweetened yogurt of 250 milligrams/deciliter in one person, 105 milligrams/deciliter in another. So checking 1-hour blood sugars is a reliable means of assessing individual sensitivity to carbs.

Many people don't like the idea of checking blood sugars, however. Or there might be times when it's inconvenient or unavailable. A useful alternative: Count carbohydrate grams. (Count "net" carbohydrate grams, i.e., total carbohydrates minus fiber grams to yield "net," or "effective," carbs, i.e., the carbs that are actually digested, not just passively passing through like fiber.) **Most people can tolerate 14 to 15 "net" grams of carbohydrates per meal and deal with them effectively.** Only the most sensitive people, for example, people with diabetes or individuals with an inherited tendency for high triglycerides, are intolerant to even this amount and do better with no more than 10 grams per meal. Then there are the genetically gifted from a carbohydrate perspective: people who can tolerate 20, 40, 50, or more grams at a sitting.

People will sometimes say things like "I eat 200 grams of carbohydrate per day, and I'm normal weight and have perfect fasting blood sugar and lipids." As in many things, the crude measures made are falsely reassuring. Glycation, for instance, from postprandial blood sugars of "only" 140 milligrams/deciliter—typical after, say, a bowl of organic, stone-ground, unsweetened oatmeal in a slender person—still works its unhealthy magic and over the long term will lead to cataracts, arthritis, and other conditions.

Humans were not meant to consume an endless supply of readily digestible carbohydrates. Counting carbohydrates is a great way to "tighten up" a carbohydrate restriction.

of health advice, who advocate that people with diabetes cut consumption of fat and, yes, eat more "healthy whole grains." I've witnessed countless diabetics follow this advice and watched them gain weight, experience increasing blood sugars and HbA1c, resulting in increased need for diabetes drugs, then insulin, not to mention experience leg edema, hypertension, acid reflux, and the myriad other effects of wheat consumption. (And just who profits from such advice? That's an entire conversation of its own. Suffice it to say that one of the biggest contributors to the American Diabetes Association over the years has been Cadbury Schweppes, the world's largest candy and soft drink manufacturer. Diabetes drug manufacturers have been quite generous, too.) It is an exceptionally common progression, one that is predicted to ensnare one in three Americans in the diabetic category in coming years. I have no question in my mind that this blunder constitutes one of the biggest nutritional crimes of the century.

Reject this advice—eat more fat and eat no "healthy whole grains"—and diabetes powerfully recedes. I've watched this happen many times.

However, if you have diabetes, there is the potential for dangerous hypoglycemia (low blood sugars) when you eliminate all things wheat and are taking diabetes medications. The risks of hypoglycemia are even greater if you eliminate wheat and restrict other carbohydrates, regardless of the source. In other words, as you become less diabetic and consume fewer foods that raise blood sugar, you may experience low blood sugars, much as a nondiabetic person taking diabetes medication might experience. For this reason, several precautions should be taken (see "Caution: If You Have Diabetes . . . " on page 48).

The Happy Wheat-Free Gastrointestinal Tract

Ever notice how having a happy gastrointestinal tract is central to feeling good overall? If you are plagued by gas, cramps, abdominal discomfort, and having to make panic runs to the toilet while making apologies to friends, it's tough to feel good. Being free from these torments, on the other hand, with well-adjusted, happy bowels, makes all-around health more likely. Well, those of you in the former category, take heart: Relief from common gastrointestinal complaints is among the most common experiences in those who enjoy wheatlessness.

Remove wheat gliadin, gluten, and lectins from your diet, and gastrointestinal health improves in a number of important ways. The dramatic relief from cramps, discomfort, and bowel urgency provided by elimination of wheat, followed by prompt recurrence with re-exposure in the majority of people, is a frequent and consistent phenomenon. In other words, eat wheat and struggle with abdominal cramps and intermittent diarrhea; eliminate wheat and experience relief for extended periods. Have a re-exposure to wheat products, purposely or inadvertently, and all the cramps, urgency, and embarrassment rush back with renewed intensity, only to recede again with stopping wheat—on again, off again, on again, off again. Unfortunately, many in the gastroenterology community deny that these associations exist because they cannot view the destruction at the end of their endoscopes and often ascribe the symptoms to anxiety or depression or dismiss you as nuts and advise an antidepressant or pill for anxiety. The fact that you can trigger symptoms with exposure and obtain relief with avoidance is sufficient proof to demonstrate a cause-effect relationship, regardless of whether some gastroenterologist "approves" or not.

Among the most common gastrointestinal experiences with wheat elimination are:

- Acid reflux. Also known as reflux esophagitis, acid reflux improves or disappears in the majority of people within days of stopping wheat. People taking drugs like Prilosec, Pepcid, Protonix, or antacids for years describe relief within 3 to 5 days of saying goodbye to wheat. I've witnessed countless people kiss their drugs goodbye after years of dependence with no recurrence of symptoms.

- Irritable bowel syndrome. Characterized by symptoms of excessive gas, cramps, and intermittent diarrhea and

constipation, as well as bouts of bowel urgency, irritable bowel syndrome symptoms also disappear in the majority within days of saying goodbye to wheat. The drugs usually prescribed for this condition provide partial relief at best. The dietary strategy for relief— eat no wheat—works like a charm in the majority.

- Improved regularity. Most people find that, minus wheat, bowel regularity is paradoxically improved. I say "paradoxically" because we've been told over and over again by health-care experts and the food industry that wheat products containing plenty of fiber promote regularity. And they do—in wheat-eating individuals. Take away wheat and regularity improves in the majority, even in people with something called *obstipation*, or severe and unremitting constipation with bowel movements delayed for up to weeks at a time. (An occasional person experiences constipation with wheat elimination, but this situation responds to restoration of bowel flora. See "What If My Colon Says, 'No Way!'?" on page 50.)

- Reduced symptoms of inflammatory bowel disease. Serious inflammatory bowel conditions—ulcerative colitis and Crohn's disease—are worsened by wheat consumption and improved with wheat avoidance. I find that the longer an individual with one of these conditions avoids wheat, the greater the relief, with substantial relief developing over extended periods of months or longer. The most common response is marked reduction in symptoms of cramps, diarrhea, and bleeding, though I have witnessed outright cure on several occasions.

I interpret the incredible ubiquity of improved gastrointestinal health with wheat elimination as evidence that this thing called modern wheat was never meant for human consumption.

Caution: If You Have Diabetes . . .

"There is not a shred of evidence that sugar, per se, has anything to do with getting diabetes."

RICHARD KAHN, PHD,
recently retired chief scientific and medical officer,
American Diabetes Association

Dr. Kahn's comment echoes conventional thinking on diabetes: Eat all the grains and candy you want; just be sure to talk to your doctor about diabetes medications.

If you eat foods that increase blood sugar, it increases your need for diabetes medications. If you reduce or eliminate foods that increase blood sugar, then it decreases your need for diabetes medications. The equation for most people with adult, or type 2, diabetes is really that simple.

But several precautions are necessary if you are diabetic and are taking certain diabetes drugs. The potential danger is *hypoglycemia,* low blood sugars (for example, less than 70 milligrams/deciliter)—as well as the uninformed objections of many doctors who have come to believe that diabetes is incurable, irreversible, and a diagnosis for life.

Some medications, such as metformin (Glucophage), pioglitazone (Actos), rosiglitazone (Avandia), and acarbose (Precose), rarely if ever result in hypoglycemia when taken by themselves. They are effective for preventing blood sugar rises but tend not to generate blood sugar lows.

However, other medications, especially glyburide (DiaBeta, Micronase), glipizide (Glucotrol), glimepiride (Amaryl), and various insulin preparations, can cause severe and dangerous hypoglycemia if taken while reducing or eliminating wheat and carbohydrates. For this reason, many people eliminate these oral drugs or slash their insulin doses by 50 percent at the start, even if it means some temporary increase in blood sugars. The key is to avoid hypoglycemia

Happy Wheat-Free Lungs and Sinuses

After eliminating wheat, an impressive number of people experience relief from common respiratory complaints, including:

- Asthma. Typically, people who previously relied on the use of inhalers to breathe experience marked reduction, occasionally elimination, of the need for them. This has happened repeatedly in both adults and children with asthma. As

as you consume less food that increases blood sugar, even if it means higher near-term blood sugars.

Other medications, such as sitagliptin (Januvia), saxagliptin (Onglyza), linagliptin (Tradjenta), exenatide (Byetta), and liraglutide (Victoza), usually do not result in hypoglycemia but occasionally can, especially if taken in combination with other diabetes drugs.

Because of the complexity of these responses, you should ideally work with a health-care provider who is adept at navigating these issues as you become less and less diabetic. The problem is that most doctors and diabetes educators *have no idea whatsoever* how to do this, as they will tell you that once you have diabetes, you will always have it and trying to get rid of it is fruitless and foolhardy (to the appreciative applause of the diabetes drug industry). So don't be surprised if you are left on your own. At the very least, you want to check to see if your doctor will work with you, and if not, at least try to find another who will. Also, frequent monitoring of blood sugars is essential. I tell my patients on the path to becoming nondiabetic that high blood sugars (though maintained below 200 milligrams/deciliter) are preferable to low blood sugars (below 100 milligrams/deciliter) in this transition period. If, for instance, you are obtaining blood sugars in the morning (fasting) of 100 milligrams/deciliter, it is time to further reduce or eliminate a medication, such as glipizide or Lantus insulin taken at bedtime.

Any person with diabetes who wants to understand the details of becoming nondiabetic would benefit from knowing about the resources of Dr. Richard Bernstein, author of *The Diabetes Solution.* More information can be found at www.diabetes-book.com. The critical issue is to understand that many people with diabetes have been told that they have an incurable condition and that a diet rich in "healthy whole grains" is essential—*advice that ensures you remain diabetic.* Do the opposite: Eliminate "healthy whole grains," especially the most dangerous grain, wheat, and limit other carbohydrates, including nonwheat grains like millet and quinoa, and diabetes unwinds itself with reduced fasting blood sugars and HbA1c in the majority.

More recently, the American Diabetes Association's former chief scientific and medical officer, Dr. Kahn, added, "Diabetes prevention is a waste of resources." Why, think of all the money that could instead go to pharmaceutical research and marketing!

asthma is among the most frequent diagnoses in emergency rooms and the disease has increased dramatically over the past 40 years, it raises the question whether the unique alpha amylase inhibitors and other new antigens (allergic triggers) from modern wheat may underlie at least some of these trends.

Compared with the obnoxious side effects of treatments like prednisone, the ill effects of wheat elimination as a potential asthma-reducing strategy are nil.

- Chronic sinus infections and sinus congestion. Many people who have struggled with sinus infection after sinus

What If My Colon Says, "No Way!"?

All of us have trillions of bacteria—"bowel flora"—living in our colons and small intestines, a necessity for life and health. For a taste of what life is like with sudden disruptions of bowel flora, witness the result on bowel habits after taking an antibiotic that temporarily reduces or eliminates bacterial inhabitants: cramps, pain, and diarrhea until they repopulate some days or weeks later.

The health implications of bowel flora are only just beginning to be appreciated. Some studies have suggested, for instance, that overweight people and people with diabetes have different bowel flora—different numbers, different species—compared with people who aren't overweight and who don't have diabetes.

People who consume wheat products also undergo changes in intestinal bacteria compared with people who don't eat wheat: They have greater total numbers of bacteria and experience changes in the species present. It means that people who *add* wheat to their diets change the composition of their bowel flora. It also means that when you *remove* all things wheat, shifts occur in the opposite direction, or at least they should.

Problem: After removing wheat, the return to a more normal, wheat-free profile of bowel flora may not occur right away. Along with the phenomena of wheat withdrawal, such as fatigue and low mood, there may be a transition period of variable duration in which you struggle with increased gas, constipation, and mild abdominal discomfort. After all, your bowels cannot create new bacteria; they have to acquire them little by little from the foods you ingest.

This delayed transition can be accelerated by adding a probiotic preparation, i.e., a preparation of concentrated bacteria that contains species of *Bifidobacterium, Lactobacillus,* and other healthy species, preferably in a total quantity of 50 billion CFUs (colony-forming units) or greater. These preparations are available in many health food stores and pharmacies. Four weeks of a probiotic and most people are back to predictable, comfortable bowel habits, with friendly bowel flora happy to do their job of assisting in digestion.

There's another layer of gastrointestinal struggles that emerge in the wheat free. This infection, having to take antibiotics for weeks or months at a time, several times per year, have experienced dramatic relief—with no stuffiness, no drainage, no sinus headaches, no sinus infections, no need for antibiotics. Likewise, chronic sinus congestion often disappears for the first time in many people.

• Chronic cough. The acid reflux caused by wheat consumption often results in acid irritation of the throat and larynx, causing a chronic and annoying cough. Conventional treatment generally involves use of prescription drugs to suppress stomach acid. I have seen this phenomenon recede with wheat elimination many times.

applies to people who've struggled with lots of gastrointestinal symptoms *before* wheat elimination, such as the cramps and diarrhea of irritable bowel syndrome, or difficulties with absorption of nutrients. These people eliminate all wheat and experience relief, but only partially. They may be left with some degree of persistent cramps and diarrhea, or poorly formed stools, sometimes with visible remnants of undigested proteins and oils. A number of conditions may account for this, including failed intestinal signaling via the signal protein, cholecystokinin (CCK), to trigger the pancreas to release digestive enzymes. Failed CCK signaling means the pancreas fails to release the digestive enzymes required to fully break down proteins, fats, and carbohydrates in foods. Incompletely digested foods result in cramps, gas, diarrhea, and failed transition in bowel flora.

Ideally, this situation is assessed by a health-care practitioner with expertise in assessing stool composition to identify the precise difficulty, but this expertise is difficult to find. A compromise is therefore to supplement pancreatic enzymes, especially the fat-digesting enzyme, lipase, that you can purchase at health food stores, and take them prior to or during every meal. If insufficient pancreatic enzyme levels are the cause of your symptoms, then a pancreatic enzyme supplement should provide partial or complete relief. Good choices include RenewLife DigestMORE Ultra and Life Extension Enhanced Super Digestive Enzymes. These can be taken along with a probiotic preparation.

Because some people experience a slow, long-term recovery of intestinal health over a long period of wheatlessness, it is worth periodically reassessing your need for the enzyme supplements, i.e., a trial of eating *without* them.

Incidentally, do not be fooled into taking enzyme preparations that purport to protect you from wheat or gluten consumption. This is absolute foolishness: There is no "antidote" to all the effects of wheat or gluten. There is only one way to protect yourself from the bowel disruptive effects of this thing: Never eat wheat again.

Happy Wheat-Free Skin

The skin can provide many clues that wheat's destruction is at work, as it represents the outwardly visible manifestation of internal body processes.

It's no news that the disfiguring skin condition dermatitis herpetiformis is cured with wheat elimination, as it is peculiar to people who also have the genetic predisposition to celiac disease. But it's all the other skin conditions attributable to wheat, from trivial to serious, that occur in people without celiac disease (or the genetic predisposition to it) that constitute the great majority of skin conditions that improve or disappear with wheat elimination.

Because the complete list of skin conditions that improve with wheat elimination is simply too long to include, here are the most common conditions that show marked or total improvement with wheat elimination.

- Seborrhea. The red, flaky rash of seborrhea, typically found on either side of the nose, other areas of the face, behind the ears, on the scalp, and in other locations, recedes in the majority of people. (In my experience, a combination of the red rash alongside the nose along with reddened cheeks and facial puffiness, especially around the eyes, is *nearly always* due to wheat.)

- Psoriasis. This raised, red, scaly rash that assumes a variety of forms can respond dramatically to wheat elimination in some, partially in others. Given the emergence of toxic drugs that cost thousands of dollars *per month* used to treat this condition, wheat removal seems almost quaint.

- Acne. Acne can recede dramatically. It makes sense when you realize that primitive hunter-gatherer (i.e., non-wheat-eating) cultures such as the Kitavan Islanders of New Guinea and Aché hunter-gatherers of Paraguay have no problems with acne, while Western cultures are plagued by it. And it's not just a problem for teenagers, since 95 percent of adults experience occasional acne breakouts as well. The cozy relationship of wheat consumption and acne is, more than likely, due to the amylopectin A of wheat, given its extravagant potential to raise blood sugar and insulin, the situation that encourages acne development.

- Dandruff. Relief from chronic dandruff is a common observation in people who go wheat free, even after years of special shampoos and salves.

- Hair loss. While we know that wheat can cause a condition called alopecia areata, or hair loss that usually develops in a patchy pattern, the thickening and regrowth of hair is something I've been seeing and hearing about more and more, as the wheat-denying experience grows.

You will be disappointed if you ask most dermatologists if the rash you've had on your arms and legs for the past 15 years could be due to wheat. As with all issues surrounding the Evil Grain, most physicians, including dermatologists, have next to no appreciation of its astounding potential for triggering multiple health conditions, including dozens, perhaps hundreds, of varieties of skin disorders.

The Happy Wheat-Free Brain and Nervous System

Under the spell of wheat, the brain is flittering, faltering, and foggy, and it kowtows to wheat's overpowering appetite-stimulating effects. This means you are potentially the unwitting victim of any food manufacturer who decides to push your appetite buttons for their gain.

Gliadin plays a leading role in creating mind effects with its opiate-like ability to penetrate into brain tissue. The immune response triggered by gliadin in genetically susceptible individuals also sets destructive brain effects in motion. The inflammatory mix-up created by wheat germ agglutinin, its ability to block the hormone leptin to provoke satiety, and the broad inflammatory battlefield generated by growing visceral fat of the wheat belly make matters worse. Is it any wonder we are able to function at all under the influence of modern wheat except through sheer force of will and plenty of caffeine?

The wheat-free brain, in contrast, is so much more focused, effective, alert, and in charge of itself.

Given the observations in schizophrenic patients that began in the 1960s connecting wheat consumption with worsening of auditory hallucinations (hearing voices), social detachment, and paranoia, it should come as no surprise that wheat elimination exerts favorable mental effects on individuals without schizophrenia. Among the observations that have been made with wheat elimination:

- Improved attention span and reduced behavioral outbursts in children with attention deficit hyperactivity disorder (ADHD) and autism.

- Cerebellar ataxia, involving deterioration and shrinkage of the cerebellum with loss of balance, coordination, and bladder control; peripheral neuropathy, or deterioration of the nerves in the legs, pelvis, and autonomic nervous system (responsible for functions like heart rate control and bladder and bowel control); and encephalopathy, destruction of the gray matter of the brain resulting in dementia, can recede with elimination of wheat, though, as with all neurological processes, they do so slowly over months and years. These conditions don't just develop out of the blue; they likely smolder and burn over many years or decades, progressively impairing the ability to concentrate, navigate a sidewalk, control your bladder, remember words, recall people's names, and, eventually, recognize your own children.

- Seizures, particularly a variety called temporal lobe epilepsy, are more frequent in people with immune markers to wheat gluten. Accordingly, removing all wheat and gluten can yield a seizure-protective effect.

Cucumbers don't affect your mind, grapefruit doesn't dissolve your brain tissue, and 16 ounces of sirloin steak doesn't ablate a lifetime of memories. But wheat does. Remove it and free your mind from its hold. Because destruction of brain tissue is a process of profound importance to an individual's health and one that does not usually pose potential for full recovery, given neurological tissue's limited regenerative capacity, if there's one thing that you can do to reduce your lifetime likelihood of seeing a shrunken cerebral cortex or cerebellum on the MRI your doctor orders, it's saying goodbye to all things wheat.

Happy Wheat-Free Joints

Along with relief from common complaints of painful, stiff, and swollen finger, hand, and wrist joints, many people experience relief from joint pain in other areas. Among the most frequent observations are:

- Reduced pain and swelling in major joints. The pain and swelling of osteoarthritis in the hips, knees, and other joints typically improve. This is most likely due to a twofold effect of wheat elimination: removal of inflammation-provoking wheat lectin and reduction of inflammation originating with the visceral fat that shrinks with wheat elimination. It is not uncommon for people to observe that,

once wheat free, despite only a modest weight loss of, say, 10 to 20 pounds, their joints experience substantially less pain and swelling. Note that cartilage cells, unique in that they lack the capacity to reproduce and the cells you have today are the same ones you had at age 18, are prone to stiffening (glycation) whenever blood sugar (glucose) rises above normal. So a lifetime of experiencing high blood sugars several times per day leads to arthritis; this effect of wheat consumption cannot be undone, as the changes induced by glycation are irreversible, but wheat elimination means that you can stop adding to the injury (and young people can avoid having it in the first place). Removing wheat and its inflammatory effect cannot, of course, rebuild lost cartilage of the "bone-on-bone" destroyed hip or knee joint, but it can reduce much of the inflammation and pain.

- Improvement in rheumatoid arthritis and other inflammatory joint diseases. We know from clinical trials that people with the autoimmune condition rheumatoid arthritis experience measurable improvement when they eliminate wheat. This effect appears to be shared by other forms of inflammatory conditions, such as lupus, psoriatic arthritis, polymyositis, and polymyalgia rheumatica, all of which improve with wheat elimination.

Unlike the relatively rapid response of gastrointestinal and other conditions, inflammatory arthritis, in all its various forms, requires a much longer period of wheat avoidance to demonstrate improvement, typically several months to a year or longer. But it sure beats years of taking nonsteroidal anti-inflammatory drugs that cause ulcers and heart attack, or a new prosthetic knee or hip joint.

Putting It All Together

Do you have celiac disease or gluten sensitivity, or are you among the majority of people without these conditions who just have no business at all eating this dietary poison?

To diagnose celiac disease, you will need the assistance of your doctor. He or she should run blood tests, particularly the test for transglutaminase antibody, which is virtually diagnostic if positive. Some physicians feel that a biopsy of the small intestine is required for positive diagnosis, an opinion I do not share, since the antibody tests are so reliable when positive. The real difficulty comes when the antibody tests are negative, yet you have all the intestinal symptoms of celiac disease; this is a situation in which the assistance of a biopsy may truly be helpful. The treatment: Eliminate all wheat and gluten-containing grains and foods.

Gluten sensitivity is really gliadin sensitivity in most cases, and tests for the gliadin antibody (blood, salivary, or stool) can be helpful here, since the degree of intestinal damage required to trigger the transglutaminase response may be insufficient and only the gliadin antibody may be detect-

able. The treatment: Eliminate all wheat and gluten-containing grains and foods.

The majority of people test negative for all antibodies, yet they still have symptoms, such as joint pain, acid reflux, cramps, leg pain, mental "fog," and appetite stimulation, that disappear with elimination of all wheat. And, lastly, there is the minority of people who perceive no improvement in any symptom with removal of all wheat. But this last group should not be fooled: They can still experience high blood sugars and glycation that lead to cataracts and arthritis, trigger small LDL particles that lead to heart attack, and inflammation, even if they feel fine. The treatment: Eliminate all wheat and gluten-containing grains and foods.

I suspect that you see where I am going with this. If nobody gets away with consuming this grain, this concoction of extreme and bizarre genetics manipulations, then the easiest, most expeditious solution for most people is simply to eliminate all wheat and gluten-containing grains and foods.

The truth is that there is simply no test—blood test, saliva test, stool test, biopsy—that identifies all the varied ways humans react to this destructive dietary invader with its myriad components that wreak havoc in a variety of ways in multiple organs.

Some will argue that it is useful to know whether you have celiac disease, since it will motivate the individual to be more meticulous in avoiding wheat and gluten if they know, for instance, that even occasional exposure, purposeful or inadvertent, can result in greatly increased risk of gastrointestinal cancer. I believe that is reasonable. In my experience, however, nobody truly gets away with consuming this thing. The long-term consequences of consuming modern wheat are often attributed to other causes, or even dismissed as being due to unknown causes, blaming the cataracts on old age, the knee and hip arthritis on wear and tear, the asthma and repeated sinus infections on allergies, the obesity and diabetes on gluttony and laziness.

Modern wheat is not a natural plant. Modern high-yield, semi-dwarf wheat does not exist in nature except for the fact that human geneticists created it. It has extensive negative and many unknown effects in humans. There is no reason to consume it.

The Wonderful Wheatlessness of Being

I know of no other nutritional or health strategy that can pack as much punch into regaining health as the elimination of this modern thing peddled to us called wheat. No other food, when eliminated, can yield such across-the-board improvements in metabolism, weight, joint and gastrointestinal health, and emotional and mental health—regardless of your degree of sensitivity.

After all, it's not wheat.

No other thing, so cleverly disguised as healthy food, is so destructive yet so ubiquitous. And no other food, when removed from the diet, yields such outsize and unexpected health benefits. Can the elimination of any other single food yield weight loss of 30, 50, 60, or more pounds? Can cutting red meat or fat yield complete relief from acid reflux, bowel urgency, joint pain, leg edema, migraine headaches, intestinal destruction by celiac disease and brain destruction by gluten encephalopathy, seborrhea, psoriasis, acne, dandruff, eating disorders, and depression? Does any other food have the capacity to manipulate behavior like the chief appetite stimulant of all, wheat gliadin?

Modern wheat is perfectly crafted for maximum damage. Eliminate this darling of nutritionists, the USDA, and "official" providers of nutritional advice, and the entire mess unwinds. You're left with normal appetite, normal weight, normal blood sugar, healthy long-lasting joints, normal blood pressure, normal bowel health, and normal mood and energy.

Look in the mirror. If you see someone with bags under the eyes, redness along the sides of the nose, and a tired and edematous pallor, well, then, you've got a case of wheat consumption on your hands. The cure is quite simple.

SUCCESS STORY

Bob Lost 78 Pounds

I guess I was a yo-yo dieter, bouncing up and down as I went on a weight-loss regimen, then lost interest and reverted to my old habits. I seemed to have a "weight comfort zone" that my body always went back to. When I read about *Wheat Belly* in September 2011, I figured I'd give it a try—on New Year's Day 2012. But on the morning of November 1, while I was getting dressed, my pants were so tight, I couldn't even close them. "Time to get a new pair of pants," I thought—but then I came to my senses. Nope, it was time to start the Wheat Belly lifestyle. No sense in waiting for January 1 to roll around—there's no time like the present.

I set a goal to be under 200 pounds by my 65th birthday—that gave me 71 weeks, at an average of less than 2 pounds a week. It certainly seemed doable, if I could manage to stick to the plan. So, at 320 pounds, I got started.

The first few days were challenging, but by the end of the first week, I was 10 pounds lighter and feeling pretty good. I lost 40 pounds the first month, and my excitement about this achievement did a lot to take away the sting of giving up all the comfort foods a Southern boy loves— biscuits and gravy, fried chicken, mashed potatoes, pasta, and bread—not to mention desserts and soft drinks.

It's been 26 weeks and counting, and so far I've dropped an average of 3 pounds a week, for a total of 78 pounds. I'm no longer diabetic, my blood pressure is down, my medications have been cut in half, and—for the first time in 30 years—all my liver function tests are normal.

It's great when friends compliment my new look, but best of all, it's amazing when my doctor says he'd gladly trade test results with me! He doesn't want to see me for another 6 months—by then I'll be close to reaching my weight-loss goal. Life is good!

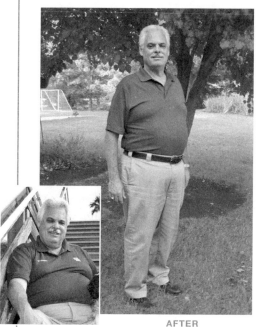

BEFORE

AFTER

ASSEMBLING YOUR WHEAT BELLY KITCHEN

BRACE YOURSELF FOR some exciting ways to reclaim your health and control over your weight yet enjoy delicious foods that, I predict, you will find *more* satisfying than their wheat-containing counterparts.

You probably already have a kitchen fairly well equipped to start this new way of life sans modern wheat. Some housecleaning will be in order, as well as shopping for some new ingredients and perhaps a few new tools, but it really just boils down to some adjustments of your prior wheat-addled lifestyle. So don't tell your husband or wife that an entire kitchen makeover with a new refrigerator, range, and sink is required!

The well-stocked kitchen that accommodates the unique aspects of cooking and preparing foods the *Wheat Belly Cookbook* way requires some new ways of thinking about foods in addition to some new ingredients to create interesting dishes to satisfy your newly enlightened wheat-free palate, all while keeping your family happy—often the toughest hurdle of all. Unavoidably, there will be relics of your prior wheat-based life that you will need to discard or give away, a necessary step for this new, healthy, slender way of life.

Let me also point out that the *Wheat Belly Cookbook* serves as a guide for everyone who wishes to eliminate wheat and gluten from their lives because wheat elimination is not just for the celiac sufferer or the gluten-sensitive; it's for everyone. The advice and recipes here are indeed appropriate for the celiac sufferer and gluten-sensitive, though additional efforts will need to be made to accomplish meticulous gluten avoidance; I will make note of that whenever appropriate.

But, before we get started on what you need to conduct your new life of wheatlessness, you first should . . .

Clean Your Kitchen!

Let's talk about purging your home of the food that caused all the trouble in the first place.

Unless you are among the most exquisitely gluten-sensitive, you do not have to literally "cleanse" your kitchen of wheat, i.e., track down every last crumb and wipe surfaces down with disinfectant. If you are among the most gluten-sensitive, then either a thorough cleaning of all utensils and surfaces and/or maintaining a set of utensils and preparation surfaces dedicated to your gluten-free lifestyle may be necessary.

Purging all evidence of this disruptive grain helps jump-start your weight loss and good health. It also helps keep you on track. At the start, most families typically have pantry shelf after shelf stocked high with wheat products, a refrigerator and freezer packed with wheat products, and snack bowls filled with wheat products. The best policy is to get rid of them—completely. Unless somebody else in the house insists on their presence and refuses to go through this process with you, get rid of them (the wheat, that is, not your spouse or family!). After all, wheat products are unnecessary for health, and saying good riddance is the most powerful and confident nutritional strategy for health you will likely encounter in your lifetime. You might give your wheat-containing discards to charity (though even that has some disturbing social implications), but don't leave them just hanging around. Remember: Wheat products contain an opiate. Just as a heroin addict hides dope in secret places and will, sooner or later, dig up the stash and get high, so will those of us in the throes of wheat with-drawal or in a moment of weakness find those hidden rolls or that bag of pretzels.

Purging your kitchen means emptying your shelves of breakfast cereals, crackers, pretzels, bread crumbs, pancake mix, pasta, macaroni and cheese mix, powdered soup mixes, canned soup, and anything else that contains wheat in some form. Clear your pantry of bread, muffins, bagels, pitas, rolls, cookies, energy bars, and pastries. Check the refrigerator for wheat-containing condiments such as soy sauce, teriyaki sauce, and salad dressings, and the freezer for breaded frozen foods, ice cream flavors like cookie dough and Oreo cookie, and frozen waffles. Look for wheat in sausage and processed meats. And don't forget the Twizzlers, granola bars, and candy—yup, wheat's there, too.

While you're at it, if overall health is your goal, think about getting rid of everything containing too much sugar or high-fructose corn syrup. I can't say, for instance, that you should eliminate wheat and then eat all the candy and drink all the soda you want, all packed with sugar and high-fructose corn syrup. This means getting rid of sugary soft drinks and desserts. (Don't worry: There are desserts in this new wheat-free world, but they will be healthy desserts, all found in the recipes in this book.) Throw away that bottle of "organic agave nectar" you thought was a healthy sweetener, as well as barbecue sauce, low-fat salad dressings, and sweet juices and drinks made with high-fructose corn syrup. Throw away that container of cornstarch, too; it was probably genetically modified anyway!

The most important job—by a long stretch—is to remove all things wheat. Remember: The gliadin protein of wheat is powerfully addictive and will pull you back.

Once you've banished all wheat-containing foods from your kitchen, it will be time to restock with healthy replacements. Here are some basic ground rules that benefit everybody.

- Read labels. Look for "wheat," "wheat flour," "gluten," "vital wheat gluten," "modified food starch," "caramel coloring," or any of the other dozens of buzzwords for concealed wheat that manufacturers slip in. (See Appendix A.) People with celiac disease and gluten sensitivity definitely need to do this, but this is also a good mind-set for everyone else to adopt to minimize exposure, especially to avoid the gastrointestinal and appetite-stimulating effects of wheat.

- Buy *single-ingredient natural foods* found in the produce aisle, butcher shop, and farmers' market that don't require labels. There are no labels, for instance, on tomatoes, portobello mushrooms, avocados, eggs, or swordfish.

- Avoid processed foods with multiple ingredients. A salad dressing you make yourself with olive oil, vinegar, and herbs is far safer than a premixed bottled dressing with 15 ingredients.

- Lose the breakfast cereal habit. There is no such thing as a healthy breakfast cereal (at least not yet). They are wheat land mines, not to mention they are also packed with corn, sugar, high-fructose corn syrup, and additives.

- Do not buy a processed or prepared food unless you can view the ingredient list. Processed meats at the deli, for instance, are frequent sources of inadvertent wheat exposure. Ask to see the label. If you cannot, pass it by.

- Don't even bother with the bread aisle or bakery. There's *nothing* there you need!

- Avoid foods made from ground meats, such as meatballs and meat loaf, as these nearly always contain bread crumbs.

- Ignore all claims of "heart healthy," "low-fat," "low in cholesterol," "part of a balanced diet," etc. These claims are there for one reason: to persuade shoppers that an unhealthy food might have some health benefit. Rarely is that true. In fact, most "heart-healthy" foods *cause* heart disease!

- Get to know your grocery stores, farmers' markets, health food stores, and anyone else selling foods in your area. To make healthy wheat-free foods, you may need some ingredients that are not sold at all mainstream outlets. Prices vary widely, so it helps to shop around and not be stuck with high prices for your everyday wheat-free ingredients.

Later on, we will discuss the specific foods you will need to purchase that will allow you to cook delicious, wheat-free, healthy breakfasts, lunches, and dinners, as well as desserts, cookies, muffins, and other baked foods.

When you're away from home, some additional strategies are helpful.

- Be careful in social situations, such as meals at the homes of family or friends, catered events, parties, etc., especially if you cannot ask what is in a dish. This can make for some awkward situations, such as when fried chicken is served for dinner at your friend's home. Be diplomatic; if necessary, perhaps even resort to the use of a white lie, such as "It looks delicious, but I have a severe wheat allergy." It spares you from sounding rude, though it might leave you hungry. It helps to not show up at such uncertain events when ravenous; eat something safe beforehand so you are not enviously eyeing everyone else's food. When there, eat what you know is safe, such as vegetables, cheese, and simple meats without sauces.

- Though it seems obvious, remember that you do not want your chicken, fish, or crab cakes breaded. Likewise, most soups contain noodles, so avoid them or ask staff beforehand. These are among the two most frequent oversights.

- People with celiac disease and extreme gluten sensitivity have to be concerned with cross-contamination issues in restaurant food preparation, such as gluten contamination of utensils or airborne contamination of food, even if no wheat or gluten was used in the preparation of the food. Most of us do not have to worry about such small exposures.

- Sandwiches, hamburgers, and wraps are off the list. An increasing number of restaurants are willing to provide a wheat-free version, such as a burger wrapped in lettuce or simply served without a bun.

- Ask for salads without croutons. Salad dressings are always suspect, so settle for the simplest—olive oil and vinegar. While it never hurts to ask the waitstaff, you cannot always count on the accuracy of the information.

- Avoid fast-food restaurants. Cooking surfaces, utensils, frying oils, etc., as well as most of the food itself all pose risk for potential contamination with wheat. Fast-food salads might be safe, but be leery of the salad dressings. For people with celiac disease or gluten sensitivity, fast food is a dangerous land mine and is best avoided.

- If you experience repeated episodes of wheat re-exposure sickness, such as nausea, bloating, diarrhea, or asthma and sinus congestion, examine everything you are doing. Look at your lipstick, stop taking the Communion wafers (or ask that they consider a wheat- and gluten-free alternative), don't eat the imitation seafood at the salad bar, and don't lick envelopes. Consider nutritional supplements and prescription drugs as a source of wheat or gluten exposure. If in doubt, contact the manufacturer. Consider following the same advice as those who know they are extremely gluten-sensitive (see "Important Reminders for the Gluten-Sensitive" on page 64).

There's no question that conducting a healthy wheat-free life represents a departure from long-standing habits. But you will be rewarded for your efforts with astounding improvements in the way you look and feel.

For those of you who are extremely gluten-sensitive, as are some people with celiac disease and its equivalents, all foods and ingredients in your kitchen, from refrigerator to pantry, should be gluten free, meaning not containing wheat or gluten sources, such as barley, rye, bulgur, triticale, and oats, but also prepared in facilities that do not handle wheat or gluten products and thereby have no potential for contamination. These products will have "gluten free" posted prominently on the package. (But remember: Many gluten-free foods are just junk carbohydrates in disguise, so be selective.) You will also have to be vigilant to avoid hidden sources of wheat and gluten exposure, such as textured vegetable protein, seitan, roux, and panko. (See Appendix A for a listing.)

Most of us who are trying to avoid wheat but are not among the most gluten-sensitive just need to look for foods and ingredients that do not list wheat or wheat-derived ingredients. For instance, with dark chocolate chips, the most gluten-sensitive will need to purchase a brand actually designated "gluten free" with no wheat, no gluten, and no potential for cross-contamination from other foods and facilities. Those of us avoiding wheat but without celiac disease or extreme gluten sensitivity can do fine with brands that are not designated gluten free but do not list any wheat or gluten equivalents on the ingredient list. The potential for cross-contamination, i.e., the presence of minor residues from, for example, airborne gluten, is rarely a problem for most of us.

So we lose all the baked wheat products from our shelves. But don't despair: In the following pages, you will learn how to create muffins, cookies, cupcakes, and pies without wheat and without gluten-free junk carbohydrates, but that are truly healthy. That's the fun part!

Some will ask, "But I don't have enough time. Can't I just buy these healthy wheat-free foods?" Unfortunately, no manufacturer has yet brought such products to the national market. It is a reflection of how little most food producers understand about nutrition when you recognize that none yet do this. There are a small number of local producers and bakers who provide such foods, and you can locate them online by searching in your area for "gluten free"— but don't be surprised if you find none. As the number of informed consumers demanding wheat-free, gluten-free products without the usual junk carbohydrate ingredients grows, food producers will introduce products to meet those demands. Just give them time: Market forces will respond.

When we remove wheat, we remove the primary ingredient for creating breads and other baked foods. So we require alternative flours to replace wheat flour. So let's start with . . .

Wheat Belly Flours

In order to create foods that look and taste like their wheat-containing counterparts yet are truly healthy, we have to be selective. We can't just choose any old ingredients. We certainly don't want to fall into the gluten-free trap of using junk carbohydrates as wheat and gluten replacements. If, for instance, you have friends who have jumped onto the gluten-free bandwagon and are reveling in their consumption of breads, pizza, and cookies made with gluten-free flours, and who insist that you, too, can eat these foods, ignore them. Follow the gluten-free path along with your friends only if you don't mind becoming overweight and diabetic, and developing cataracts and arthritis. Yes, that's how bad the conventional gluten-free foods made with junk carbohydrates are.

I have several basic requirements for anything we choose to use as flour in recipes. Our flour and meals must be:

- Wheat free and gluten free

- Free of conventional gluten-free junk carbohydrate ingredients—no cornstarch, potato starch, tapioca starch, or rice starch, the ingredients contained in most commercial gluten-free products that raise blood sugar levels even higher than wheat flour does, trigger growth of visceral fat, and add to inflammation

- Low in carbohydrate exposure. Otherwise, we'll have high blood sugar levels and other undesirable phenomena. The dried, pulverized starch in flours can be especially destructive because the fine consistency exposes a large amount of surface area that results in rapid breakdown to blood sugar. So we need to strictly limit our exposures to carbohydrates in powdered form. The more healthy fat, protein, and fiber, the better!

This means that rye, barley, oats, triticale, bulgur, and barley flour won't work due to immune cross-reactivity with wheat gluten. It also means that some alternative flours such as amaranth, teff, millet, chestnut, and quinoa can be crossed off the list because of excessive carbohydrate exposure (except when limiting carbohydrate exposure may not be as important, as in snacks or desserts for kids). While many gluten-free cookbooks, recipes, and commercially produced products promote use of these alternative gluten-free grains, they pose potential problems of their own. Let's not

(continued on page 66)

Important Reminders for the Gluten-Sensitive

People with celiac disease or equivalents, such as neurological impairment or dermatitis herpetiformis, and those with gluten sensitivity need to be meticulous in avoiding wheat, gluten, and nonwheat gluten sources such as barley, rye, triticale, bulgur, and oats. (Yes, not all gluten-sensitive people have reactions to the avenin protein in oats, but oatmeal and oat bran still cause your blood sugar levels to skyrocket. So kiss oats goodbye and you'll be better off.) Not only is meticulous gluten avoidance necessary to avoid such things as violent bowel reactions, but it is also important to avoid the many-fold higher risk of gastrointestinal cancers and progressive neurological impairment that comes from even occasional exposure.

So, unlike most of us non-gluten-sensitive folk who may experience "only" a bout of diarrhea, mental "fog" and fatigue, or hand pain for several days, genuinely gluten-sensitive people can experience dire long-term consequences and should make every reasonable effort to avoid exposures, purposeful or inadvertent.

Some important strategies to keep in mind above and beyond just avoiding wheat include:

- Getting *everyone* in the house to be free of wheat and gluten really helps make life easier. It reduces exposure to tempting foods, and it reduces potential for contamination. Don't forget that your dog, cat, or other pet should also be consuming wheat- and gluten-free foods; dishing out their food is otherwise a potential exposure.

- If getting everyone in the house to give up wheat and gluten is not possible, a diplomatic but firm segregation of foods, utensils, and cooking surfaces will be necessary. (The most extremely gluten-sensitive individuals cannot even tolerate this, however.) Separate pots and pans, serving tools, and even plates, glasses, and utensils are necessary for many people.

- Help educate others that living a wheat- and gluten-free lifestyle is not just some food neurosis. It is how you manage *a disease condition,* just as someone with cancer requires chemotherapy. *Never* feel guilty about having to inform others about your needs.

- In a household in which there is segregation of foods and utensils, label foods so that you know which container of hummus, for instance, has had wheat-containing pita chips dipped into it. All it takes is someone buttering a slice of bread and then dipping the same knife into the peanut butter jar, contaminating the peanut butter that you thought was confidently gluten free, to trigger a disaster. Avoid sharing foods such as butter, nut butters, preserves, cream cheese, dips, and spreads, because the knife or food that contacts them may be contaminated.

- Eating outside the home is especially hazardous. Thankfully, some of the more progressive restaurants truly understand the concepts of gluten cross-contamination, a trend that will spread, given the rapidly growing interest in eating a wheat- and gluten-free diet. A restaurant meal prepared using a pan previously used to sauté breaded tilapia is all it takes to go down the wheat re-exposure path. Adhere to this simple rule: If in doubt, don't.

- If you choose to take your chances at a restaurant, be especially careful to avoid breaded meats, foods fried in oils also used to fry bread crumb–coated or other wheat-containing foods, gravies, salad dressings, and most desserts. The most extremely gluten-sensitive, however, should not take even these risks.

- Check with the manufacturer of every prescription drug or nutritional supplement you take and make sure it is gluten free.

- With rare exceptions, avoid fast-food restaurants. Sure, the salad may be gluten free and the salad dressing, too, but cross-contamination from buns and cookies prepared just a few feet away, or prepared using incompletely cleansed equipment, is all it takes to invite an exposure. Cross-contamination is the hurdle that many restaurants, fast-food and otherwise, have struggled with and the reason why many are reluctant to declare any of their dishes gluten free.

- Be aware that gluten exposure can come via vehicles other than foods, including drugs, nutritional supplements, lipsticks, chewing gums, shampoos, creams, and cosmetics. If in doubt, check with the manufacturer, but don't be surprised if the answer you get is the usual corporate-speak and/or a disclaimer that they cannot guarantee something is gluten free because of potential cross-contamination.

- Cross-contamination can occur even in single-ingredient foods during preparation, packaging, or display; for example, be wary of bulk bins at the grocery store, salad bars and food bars, and slicing meat with the same knife used to cut a sandwich.

Let's face it: We live in a world dominated by this thing called wheat. Inadvertent exposures *will* occur. You can only do your best to keep exposures to an absolute minimum.

replace a problem food—wheat—with another problem food.

The choices below constitute our range of healthy options. As you will see, it's quite a diverse list. You will find that different flours or meals are best suited for different applications. Almond flour, for instance, made from blanched almonds and ground to a fine consistency and (sometimes, not always) pressed to reduce oil content, is capable of making light, cakelike dishes, while pecan and walnut meals tend to be coarse and heavy, best for pie and cheesecake crusts.

It's also helpful to learn how to combine and mix the various flours and meals. One of my favorite workhorse combinations is a mix of 12 parts almond meal, 4 parts ground golden flaxseed, and 1 part coconut flour (for example, 1½ cups almond meal, ½ cup ground golden flaxseed, and 2 tablespoons coconut flour). Others have succeeded with less almond meal, more coconut flour, and more eggs. Some experimentation may be required, especially if you switch one meal or flour for another or when you try unique combinations. This may modestly affect how much moisture (for example, coconut milk, sour cream, or water) you need, as well as baking time.

All flours should be stored in the refrigerator or freezer in an airtight container to slow oxidation; this is necessary because they are ground with a lot of surface area exposed. (If you consume oxidized foods, you get oxidized also!) For the same reason, try not to store them for longer than 4 weeks. Alternatively, buy your nuts and seeds whole and grind them as you need them. A food processor, a high-quality food chopper, or a coffee grinder will work, grinding a batch of whole nuts or seeds down to a meal or flour within 30 to 60 seconds. Grind only to a meal or flour consistency, as grinding further will yield nut or seed butters. (If you inadvertently grind to a nut or seed butter, however, all is not lost: Nut and seed butters are useful, too, for a variety of purposes.)

Nut and seed flours are healthy. They are wonderful sources of monounsaturated fats (similar to that in olive oil), protein, and fiber. Because of the dense nature of nuts and seeds, they are also filling, much more so than grain flours. And, of course, none of these meals and flours contain anything that stimulates appetite!

Almond Meal and Flour

Almond meal and flour are the most versatile, tasty, and available of all the healthy choices we have. Almond meal and flour are our workhorses for creating nearly any muffin, cookie, or cake.

Many people, unfamiliar with the flourlike taste and texture of ground almonds, are delighted at the prospect of re-creating familiar wheat flour–based baked goods with a truly healthy replacement. Not only does this flour or meal lack the appetite-stimulating gliadin protein of wheat, immune response–activating gluten, blood sugar–raising amylopectin A, and intestinally disruptive wheat germ agglutinin, but almonds are also healthy in their own right. Full of healthy monounsaturated fat, proteins, and fibers, almonds can do nearly everything wheat flour can do, though some tweaks need to be made in baking techniques.

First, some clarification on almond "meal" versus "flour." Most commonly, almond meal refers to the product that results from grinding whole almonds, including skin, while almond flour refers to ground blanched almonds, that is, with the skin removed prior to grinding. Some manufacturers also press the almond flour to reduce oil content. (Not all manufacturers adhere to this distinction. Bob's Red Mill, for instance, labels its product, ground from blanched almonds and unpressed, "almond meal/flour.") Almond flours are tougher to find and cost a bit more. I'll use almond flour, however, when an especially light texture is desired, such as in a birthday cake or a French financier cake. Personally, I prefer the coarser meal with skins left on, as it provides a nut source of fiber, among the best sources of fiber in the diet.

Almond meal and especially almond flour are more costly than wheat flour. It therefore really pays to shop around, as prices vary across a wide range. (In Milwaukee, where I live, prices range from $3 per pound to $18.99 per pound, averaging around $12 per pound.) Popular national brands are Trader Joe's (very economical) and Bob's Red Mill. If you grind your own almond meal, you can generally purchase bulk almonds for $3 to $6 per pound from the big-box stores like Sam's Club and Costco, or nut wholesalers and retailers.

Coconut Flour

Coconut flour has a delightful, cakelike scent. It contributes a fine, though dense, texture when added to nut meals and flours. Coconut flour is unusually rich in fiber, nearly 40 percent by weight.

Coconut flour is best and most safely used to modify the texture and flavor of nut meals. Only occasionally is it useful as a stand-alone flour, such as a thickener for gravy, as it tends to be very hygroscopic, or water-absorbing, so much so that it can actually lodge in the throat because it soaks up all the moisture in the mouth and throat. So be sure to use it in a mixture with other flours, such as in the recipes in the Wheat Belly Bakery chapter. Its fine texture also makes it useful for "breading" fish, poultry, and meats.

Coconut flour is especially wonderful as a thickener. It is my number one choice to thicken gravies and soups in place of cornstarch, wheat flour, and other thickeners. If a slight coconut flavor shows through (which usually does not happen), add a bit of onion powder, garlic powder, or other herb or spice. This generally masks the bit of coconut flavor. Add coconut flour sparingly when using it to thicken gravies or sauces, as its water-absorbing tendency makes a little bit go a long way. When making gravy, for instance, add 1 teaspoon at a time to the drippings, stirring and waiting for a full minute before adding more. You will be surprised how much a small quantity will thicken over time.

Garbanzo Bean (Chickpea) Flour

Most bean flours are too high in carbohydrate content for our purposes. Garbanzo bean, or chickpea, flour is an exception. While it is a bit higher in carbohydrate content than most other meals and flours listed here, usually around 12 to 13 grams of "net" carbohydrates per ¼ cup flour, it is useful to lighten nut flours or occasionally as a stand-alone flour when you are not that interested in limiting carbohydrate content, such as when you're preparing foods to serve to friends or children. Garbanzo bean (chickpea) flour is best mixed with other meals and flours to give the nut meal or flour a bit of lightness, such as a 3:1 mixture of almond meal to garbanzo flour.

Bob's Red Mill has both a garbanzo bean flour and a garbanzo/fava bean mixture, both similar in composition and baking characteristics.

Ground Golden Flaxseed

Like coconut flour, ground flaxseed is best used as an addition to nut meals and flours. Used by itself for baking, it tends to yield too crumbly a texture, so successful baking usually requires mixing the flaxseed with other meals or flours. It is a great way to add soluble fiber to a recipe, as well as linolenic acid, the plant-sourced omega-3 fatty acid.

The most baking-friendly variety of flaxseed is the golden, not the brown.

Golden flaxseed yields finer flour that provides excellent texture in baked products. I will often use ground golden flaxseed in a five-to-one ratio with almond meal or flour, such as, 2½ cups ground almonds to ½ cup ground golden flaxseed. Both the ground golden and brown flaxseed are especially useful as "breading" for meats, poultry, and fish, either alone or mixed with a nut meal or coconut flour (with added salt, pepper, herbs, and spices).

Flaxseed can be purchased already ground or as whole seeds that need to be ground. Store flaxseed, especially if ground, in an airtight container in the refrigerator or freezer to prevent oxidation of the oils, and try to use it within 4 weeks.

Be sure to drink plenty of water when you include flaxseed in your recipes, as it is highly water-absorbent in your gastrointestinal tract. With proper hydration, flaxseed promotes bowel health and regularity; without good hydration, it can cause a nasty case of constipation.

Hazelnut Meal

Hazelnut meal provides an alternative to the workhorse almond meal and flour. However, it's pricey and tougher to find.

I've found hazelnut very similar to almonds in baking behavior, but it doesn't seem to provide any specific advantages.

Pecan Meal

Pecan meal can be used as a replacement for almond meal, though it yields a denser, coarser meal. It is most useful for pie and cheesecake crusts to replace graham crackers. Pecan meal will work in dishes in which a dense texture is acceptable, such as cookies and muffins, but not for foods requiring a light texture, such as cakes.

Pumpkin Seed Flour

Pumpkin seeds are rich in linolenic acid (similar to that in flaxseed and chia) and magnesium, as well as fiber. These seeds provide unique and surprisingly forgiving flour (meaning you can goof up and it will allow some leeway).

I have never seen pumpkin flour sold, so I grind it myself. The soft seeds are easy to grind, requiring just seconds to yield a fine flour. Due to high oil content, the resulting flour is moister than most other nut and seed flours. There are no recipes in this cookbook based on pumpkin flour, but I suspect there are many ways to use this underutilized seed flour.

Sesame Seed Meal

If you can find bulk sesame seeds, you will find that they make a fairly baking-friendly flour. While brown sesame and the lighter sesame seeds can both be used, the lighter variety is preferred, as it yields less bitterness.

Sesame seed meal is best used in dishes that contain flavors of cheeses, peppers, onions, and salt, though it can also be used in ways similar to that of almond meal and nut meals and flours. I like mixing a bit of the whole seeds in with the ground meal to yield some crunchiness.

Sunflower Seed Meal

Sunflower seed meal is an underappreciated ingredient in baked products. I have never seen preground sunflower seed meal, so you will more than likely have to grind it yourself in your food chopper, food processor, or coffee grinder. Sunflower seeds are generally lower in cost than most other nuts and seeds and therefore provide an affordable way to extend use of more expensive meals and flours by adding, for instance, ½ cup of ground sunflower seeds to 1 cup of ground almonds.

Sunflower seed meal provides a heavier, chewier end product that is best suited to yield crispy cookies, but not very friendly for making lighter dishes such as cakes.

Walnut Meal

Like pecan meal, walnut meal is most useful in situations where a coarse grind is desired, such as in pie and cheesecake crusts. It can be used interchangeably in recipes that call for almond meal or flour, but will yield a heavier, darker texture in the end product. Walnut meal, like pecan meal, is not well suited for dishes in which a light texture is required, such as in cakes.

Wheat Belly–Friendly Oils

We shun wheat. We also don't indulge in junk carbohydrates, such as those in most gluten-free foods, junk foods, and candy.

So where do our calories come from? Corollary to the no-wheat, limited carbohydrate approach is to not limit fats.

Problem: Fats vary in health effects, from great to bad. So what fats and oils are best?

Let's agree that saturated fats are not bad, despite 40 years of misguided vilification. The original studies that were used to justify cutting saturated and total fat for cardiovascular health were flawed and misinterpreted, with recent expert reviews arguing that there are no cardiovascular benefits to reducing saturated or total fats in the diet. When humans roamed the earth naked, unwashed, and hungry for their next meal, they consumed the saturated fat in wild game. They did not consume liquid vegetable oils popular in the 21st century, such as corn oil, safflower oil, and mixed vegetable oils, and they certainly did not hydrogenate them to yield destructive trans fats.

The latter 30 years of the 20th century were spent advocating consumption of polyunsaturated oils. As with many nutritional strategies of that era, this also backfired. Polyunsaturates like those in margarine (often also hydrogenated) not only failed to be an improvement on the saturated oils they were meant to replace, but had adverse health effects all their own, specifically activation of inflammatory responses when consumed in large quantities. The one exception: polyunsaturated omega-3 fatty acids from fish, EPA and DHA, and that from plant sources like flaxseed and chia seeds, linolenic acid. The evidence is quite solid: Omega-3 fatty acids, especially the EPA and DHA from fish sources, provide extravagant health benefits, including reduction in heart attack risk.

Besides fish oil—not terribly compatible with day-to-day cooking beyond eating fish—what oils fit comfortably in this wheat-free lifestyle for health? Here are your choices.

- Coconut oil—Formerly demonized because of its saturated fat content, coconut oil is truly among the most versatile, cooking-friendly, heat-tolerant, and healthy of the oils we have to choose from. Not only is coconut oil rich in wrongly accused saturated fat, it is especially rich in the medium-chain triglyceride lauric acid, which constitutes 48 percent of all the fat in coconut oil. Lauric acid is especially interesting, as it has been associated with weight loss via its unique capacity to mobilize fat stores and accelerate weight loss.

- Extra-virgin olive oil—Delicious, aromatic, and rich in antioxidants and healthy polyphenols, extra-virgin olive oil, treasured by Mediterranean cultures for centuries, is a cornerstone of cooking in the Wheat Belly lifestyle. Rich in monounsaturates, olive oil is one of the several healthy components of the Mediterranean diet. Extra-virgin olive oil deserves an especially prominent place on your shelf.

- Flaxseed oil—Rich in the plant-sourced omega-3 fatty acid, linolenic acid, flaxseed oil is an especially healthy oil. It has, however, a strong nutty flavor and can be slightly bitter, limiting its usefulness. The linolenic acid in flaxseed oil is unusually oxidation-prone, so this oil is best stored in an airtight container in the refrigerator. Flaxseed oil is best used when its taste is compatible with the dish being prepared, such as dishes that have a vegetal taste.

- Extra-light olive oil—The extra-light version of olive oil lacks the pungent aroma and vegetal taste of extra-virgin olive oil. While lacking many of the healthful components of the extra-virgin variety of oil, such as polyphenols and antioxidants, the extra-light version allows you to take advantage of the rich monounsaturated form of oil without the unique taste and smell of olive oil when it might be undesirable, such as in a brownie or cupcake recipe.

- Walnut oil—Another rich source of the plant-sourced omega-3 fatty acid, linolenic acid. Walnut oil is very baking compatible.

- Avocado oil—A little tougher to find and more expensive, avocado oil provides a rich taste and texture that is useful for any recipe in which a rich though somewhat vegetal taste and scent are not objectionable, especially the more pungent unrefined avocado oil. Avocado oil is great for cooking, given its high smoke point and overall healthy characteristics. Like the avocados it comes from, avocado oil is rich in healthy monounsaturated oils. Its light green color along with its slightly vegetal,

nutty flavor makes it a great accompaniment to salads or vegetables.

- Butter—Butter raises some confusing and complex issues. First of all, there is nothing wrong with the fat in dairy products. So fat-free, 1%, 2%, or full-fat have no bearing on health for most of us. Likewise butter: Its high dairy fat content is *not* an issue, despite its tainted reputation for the past 40 years. But butter is not perfect. It shares the same problem as other dairy products: unusually vigorous provocation of insulin release from the pancreas, a so-called *insulinotropic* action. For this reason, it is worth using butter lightly and not smothering foods in oodles of butter. Many dairy producers also use bovine growth hormone to increase milk production in their cows; look for organic butter to avoid this issue.

Armed with a collection of coconut oil, extra-virgin olive oil, flaxseed oil, extra-light olive oil, walnut oil, avocado oil, and organic butter, you will be well equipped to start on your wheat-free journey to better health. And use as much as you like!

Converting Wheat-Containing Recipes to Wheat-Free Recipes

Perhaps there's that favorite recipe for rhubarb-pineapple upside down cake that your grandmother passed down to you and that has been part of family tradition for generations. You want to keep baking this recipe but don't want all the health sacrifices required to consume modern wheat. So how to convert this wheat-containing recipe to a wheat-free counterpart?

Nearly all recipes based on wheat flour can be converted to healthy and delicious nonwheat equivalents. But there are no hard-and-fast rules to follow to make the conversion. Some experimentation may be required, so attempt your conversion when not pressed—definitely not an hour before dinner guests arrive!

In baking with alternative flours, leavening can be a factor, especially in cakes, quick breads, and pancakes, because they lack the structure created by gluten. Start by adding one more egg than called for in the recipe. Separate the eggs and beat the egg whites with cream of tartar (¼ teaspoon per 2 egg whites) until soft peaks form; then fold them into the batter along with the yolks. This will add body and height.

I obtain the best results using predominantly almond flour, which provides the body and structure, at about 75 to 80 percent of the total flour recommended in the recipe, with the addition of ground golden flaxseed, which lends a mild and slightly sweet flavor, and coconut flour, which tightens the recipe and absorbs some of the fats from the almond flour, to make up the remaining quantity of flour called for in the recipe. Recall that almond flour made from blanched almonds is preferred when a

lighter texture is desired, while the almond meal ground from whole nuts works well when a coarser texture is desired. Alternatively, also using almond flour as the predominant flour, add ground golden flaxseed and garbanzo bean (chickpea) flour, which tightens like coconut flour but lends a savory flavor instead of a sweet flavor.

The key is to experiment with your recipe until you get it right. I find that after a couple of tries, I generally have a very satisfactory result. And rarely do you have to toss your failed experiments out.

Sweeteners: What You Need to Know

Over the years, most of us have been terribly overexposed to sweeteners, especially sucrose (table sugar) and high-fructose corn syrup. Growing up with Fruit Loops and Ring Dings, as well as low-fat, high-sugar cookies and sugared soft drinks, most of us spent many years beating up our poor, vulnerable pancreases, organs that have limited capacity for such a sugar/carbohydrate onslaught.

Being wheat free dramatically reduces junk carbohydrate exposure, but we don't want to eliminate one problem—wheat—only to replace it with another problem—lots of sugar. It sure is nice, though, to have some cookies or muffins that have some sweetness without having to suffer all the sugar-related consequences. That's where some of the nonnutritive sweeteners come in handy. (Some call these artificial sweeteners, but that's not entirely true. Stevia, erythritol, and xylitol, for instance, are natural sweeteners but provide few to no calories.)

There are four nonnutritive sweeteners compatible with the *Wheat Belly Cookbook* program that have proven to be relatively benign and useful for inclusion in our recipes: stevia (or the stevia isolate, rebiana), erythritol, xylitol, and sucralose (Splenda).

Each sweetener yields a slightly different end product. Xylitol, for instance, is very baking friendly and adds a bit of browning to the exterior of breads and muffins, while Truvía (rebiana and erythritol) provides a bit more "rise" in wheat-free bread and muffins than stevia. Note that the recipes in the *Wheat Belly Cookbook* may change a bit if you switch sweeteners, rising more or less with a change, for instance. The key for most cooks is to choose a sweetener and a brand you like for its taste and baking characteristics, then stick with it for most, if not all, of your sweetener needs.

Be aware that nonnutritive sweeteners, due to their sweetness, have the potential to increase appetite and, in susceptible individuals, increase insulin modestly. To minimize these effects, it is wise to use these sweeteners sparingly, adding only enough to make your recipe slightly and pleasantly sweet. Thankfully, the majority of people who are wheat free experience a heightened sensitivity to sweetness, and the need for sweeteners of any sort diminishes over time. While an occasional person experiences heightened desire for food or a slowing or stalling of weight loss with use of these sweeteners, most of us do not, and weight gain with use of stevia and the other sweeteners specified here is generally not an issue, especially in the world of the wheat-free absent the appetite-stimulant wheat protein, gliadin.

There are a growing number of sweeteners (not used in these recipes) that are among the important no-no's. Most of these are problems because of fructose exposure. Fructose is proving to be a real problem sweetener, as it is metabolized through an entirely different liver pathway from glucose and can result in higher insulin and blood sugars (though delayed, not immediate), weight gain in visceral fat, higher levels of triglycerides, and provocation of the dreaded small LDL particles that cause heart disease. Problem sources of fructose include, from worst on down, agave nectar, maple syrup, honey (yes, it has good things in it, too, but too much fructose), high-fructose corn syrup, and sucrose. Other problem sweeteners include many new sweeteners that are trying to hide behind various "natural" claims, such as coconut sugar. If you absolutely must use a fructose-based sweetener, then the darkest honeys are among the best choices, but use them sparingly.

The sugar alcohols outside of erythritol and xylitol, such as mannitol, sorbitol, and maltitol, generate substantial gas, cramps, and diarrhea, not to mention increase blood sugar, and are therefore not recommended, since most of us don't relish the prospect of diarrhea with dessert.

Stevia

Most of the *Wheat Belly Cookbook* recipes that require a sweetener were prepared using some form of stevia. It is a versatile and safe sweetener, useful for nearly all recipes in which some level of sweetness is desired without the caloric burden.

Stevia plants are naturally sweet, often called sweet leaf. Some people grow the plants and chew the leaves for their sweetness or add the leaves to recipes. "Stevia extracts" are usually a mixture of naturally occurring sweeteners from stevia leaves.

Stevia extracts have been available in the United States for years as a "nutritional supplement." Stevia recently received a boost into mainstream use with the FDA's "Generally Recognized as Safe," or GRAS, designation in 2008 for its rebaudioside component, also known as rebiana. Agribusiness giant Cargill launched its Truvía brand, which contains rebiana with erythritol, while PepsiCo launched PureVia, a combination of erythritol, rebiana, and a small quantity of the sugar isomaltulose.

Stevia is widely available as powdered and liquid extracts. Powdered extracts are made with added inulin or maltodextrin to add volume or to mimic the look and feel of sugar. Powdered stevia made with inulin is preferred over that made with maltodextrin. Inulin is a benign additive with no potential for raising blood sugar, nor gastrointestinal havoc. The powdered Sweet-

Leaf and Trader Joe's brands, both widely available, are made with inulin. Inulin is often regarded as a "prebiotic," i.e., inducing positive changes in bowel flora for bowel health, and it's therefore also included in many probiotic/prebiotic preparations. Maltodextrin is produced from corn or wheat and may therefore represent a potential source of wheat gluten exposure for people who are extremely sensitive. A polymer of glucose molecules, maltodextrin is added in large quantities to bulk up the stevia so that it can be used cup-for-cup like sugar, but it also then becomes a source of needless carbohydrate calories. The Stevia in the Raw brand made with maltodextrin lists fewer than 2 calories per teaspoon on its nutritional composition, but note that 2 calories per teaspoon equates to 96 calories per cup, or a total of up to 24 grams of carbohydrates per cup. Carbohydrate exposure is therefore a concern when large quantities are used. Maltodextrin occasionally can be responsible for gas, cramps, and diarrhea, too. Pure powdered stevia without a bulking agent is also available; the KAL brand is one example. Because it is pure stevia and more concentrated, it is also more expensive.

Liquid stevia extracts are highly concentrated with little else but stevia and water. My favorite is the KAL brand, which is often sold in health food stores. It is highly concentrated, almost viscous in thickness. SweetLeaf is another excellent brand.

Because of the variety of ways stevia is purified and packaged, you will need to adjust the volume of powder or liquid depending on the preparation. Most manufacturers provide advice on what quantity matches the sweetness of sugar. The Sweet-Leaf brand, for instance, claims that two drops of its Stevia Clear liquid extract equals 1 teaspoon of sugar, while some other brands require five drops for equivalent sweetness. Likewise, inulin- or maltodextrin-based stevias all vary in sweetness, so consult the manufacturer's recommendation.

Also, the presence of other ingredients such as erythritol or maltodextrin can influence how various recipes respond; some experimentation may therefore be necessary, especially when trying a new brand of sweetener in a recipe. Whenever possible, especially when trying a new sweetener preparation or a combination of sweeteners, it helps to taste your batter or dish before cooking to gauge sweetness.

Some people experience a bitter aftertaste with stevia. The stevia glycerite form, such as the Now brand, is less bitter. Bitterness can also be reduced by combining other sweeteners, such as erythritol, or using an erythritol/rebiana mixture such as Truvía. Adding a very small amount of fruit sugar can help, too. Make a paste of a tablespoon or two of raisins, apricots, or dates in a food chopper or food processor and add it to the recipe along with stevia.

Erythritol

Erythritol is a naturally occurring sugar alcohol—a carbohydrate with an OH group attached and thereby labeled an alcohol, though it has nothing to do with ethanol (the alcohol in a martini or glass of wine). Erythritol is found in gram quantities in fruit. In commercial production, erythritol is produced from glucose with a process using yeast. Unlike with the sugar alcohols mannitol, sorbitol, and maltitol, gas and bloating generally do not occur with erythritol unless large quantities are ingested (20 to 30 grams or more, or about 5 or more teaspoons). Erythritol is a useful and safe sweetener for many or most of the *Wheat Belly Cookbook* recipes.

More than 80 percent of ingested erythritol is excreted in the urine, and the remaining 20 percent is metabolized by bacteria in the colon. For this reason, it yields no increase in blood sugar even with a "dose" of 15 teaspoons all at once. There are fewer than 1.6 calories per teaspoon in erythritol. Limited studies have demonstrated modest reductions of blood sugar and hemoglobin A1c (a reflection of the previous 60 days' blood sugar) in people with diabetes who use erythritol.

Erythritol is somewhat less sweet than table sugar. It also causes a unique "cooling" sensation, similar to that of peppermint, though less intense. It may therefore confer a modest cooling sensation to your baked products.

Xylitol

Like erythritol, xylitol is a form of sugar alcohol, i.e., a carbohydrate with an OH group attached. Xylitol is found naturally in fruits and vegetables. It is also produced by the human body as part of normal metabolism. Many of the Wheat Belly Bakery recipes were tested using xylitol with excellent results.

Teaspoon for teaspoon, xylitol is equivalent in sweetness to sucrose. It yields approximately half the calories of sucrose and, because digestion occurs in the intestine rather than the stomach, triggers a slower and less sharp rise in blood glucose than sucrose does. Most people experience a minimal to small rise in blood glucose with xylitol. In one study of slender young volunteers, for instance, 6 teaspoons of sucrose increased blood sugar by 36 milligrams/deciliter, while an equivalent quantity of xylitol increased it by 6 milligrams/deciliter. Interestingly, studies have demonstrated other health effects, including prevention of tooth decay and ear infections in children, due to xylitol's effects on inhibiting bacterial growth in the mouth. Most people do not experience gas and diarrhea unless large quantities (for example, 20 to 30 grams or more, or about 5 teaspoons or more) are consumed.

Xylitol can be used interchangeably with sugar in recipes, i.e., cup for cup the same as sucrose. It also is the least likely to alter baking characteristics.

Pure xylitol is moderately priced, running about $7 per pound. While it has traditionally been produced from birch trees, more recent large-scale production uses corn as its source.

Sucralose

Sucralose is manufactured from glucose by adding chlorine atoms. It has become the most popular artificial sweetener in the world, known to most Americans as Splenda.

Sucralose is very baking compatible, not changing in taste or texture with baking. Sucralose does a pretty good job of mimicking the taste and feel of sugar in recipes. The various forms of sucralose are usually combined with maltodextrin, such as in Granulated Splenda, and therefore pose some of the concerns listed above, including occasional abdominal complaints such as bloating and gas and potential carbohydrate exposure of 0.5 gram carbohydrate per level teaspoon or 24 grams per cup, yielding 96 calories per cup. Carbohydrate content is therefore a potential issue when large quantities are used. Like stevia, sucralose is also available as a liquid without maltodextrin (though tough to find).

Although sucralose has proven to be safe in worldwide consumption with no formal reports of adverse health effects, there have been plenty of anecdotal reports of potential adverse effects. There's the theoretical effect from the chlorine molecules contained within the sucralose molecule and limited animal evidence suggesting alteration of bowel microorganisms with ingestion of large quantities; this has not been reproduced in humans.

So some people like and trust sucralose, while others do not. Make your own choice.

A Wheat Belly Shopping List

Once you've cleared your kitchen shelves of wheat-containing products, you will need to repopulate them with essentials that allow you to navigate a wheat-free diet easily and conveniently. These foods form the backbone of a healthy wheat-free lifestyle and provide the basic ingredients necessary to create the unique recipes that fit this approach.

The safest, healthiest wheat-free, gluten-free foods that should fill your cupboards and refrigerator are natural, single-ingredient foods from the produce aisle, farmers' market, green grocer, butcher, or your garden. You can be absolutely certain, for instance, that the cucumber, kale, spinach, or lamb chops you purchased are free of any trace of the evil grain.

Outside of single-ingredient natural foods, you have to read labels. Obviously, avoid anything with "wheat," "gluten," or any of the dozens of secret code words for wheat products on the label. You can only try to do your best to avoid the dietary land mines. As anyone with celiac disease or extreme gluten sensitivity will attest, everyone experiences inadvertent exposures; given the ubiquity of wheat, you can only minimize exposure. It really pays to try, however, as many of us have tumultuous re-exposure reactions that can last days to weeks. If there is any doubt, consult a product's Web site and/or contact the manufac-turer. If the information is still unclear or the manufacturer takes the common default position of saying "it's a wheat- and gluten-free product but not produced in a gluten-free facility," then those of us just avoiding wheat are likely able to consume it safely, but the extremely gluten-sensitive should be especially careful and perhaps avoid the item.

Cross-contamination, i.e., possible wheat contamination of a food that contains no wheat but was produced in a facility that also produces wheat products, provides a potential problematic exposure for only the most gluten-sensitive among us. In other words, the issue of cross-contamination is raised if no wheat- or gluten-containing ingredients were used in the preparation of the food, but it was produced in a facility (farm, factory, kitchen) that also prepares foods made with wheat/gluten. Very gluten-sensitive people should avoid this uncertainty. For most of us, however, the minuscule potential exposure is not an issue.

Wheat- and gluten-free foods tend to be more costly, enjoying none of the government subsidies that wheat and corn receive. It really pays to shop around, as prices vary widely, as much as fourfold. For instance, for ground almonds, I've paid anywhere from $3 per pound to $18.99 per pound. Sure, an expensive brand might yield a slightly finer flour, but I've had many excellent muffins and cookies made with the $3-per-pound variety.

Note that some foods, such as flaxseed, chia, and nut meals, are best purchased and used within 4 weeks to minimize oxidation of the oils, especially if purchased preground. Store in airtight containers in the refrigerator or freezer once ground.

Almond meal, almond flour. Our workhorse wheat flour replacement, almond meal ground from whole almonds and almond flour ground from blanched almonds work in virtually all *Wheat Belly Cookbook* baked recipes that call for a nut meal or flour. Anyone unfamiliar with almonds used in this fashion will be pleasantly surprised at the light and non-nutty taste that it yields. Reserve almond flour for occasions when the lightest texture is desired, such as when baking a layer cake or pound cake. Use the coarser, less costly, and more widely available almond meal for everyday use.

Almond milk, unsweetened. Thinner than cow's milk, almond milk is useful for drinking and baking, and as the milk in grainless "granolas." Almond milk is the strained liquid from pulverized almonds. If you're really ambitious and want to make your own, puree whole almonds and then strain the liquid through cheesecloth, diluting it with water to the desired thickness; save the pulp for baking. Avoid the sweetened varieties and instead control the degree of sweetness yourself.

Baking powder. While flours and meals that don't contain wheat do not rise as much as wheat flours, baking powder can help rise just a bit. Look for gluten-free and aluminum-free preparations, or just make your own by combining cream of tartar and baking soda, 2:1; store in an airtight container.

Cauliflower. Cauliflower is worth keeping on hand fresh when you are anticipating a replacement for mashed potatoes, rice, or stuffing or dressing.

Cheeses. Keep a variety on hand, including Parmesan, mozzarella, and ricotta. Grated Romano and Parmesan are great to keep handy to add life to Italian dishes. Flatbread recipes made with nut meals and flours also do best with added cheese ground down to a granular consistency, as the melted cheese mixed into the dough confers flexibility and sturdiness to the somewhat crumbly nut meal texture.

Chia seed. Chia is an optional, though interesting, seed. Many people like adding it to smoothies or grinding it into flour and using it as a secondary baking flour, perhaps adding it to almond meal, for instance. Its peculiar capacity to expand when exposed to water makes it useful to create puddings and mousses.

Chocolate. One hundred percent or unsweetened chocolate, i.e., cacao with cacao butter but no sugar, is useful anytime and anywhere you want a rich chocolate taste. Ghirardelli and Baker's are two widely available brands. Unlike with ready-made chocolate, you can determine just how much sweetness you desire by adding your own sweetener to melted chocolate, since you are likely to require very little the longer you are wheat free.

Chocolate chips. Look for the semisweet, dark, or 60 percent cacao chocolate chips to minimize sugar content, while avoiding those made with milk chocolate. Most of the darkest chocolate chips will have around 8 grams "net" carbohydrates (total carbohydrates minus fiber) per 15-gram serving. Extremely gluten-sensitive people should look for gluten-free chips.

Cocoa powder, unsweetened. Ghirardelli, Scharffen Berger, Hershey, and Trader Joe's are excellent brands that are widely available. Using cocoa powder instead of ready-made chocolates ensures that you control the amount of sweetness.

Coconut, shredded and unsweetened; coconut flakes. Unless you are among those with a distinct aversion to coconut, unsweetened coconut is a wonderful way to add texture, chewiness, and flavor to a variety of breads, muffins, and other baked foods. It's also surprisingly rich in fiber and potassium.

Coconut flour. Coconut flour, which is the flour that results from grinding dried coconut meat, is a staple of the wheat-free kitchen. While few recipes work well with coconut flour as the stand-alone flour, it is most commonly used to help yield a finer texture when added to nut flours and meals, which tend to be coarse and crumbly when used by themselves. Store coconut flour in an airtight container, as it is very water absorbent.

Coconut milk. Thicker varieties of coconut milk, usually sold in cans, are used anytime sour cream is called for in a recipe or whenever a thickener is desired. The recently released carton varieties are used anywhere you'd use milk, such as in coffee as a whitener, for cereal, or in baking when a less thick liquid than canned coconut milk is needed. Note that using the carton milklike variety will yield a thinner batter if used in place of the thicker canned version. Anyone wishing to avoid the bisphenol A of cans may use the carton version, but add shredded or flaked coconut pulverized in your food chopper or food processor to thicken it. Alternatively, you can make coconut milk in any consistency by grinding down the coconut meat with water and straining the coarse remains. (As of the printing of this cookbook, only the Native Forest brand has declared its canned coconut milk BPA-free and organic.)

Cream of tartar. Cream of tartar is the common name for potassium bitartrate, found in wine and grape juice. It is one of the components of baking powder and is especially useful to stiffen egg whites for a lighter, fluffier end result (use ¼ teaspoon per two egg whites), as in bread recipes where "rise" is desired. Combined 2:1 with baking soda, it will yield homemade baking powder minus the aluminum contained in many commercial preparations.

Dried fruit. Dried apricots, cranberries, currants, blueberries, strawberries, dates. Always buy the unsweetened variety, as those soaked in sugar or high-fructose corn syrup can present a substantial sugar load.

Eggs. Everyone has eggs, but you are going to be needing a lot more! If budget permits, look for organic eggs obtained from free-range chickens. (They're often green, blue, or brown, depending on the breed, and they have deeper yellow yolks along with a richer taste.)

Extracts. Natural almond, coconut, vanilla, and peppermint extracts are useful expedients for jazzing up a variety of cookies, muffins, and other dishes.

Flaxseeds. Purchased either preground or whole that you grind yourself, flaxseeds are a fiber-rich, linolenic acid–rich (plant-sourced omega-3) staple of multiple baked products and cereals in your new wheat-free diet. The most baking friendly is the golden variety, rather than the brown. It is the fiber of choice for those of you searching for bowel regularity in a wheat-free world.

Ground nut meals. These include ground almonds, pecans, walnuts, and hazelnuts.

Guar gum. An optional thickener, guar gum is useful to make wheat-free baked products when improved cohesiveness and stiffness is desired; for example, use ½ teaspoon per cup of almond meal. It is also useful for making ice cream or iced coconut desserts.

Nut and seed butters. Almond butter, peanut butter, and sunflower seed butter can be purchased as preground butters, or you can make your own by grinding the whole nuts in your food processor.

Nuts. You'll want a supply of raw almonds, pecans, walnuts, pistachios, hazelnuts, macadamias, and Brazil nuts on hand, plus chopped walnuts or pecans for baking.

Oils. Focus on extra-virgin olive, coconut, avocado, flaxseed, walnut, extra-light olive oils, and organic butter.

Seeds. Raw sunflower, raw pumpkin, sesame, and chia seeds are underutilized. They can be ground into flours and used in baking, used whole in nongrain "granola," or included for crunch in cookies and bars.

Shirataki noodles (in the refrigerated section). These are the noodles and pasta replacements made from the konjac root that pose virtually no carbohydrate challenge. While shirataki noodles can be used in any recipe that calls for noodles or pasta, they work best in Asian dishes. Shirataki is packaged in liquid in single-serve bags, usually found in the grocery store refrigerator. It needs to be drained, briefly rinsed (don't mind the slightly fishy odor), and then boiled briefly to warm.

Sweeteners. Liquid stevia, powdered stevia (preferably with inulin, not maltodextrin), powdered erythritol, Truvía, and xylitol are the best choices. The widely available Splenda is another choice, provided you have no personal sensitivity to it.

Xanthan gum. This is an optional thickener, useful for making nonwheat doughs sturdier and more cohesive. Use ½ teaspoon per cup of almond meal or other nut/seed meal. It is also useful for making ice cream or iced coconut desserts.

It helps also to keep a well-stocked pantry of different vinegars (white, rice, red wine, balsamic—watch the sugar!—and infused); a variety of dried herbs and spices, as well as fresh herbs like basil, oregano, and cilantro; fresh garlic and shallots; and a variety of mushrooms (cremini, shiitake, portobello).

While not specified in the recipes, as often as budget and availability permit, meats such as beef, turkey, chicken, and pork should be obtained from trusted sources that are organic, specify "free-range" or "pasture-fed," do not use hormones to accelerate growth. Likewise, whenever possible, fish should be wild, not farmed, since farmed fish have been shown to have altered proportions of fats (more omega-6).

If you include dairy products in your diet, such as cheese, sour cream, butter, cottage cheese, yogurt, and milk, as often as budget permits, choose organic sources that do not contain bovine growth hormone.

Kitchen Tools

Don't panic! Most of the tools and appliances required for your new wheat-liberated lifestyle are the same as those you already have in your kitchen. Besides a good scrub if you've been preparing wheat-containing dishes, your current utensils will serve your new needs just fine except for the few that have porous surfaces, especially wooden spoons and cutting boards—consider replacing them.

Gluten-sensitive people should consider an extra-thorough scrub before using a blender, a food chopper or processor, pots, pans, dishes, and utensils. If the entire household is not giving up wheat and gluten, then strongly consider purchasing duplicates of frequently used items, such as pots, pans, and a food chopper, and especially any device with multiple surfaces, cracks, or joints where nasty crumbs can hide, even if you cannot see them. Your own set of porous wooden spoons, cutting board, and other utensils is a must. You may have to point out to the wheat-eaters in your home that none of your utensils should be used by them. It may therefore be helpful to purchase products that are visibly different, such as having a different color scheme.

For all of us, a few small additional changes or adjustments might be required.

Muffin pan. Pans with small- to medium-size cups work best, rather than the large or super-large cups. One of the hurdles with wheat-free baking is getting the interior of nut- or seed-based meals and flours to bake along with the exterior. (If you must use a muffin pan with large cups, consider using less batter to make a less tall muffin or baking a bit longer at a lower temperature.)

Muffin cups. Paper muffin cups will spare you the hassle of cleaning your muffin pans. Also consider reusable silicone muffin cups.

Electric hand mixer. A handheld mixer is invaluable to quickly whip your egg whites. Because wheat-free baking does not rise like wheat-based baking, we often try to increase the lightness of our baked products by whipping egg whites first (cream of tartar also helps).

Food chopper/food processor. Food processors are wonderful devices that allow you to chop, reduce nuts and seeds into

Replacement Ingredients for Other Food Sensitivities

If you are sensitive to:	Consider replacing with:
Almonds	Chia seed meal, garbanzo bean (chickpea) flour, pecan meal, pumpkin seed meal, sesame seed meal, sunflower seed meal, walnut meal
Butter	Avocado oil, coconut oil, extra-light olive oil, walnut oil
Eggs	Applesauce, chia seeds, coconut milk (canned variety), Greek yogurt (unsweetened), ground flaxseed, pumpkin puree, tofu (from non-GMO soy)
Milk	Almond milk, coconut milk (carton variety), hemp milk, soy milk (from non-GMO soy)
Nuts	Chia seeds (whole, flour), garbanzo bean (chickpea) flour, pumpkin seeds (meal, butter), sesame seeds (whole, flour), sunflower seeds (meal, butter)
Peanut butter	Almond butter, hazelnut butter, sunflower seed butter
Sour cream	Coconut milk (canned variety)

meals and flours, and puree fruits to use as a sweetener. But I have to admit it: When it comes to cleaning up, food processors, in my experience, are a major pain. For this reason, I love the KitchenAid food chopper. At around $40, it is worth its weight in gold, with a powerful motor that allows you to handle nuts, seeds, and veggies without blinking an eye, and cleanup is a snap. Some of the other brands use weaker motors that stall with heavy grinding, such as when you're grinding nuts.

Ice cream maker. An optional device, though quite helpful if you are a fan of iced desserts but don't want the sugar/carbohydrate exposure typical of store-bought versions. Electric devices are a lifesaver. I still have memories of using a hand-operated device, rotating the crank for hours! Hav-

ing your own ice cream maker will also open up a world of unique flavors for your coconut milk–based ice "creams."

Waffle maker. While there's little use for a bread maker any longer when living a wheat-free lifestyle, a waffle maker comes in handy to make wheat-free waffles.

Whoopie pans. In the past, I ignored these shallow muffin pan–like devices to make "whoopie pies," dismissing them as unnecessary for us wheat-liberated folk. However, I've come to recognize that the extra-shallow cups of the whoopie pans are perfect for less sturdy wheat-free doughs, delivering more uniform heat than just baking freestanding dough on a baking sheet. These pans are especially useful to make small biscuits or breads.

Wooden picks. If you plan on doing

some wheat-free baking, you will need a generous stock of wooden picks, or toothpicks, to test doneness. One of the hurdles of wheat-free baking is getting the interior to cook along with the exterior. Unlike wheat-based products that bake more uniformly, denser wheat-free baked products will often be cooked on the outside but remain uncooked on the inside. It really pays to have a wooden pick ready to test the interior by inserting it to see if it withdraws dry. If it does, the baked product is probably cooked on the inside. If the wooden pick withdraws with some batter attached, bake a bit longer.

Some Additional Wheat Belly "Ground Rules"

The Wheat Belly approach, of course, involves avoidance of this most flagrantly unhealthy of dietary ingredients, modern high-yield, semi-dwarf wheat. But there is more to a healthy diet and lifestyle than avoiding wheat. In other words, if I asked you to avoid wheat but eat all the jelly beans and drink all the vodka you wanted, that is not a good strategy for overall health, either. Avoiding wheat is the most powerful nutritional strategy I have ever witnessed, but achieving ideal health calls for more than avoiding wheat.

For that reason, when navigating through your choices of foods or following the recipes included in the *Wheat Belly Cookbook*, be aware of several additional basic issues important to overall health.

- Meats should be uncured and unprocessed and not contain sodium nitrite. Sausages, pepperoni, bacon, salami, and other processed meats often contain the color-fixing and antioxidative chemical sodium nitrite, which has been linked to gastrointestinal cancers. Instead, look for meats that are processed naturally and do not contain sodium nitrite. Of course, also look for no wheat or other hidden wheat-containing ingredients.

- Choose organic dairy products. Because the use of bovine growth hormone dominates in many commercial high-volume dairies, avoid it by choosing milk, sour cream, cheese, yogurt, and butter from organic producers who do not use this chemical growth stimulant.

- Choose the least processed foods. I've said this before, but it bears repeating. One lesson we've had repeated occasions to learn over the past 40 years is that we cannot trust manufacturers of Big Food to decide for us what is healthy and what is not. Artificial colorings are added, sodium benzoate and other preservatives are added, excessive sweeteners are used, hydrogenated oils are added, etc. Your best bets for healthy foods include your own garden, the local CSA or farmers' market, and the peripheral aisles of your grocery store, such as the produce section and the butcher.

- Avoid fructose-containing sweeteners. The most common culprit is high-fructose corn syrup, which is put into virtually every processed food by manufacturers. Sucrose, or table sugar, is 50 percent fructose, so it's not too different from high-fructose corn syrup and should therefore also be minimized. Beware of some of the new "healthy" sweeteners that are really nothing more than sources of sucrose or fructose. The worst offender among fructose-rich sweeteners is agave (90 percent fructose), which is, unfortunately, popular among people following gluten-free diets due to the incomplete understanding of nutrition by gluten-free food manufacturers and authors of gluten-free cookbooks. Honey and maple syrup are also rich in fructose, so use them sparingly, if at all.

- Choose organically grown vegetables and fruits whenever availability and budget permit. This is most important when the exterior is consumed, as with blueberries and broccoli, for example. If the exterior is not consumed, as with bananas and avocados, it is not as important, though pesticides and herbicides can still penetrate into the interior. At the very least, if you cannot choose organic, rinse the produce thoroughly in warm water to minimize pesticide/herbicide residues, such as perchlorates that can block thyroid function.

- Minimize exposure to bisphenol A (BPA). A compound found in polycarbonate plastics (clear, hard plastics with recycling code number 7) and the resin lining of cans, BPA is suspected of exerting endocrine disruptive effects leading to congestive heart failure, diabetes, thyroid dysfunction, and weight gain. This may be a problem with our use of canned coconut milk. Although a handful of manufacturers have declared that they are converting to BPA-free cans, most remain potential sources of contamination. (The Native Forest brand is now the first to declare a BPA-free can.) Unfortunately, I have never seen cooking-grade, thick coconut milk in anything but cans. Alternatives include making your own coconut milk from raw coconuts or using carton coconut milk or water and putting it in your food chopper or processor with shaved unsweetened coconut to thicken. Let's hope that more manufacturers convert to BPA-free lining. In the meantime, it will be worth watching the organic producers of coconut milk, as they will likely be among the first converting to BPA-free packaging.

- Avoid soft drinks, carbonated beverages, and juices. Carbonation erodes bone health (acid-base effects: carbonic acid is neutralized by extracting calcium salts from the bones), while juices and soft drinks are simply too rich in sugar. If you must drink fruit juice (for example, pomegranate juice for its health benefits), be sure it is 100 percent juice (not fruit "drinks" usually made with high-fructose corn syrup with a little added juice) and consume it in small quantities (no more than 2 to 4 ounces). Instead, drink water (squeeze some lemon or lime into it; keep a filled water pitcher in the refrigerator with a few slices of cucumber, kiwifruit, mint leaves, or orange), teas (i.e., brewed from the leaves of the *Camellia sinensis* plant), infusions ("teas" brewed from other leaves, herbs, flowers, and fruits), unsweetened almond milk, unsweetened coconut milk (the carton variety from the dairy refrigerator), coconut water, and coffee.

- Avoid sources of hydrogenated oils. Hydrogenated oils, or trans fats, that are used in processed foods are unquestionably a contributor to heart disease, hypertension, and diabetes. The worst culprit is margarine, which is made with vegetable oils hydrogenated to yield a solid stick or tub form, but many processed foods, from cookies to sandwich spreads, contain hydrogenated oils.

- Minimize your exposure to high-temperature cooking. Any method of cooking that employs temperatures that exceed 450°F (230°C) will provoke undesirable reactions in foods called *glycation* or *lipoxidation* reactions between carbohydrates and proteins with the fats in foods. These reactions develop with deep frying (not sautéing, a relatively low-temperature process), broiling, and any form of cooking that involves

charring the surface. Glycation and lipoxidation contribute to hypertension, the formation of cataracts, arthritis (glycation of cartilage), heart disease, and cancer.

If that seems like a daunting list, just remember that the simplest, least processed foods are generally the healthiest. The tomato you picked from your backyard garden is a far cry healthier than a "heart-healthy" breakfast cereal. Stick with real foods that require no labels and are least processed by manufacturers, foods you are confident are safe to serve to your family.

Wheat Belly Cookbook Happy Hour: Stocking the Wheat Belly Bar

Having a glass or two of wine, or a beer or cocktail, is perfectly in line with the healthy wheat-free lifestyle—if you are selective. (More than two glasses of wine or two cocktails, or more than one higher-carbohydrate beer, however, and weight loss is stalled, with metabolic distortions driven by increased triglycerides.)

There are many choices for alcoholic beverages in the wheat-free world, though many wheat-containing drinks are unquestionably best kept off-limits. Most beers, for instance, are brewed from wheat and barley and share at least some of the adverse potential of wheat-containing foods, including triggering of appetite, inflammation, and gastrointestinal distress and destruction. But there are indeed beers that will satisfy most beer lovers with none of the health hassles.

A simple rule of thumb to minimize exposure to wheat and gluten: Stick to the simplest version of liquor. For example, simple traditional Smirnoff vodka is gluten free. But add some Bloody Mary mix and it now contains residues of wheat and gluten, not to mention high-fructose corn syrup. If you can't see what is being poured, as in mixed drinks or at a social event, then don't

A Quick Word about Wheat Belly Sustainability

"Now wait a minute, here!" you might say. Notions of sustainability from the guy who advocates a potentially resource-intensive lifestyle minus wheat, a highly mechanized, mass-produced commodity that, given its agricultural efficiency, is among the most sustainable of foodstuffs (or so they say)?

The practice of widespread reduced consumption of wheat products has not been around long enough and on a large enough scale for us to know precisely what impact it will have on resource consumption. My prediction: *It will dramatically reduce our ecological footprint.*

But how?

Given the 440 fewer calories consumed per day by those who avoid wheat, we potentially consume fewer resources by eliminating wheat. Perhaps we consume more meat, oils, eggs, and vegetables, but we consume considerably fewer calories. Beyond this, if we weigh, say, 30, 40, or 150 pounds less, we consume less fuel to get us around, whether it's by car, plane, or other means of transportation.

In terms of consumption of health-care resources, we wheatless folk have fewer visits to the doctor for high blood pressure, acid reflux, hypertension, leg edema, and the myriad other complaints of the wheat-eating. We take fewer drugs, make fewer emergency room visits, and develop fewer long-term chronic illnesses, from diabetes to cancer to heart disease.

I'm willing to make some sacrifices for sustainability. But I am not willing to sacrifice my health and live a lifetime of overweight or obesity, acid reflux, and arthritis, dragging from day to day, and consuming more resources in the health-care system.

So, on balance, is being wheat free more sustainable and softer on the environment? We don't have formal data, but given the common sense and fairly marked *overall* reductions in the environmental footprint we wheat-free people make compared to the wheat-consuming, my prediction is that we will come out way *behind* in resource consumption.

Beyond elimination of wheat, there are other ways you and I can contribute to the cause of sustainability. We can:

drink it. Stick to the simplest drinks that you know are wheat- and gluten-safe.

Beer

Ales, beers, malt liquors, and lagers—all wheat-based—are out. But this does not mean you can't still enjoy an occasional beer. In addition to those listed below, I have seen some microbreweries starting to jump on the wheat-free bandwagon, brewing beers from sorghum, chicory, and other nonwheat ingredients. Watch out for

- Buy local ingredients whenever possible. I live in Wisconsin, and I can obtain spectacular produce in late spring and summer. Dairy products like cheese are wonderfully abundant (though even here I have to determine whether it is organic). Shop farmers' markets and vegetable and fruit stands, and subscribe to community-supported agriculture (CSA) to obtain produce and animal products directly from the source, with whom you can verify issues like no use of bovine growth hormone and the humane treatment of animals.

- Eat what you purchase and prepare. If you make more than you require for the short term, freeze it. Most *Wheat Belly Cookbook* dishes are perfectly fine stored in the freezer for long-term storage.

- Buy organic. High-volume commercial agriculture has a higher environmental price. Whenever available and your budget permits, purchase the organic option of vegetables, fruits, dairy, and meats.

- Grow your own vegetable garden. Not only is it energy saving, it is also satisfying and delicious to slice your own tomatoes, cucumbers, and peppers. Think about planting some fruit trees in your backyard, such as apple, peach, and cherry. Even just growing your own herbs such as basil and oregano in a window shelf planter is a great way to reduce reliance on energy-consuming producers.

- Compost. Don't let grass clippings, vegetable peels, fruit cores, and coffee grounds end up in the trash. Pile them onto your compost pile and decrease your contribution to waste and reduce the need for synthetic fertilizers for your garden.

Surely, a world of slender, healthy, nonwheat-consuming people is more resource efficient than a world of overweight, high-calorie-consuming, unhealthy people who rely on the medical system, medications, and procedures for health.

barley if you are among the most gluten-sensitive.

Bard's Gluten-Free Beer. Brewed from 100 percent sorghum without barley, this beer is truly gluten free. As with many of the gluten-free beers, however, it can present an excessive carbohydrate exposure if more than one beer is consumed (14.2 grams of carbs per 12-ounce bottle).

Bud Light. This Anheuser-Busch beer is brewed from rice but also with barley malt. The most severely gluten-sensitive should therefore not indulge in this beer because of the potential immune cross-reactivity of barley and wheat gluten. But those of us just avoiding wheat but without gluten sensitivity can safely consume this brand without exposing ourselves to the undesirable effects of wheat. One 12-ounce bottle contains 6.6 grams of carbohydrate.

Green's Gluten-Free Beers. UK brewer Green's provides several gluten-free choices made from sorghum, millet, buckwheat, brown rice, and "deglutenised" barley malt. The carbohydrate content of these beers is slightly less than most others, ranging from 10 to 14 grams per 330-milliliter bottle.

New Grist. Brewed from sorghum, New Grist beer tastes more like a hard cider than a beer. The carbohydrate content is a moderate 14.2 grams per 12 ounces.

Redbridge. Another Anheuser-Busch beer, Redbridge is brewed from sorghum and is not brewed with wheat or barley and is therefore confidently gluten free. The

carbohydrate content is a bit high at 16.4 grams per bottle; more than one beer and carbohydrates begin to stack up.

Wine

Wine is as close as we can get to a nearly perfect wheat- and gluten-free haven, regardless of varietal or vintage. Combined with the probable health effects that derive from light wine drinking (no more than two 4-ounce glasses per day) due to the combination of alcohol, anthocyanins (wine constituents that provide the red-purple color), and resveratrol, wine drinking is proving to be one of those things that are truly both pleasurable and healthy.

The only stumbling block is the occasional use of gluten as a clarifying agent. Ever since bovine spongiform encephalopathy ("mad cow disease") called the use of gelatin as a wine clarifying agent into question, winemakers have sought nonanimal alternatives. Gluten has emerged as one such possibility, though very few winemakers use it. Even less commonly, a paste containing wheat flour is used to seal the barrels used to age wines.

Thankfully, the presence of truly meaningful quantities of gluten (generally defined as 20 parts per million or more) is rare, and only the most exquisitely gluten-sensitive among us are likely to experience a reaction. While gluten can be detected at low levels in wines in which gluten has been used as the clarifying agent, it is unlikely to achieve the level required to generate an immune response in the great majority of gluten-sensitive people. While we do not have a broad survey of residual gluten content in the many wines on the market, it is likely that there are few, if any, that contain sufficient immunoreactive gluten. The majority of us who are avoiding wheat but are not among the most exquisitely gluten-sensitive do just fine with wine, gluten-treated or no.

Wine coolers are a bit different, however, in that they typically contain barley malt and should be avoided by the gluten-sensitive.

Liquors and Liqueurs

The process of distillation should theoretically remove all gluten residues in the finished product. Nonetheless, many gluten-free people will tell you that they still react, sometimes violently, to "gluten-free" liquors brewed from wheat and gluten cross-reacting grains. And, at least anecdotally, this also seems to happen to those of us who are not among the most gluten-sensitive but are just trying to avoid wheat. (I've personally had trouble with wheat-based vodkas.)

It's helpful to know which liquors are brewed from wheat and related grains and avoid them, and only allow exposure to liquors distilled from safe sources such as grapes, potatoes, and corn.

Brandy and cognac. Because brandies and cognacs are distilled from wines that, of course, are pressed from grapes, they should be confidently free of wheat and gluten. This includes Grand Marnier (*ugni*

blanc grapes and oranges), Courvoisier (*ugni blanc* grapes), and Rémy Martin (Grande and Petite Champagne grapes). The rare exceptions are some brands that add caramel coloring, such as Martell.

Liqueurs. These are truly a mixed bag of ingredients, but few have gluten exposure potential. Safe liqueurs without wheat or gluten residues include Kahlúa (contains dairy), fruit liqueurs such as Triple Sec and Cherry Kijafa, Amaretto di Saronno, and Bailey's Irish Cream. The most gluten-sensitive may have to avoid those blended with whiskey, as the source of the whiskey is often not specified.

Rum. Rum is distilled from sugarcane and so should not contain any residues of wheat or gluten proteins. Of course, be cautious of any flavored or spiced rums, which run the risk of a gluten-contaminated ingredient. However, the wheat-avoiding among us (but not the exquisitely gluten-sensitive) should have free choice among the many rums of the world.

Vodka. Avoid vodkas brewed from wheat. Wheat-sourced vodkas include Absolut, Grey Goose, Ketel One, SKYY, Stolichnaya, and Van Gogh (wheat, barley, corn). Nonwheat but gluten-containing grain-sourced vodkas include Belvedere (rye) and Finlandia (barley).

Vodkas prepared from grapes, potatoes, or corn and usually free of any wheat or gluten proteins include Chopin (potatoes), Cîroc (grapes), and Smirnoff (corn). However, note that, given the incredible variety of some of the flavored offerings that keep pouring out onto the market, you may have to investigate a specific brand to be sure. In general, you are safest with simple unflavored vodkas, as opposed to flavored or blended vodkas.

Whiskey. Because whiskeys are distilled from the mash of rye, barley, wheat, and corn, most whiskeys are off our list for those who are gluten-sensitive. To my knowledge, no whiskey has tested above the proposed 20 parts per million cutoff that the FDA considers the threshold for safety for people with celiac disease and gluten sensitivity. But there are just too many people who appear to react to whiskeys distilled from rye, barley malt, and wheat. This means that consuming many popular whiskeys, such as Jack Daniel's (barley, rye, corn), Jameson (barley), and Bushmills (barley), could put you at risk of a gluten reaction.

Many of the whiskeys that are brewed from nonwheat, gluten-free grains originate from boutique distillers such as Koval Distillery (millet), Queen Jennie Whiskey from Old Sugar Distillery (sorghum), Roughstock Montana Sweet Corn Whiskey (corn), and 303 Whiskey (potatoes).

The world of alcoholic beverages is incredibly varied and rich, changing frequently to accommodate modern tastes. It helps to be on the lookout for any change in your drink(s) of choice, always vigilant for something new and possibly gluten-containing.

Next: The Recipes!

After all this talk of eat this and don't eat that, I hope you are eager to jump into your new wheat-free lifestyle to enjoy some of the wonderful dishes that are possible.

All the recipes in the *Wheat Belly Cookbook* are specifically designed not to cause weight gain or visceral fat accumulation, not to trigger appetite, not to cause high blood sugar or glycation, not to increase triglycerides or cause formation of small LDL particles that cause heart disease—all the effects caused by wheat. In short, all the recipes presented here are healthy.

This means that, rather than having a sandwich or a brownie that causes weight gain, makes you hungrier, and messes up metabolic patterns such as blood sugar and triglycerides, you can instead have a big, thick Reuben sandwich, three slices of pizza, or several brownies with none of the usual wheat-based concerns. You can just eat and enjoy!

This conversion of unhealthy fattening foods into healthy nonfattening foods introduces some interesting opportunities, such as eating cupcakes for lunch or cheesecake for breakfast. If these formerly indulgent foods are converted to healthy versions without undesirable health implications, you can enjoy them without guilt or worry.

On with the recipes!

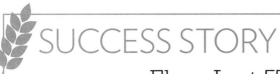

SUCCESS STORY

Elana Lost 57 Pounds

Lots of things conspired to make me put on the pounds. First there was a bout of postpartum depression after the birth of my first child. During my stay in that black hole of despair, I subsisted mostly on candy and sandwiches and put on about 45 pounds that just didn't want to come off. Then there was a move from Sweden to my husband's home country of Iceland, farther north than I'd ever been before. I was alone, friendless, and unable to communicate well in the new language. I munched antidepressants and packed on more pounds every winter. At my heaviest, I weighed about 260 pounds. Nothing fit, and I was always tired. In the summertime, I'd go off the medication and lose 20 pounds without even trying, but they'd all come back—sometimes bringing friends—the following winter.

I tried everything. I used a SAD (seasonal affective disorder) lamp; I tried to eat healthy, whole grain, organic food; I took daily walks and went swimming every morning in our neighborhood pool. I'd lose a few pounds—but not enough to make a difference.

Finally, in January 2011, I went full-out wheat free, low carb, high fat—the *Wheat Belly* way. I was very diligent, and the pounds just melted off. My starting weight was 226 pounds; my waist, 46 inches. After just a month, my weight dropped to 217 pounds and my waist to 39 inches.

My life seemed to open up before me like a flower. I slept better and woke up rested and smiling, eager for the day ahead. My dry hair, dry skin, and brittle nails were all of a sudden strong and healthy. My gums stopped bleeding, and my belly started to behave very well. My horrible PMS symptoms vanished, and my chronic knee pain disappeared.

I'm about to turn 47. Today I sail along with a low daily carb intake, all from veggies, cream, nuts, and berries. I eat wheat like I drink alcohol—very seldom and only if I'm willing to pay the price the next day. So far I've dropped 57 pounds, and my waist size has shrunk to a little over 30 inches—I look really good in a skirt these days! I'm so happy and so thankful that I've started this wheat-free journey!

PART 2

WHEAT BELLY COOKBOOK RECIPES

Okay: Time to get down to some wheat-free cooking, baking, and eating!

In many ways, cooking, baking, and eating wheat free means being able to enjoy meals, snacks, even desserts with none of the usual concerns of conventional foods. Have some cupcakes or muffins and don't worry about weight gain or other effects. In some ways, it turns the whole notion of breakfast, lunch, dinner, and snack foods topsy-turvy, converting formerly unhealthy foods like cheesecake or cookies into healthy foods that fit into any meal or occasion. Have cookies for breakfast!

My list of criteria for including the various recipes in this book was quite straightforward. All recipes must be delicious but also wheat free and possible to create using gluten-free ingredients when appropriate (see below), limited in carbohydrate and sugar exposure, and otherwise healthy. It means that you will find no cornstarch, agave nectar, hydrogenated oils, high-fructose corn syrup, or added food colorings in these recipes. Nor will you find the junk carbohydrates typically used in gluten-free foods. I also focused on primarily providing recipes that are traditionally wheat-containing, now converted to a wheat-free, healthier, and slimming version.

For the sake of minimizing repetition, I've used several conveniences in describing these recipes. These descriptive conveniences include:

• If you have celiac disease or have known gluten sensitivity, then only use ingredients that are known to be gluten free. If you do not fall into either of these two groups, then avoid foods containing any wheat ingredients, including hidden sources (see Appendix A), but not explicitly gluten free.

- When sweeteners such as stevia are used, some recipes specify a quantity, for example, 4 drops of liquid stevia. However, given the wide variation in sweetness among different brands, this should only serve as a starting place. You may need to adjust to the sweetness of your specific brand. It always helps to taste your batter or dish before cooking.

- When "coconut milk" is specified, I am referring to the thicker variety generally purchased in cans, rather than the thinner variety meant to be consumed like milk and often found in the dairy refrigerator of the grocery store. The canned variety usually has the consistency of sour cream and adds body to recipes, whereas the thinner carton coconut milk is more useful to thin dishes.

- Follow this simple rule when baking: Combine dry ingredients such as almond meal, coconut flour, and baking soda, and combine wet ingredients separately. Only then combine wet and dry mixtures. This means that if a powdered sweetener is used, add it to the dry mixture. If a liquid sweetener is used, add it to the wet mixture. This is not specified in each recipe, but it's an important step to obtain the best quality in your baking.

- Factor in your own unique dietary sensitivities. If you are dairy intolerant, consider the various dairy alternatives, such as coconut milk (canned) in place of sour cream or Greek yogurt. If you're allergic to almonds, try ground walnuts. A listing of possible replacement foods can be found on page 82.

- If you have any unique health conditions, such as a history of calcium oxalate stones for which a low-oxalate intake may be required, or a history of gout for which a low-purine diet may be required, discuss the advisability of any of the recipes listed here with your doctor beforehand.

The wheat-free lifestyle is, in some ways, a work in progress. It has only been around for a relatively few years, and we need to continually seek out new ways to make it better. If you improve on any of the *Wheat Belly Cookbook* recipes presented here, or if you develop your own variations, please share them with me and my blog followers. You can find an entire world of wheat-free eating ideas on the Wheat Belly Blog at www.wheatbellyblog.com.

BREAKFASTS

FRENCH TOAST

PREP TIME: 10 MINUTES | **TOTAL TIME:** 20 MINUTES

Makes 6 servings

Thought you'd never have French toast again? Well, here's the solution.

You'll need some of the Basic Bread from the recipe on page 225. Slice the bread ½ to ¾" thick. You will find that the end result is a bit heavier than traditional French toast made from wheat-based bread, as with many wheat-free dishes, but this variation is wonderfully simple and pleasurable with none of the unhealthy consequences of the "real" thing.

Serve with unsweetened Greek yogurt or whipped cream and blueberries, raspberries, or strawberries; fruit butters such as apricot or pumpkin butters; or sugar-free maple syrup, preferably sucralose-based and not sorbitol-based to avoid the blood sugar–increasing effects of sorbitol, not to mention the awful gas and cramps typically caused by some sugar alcohols.

1 **large egg**

¼ **cup coconut milk, almond milk, or milk**

1 **teaspoon ground cinnamon**

2 **tablespoons butter or coconut oil**

6 **slices Basic Bread (page 225)**

In a shallow bowl, whisk the egg. Add the milk and cinnamon and whisk until blended.

In a large skillet over medium heat, heat the butter or coconut oil.

Carefully dip the bread in the egg mixture, coating both sides. Place in the skillet and cook, for about 5 minutes, turning once, or until golden. Repeat with the remaining slices.

PER SERVING: 224 calories, 9 g protein, 8 g carbohydrates, 19 g total fat, 7 g saturated fat, 3 g fiber, 339 mg sodium

WHEAT-FREE PANCAKES

PREP TIME: 15 MINUTES | **TOTAL TIME:** 30 MINUTES

Makes 14 pancakes (4" diameter)

Of all the wheat-free, healthy recipes I've tried, this is my family's favorite. You'll find these almond meal–based pancakes to be a very close approximation of the flour-based variety. They are wonderfully filling; few people can eat more than 3 or 4 medium-size pancakes.

I'd forgotten how much I missed pancakes until I sat down one Sunday morning to a stack, butter between the layers, topped with (sugar-free) maple syrup—but followed by none of the fogginess, sleepiness, and abdominal distress that always followed wheat flour pancakes. Top pancakes with sugar-free maple syrups, but avoid the kind that contains sorbitol, since this sugar alcohol increases blood sugar and usually causes horrendous gas and diarrhea. Sucralose-based maple syrups are made by Walden Farms and DaVinci. Torani and DaVinci also make berry-flavored sucralose-based syrups that are great for drizzling on Wheat-Free Pancakes. If you are averse to sucralose, try blueberries or other berries with whipped cream, a dollop of Greek yogurt, or some fruit butters (for example, apricot, apple, cranberry, pumpkin—just watch the sugar!).

3 cups almond meal

1 tablespoon ground flaxseeds

½ teaspoon sea salt

½ teaspoon baking soda

3 large eggs

¾ cup unsweetened almond milk, light coconut milk, or milk

2 tablespoons extra-light olive oil, walnut oil, coconut oil, or butter, melted

In a medium bowl, combine the almond meal, flaxseeds, salt, and baking soda.

In a large bowl, whisk the eggs. Add the milk and oil or butter and whisk thoroughly.

Gradually whisk the flour mixture into the egg mixture. The consistency should be similar to that of conventional flour-based batter; if too thick, add 1 or more tablespoons of milk or water until of desired consistency.

Lightly oil a large skillet and heat over medium heat. For each pancake, pour ¼ cup of batter onto the griddle. Cook for 3 minutes, or until bubbles form and the edges are cooked. Turn and cook for 3 minutes, or until the underside is lightly browned. Repeat with the remaining batter.

Almond meal pancakes can be delicate; if you encounter difficulty turning them, release all the edges first and then turn.

Note: You may use this batter to prepare waffles. Simply cook according to the manufacturer's directions.

PER PANCAKE: 175 calories, 7 g protein, 5 g carbohydrates, 15 g total fat, 1.5 g saturated fat, 3 g fiber, 124 mg sodium

COCONUT FLAPJACKS

PREP TIME: 15 MINUTES | TOTAL TIME: 30 MINUTES

Makes 4 servings (4 pancakes per serving)

Here's another simple variation on pancakes, in addition to the recipe for pancakes on page 96.

For many people, sitting down to a Sunday breakfast means enjoying a big stack of pancakes with butter and maple syrup, only to fall asleep an hour later, battle with mental "fog" for hours afterward, and then deal with the pound of weight gain that inevitably follows. All of us wheat-free folk want nothing to do with such wheat-related phenomena.

So what a surprise that you and I can re-create this traditional American breakfast, but without the sleepiness, fog, or weight gain! And it's no more difficult than whipping up the pancake batter the old way.

¼ cup coconut flour	½ cup water
¼ cup almond meal	1 teaspoon vanilla
1 teaspoon baking soda	2 tablespoons butter, melted
3 eggs	1 tablespoon xylitol or ⅛ teaspoon liquid stevia or to desired sweetness (optional)
½ cup almond or carton-variety coconut milk	

Preheat a griddle over medium heat. In a large bowl, combine the coconut flour, almond meal, and baking soda.

In a small bowl, whisk the eggs. Add the milk, water, vanilla, butter, and xylitol or stevia (if using), and whisk well.

Pour the egg mixture into the flour mixture and stir until combined.

Grease a skillet or griddle and heat over medium heat. For each pancake, pour ⅛ cup of batter onto the griddle. Cook for 2 to 3 minutes, or until bubbles form and the edges are cooked. Turn and cook for 2 minutes, or until the underside is lightly browned. Repeat with the remaining batter.

Serve hot.

PER PANCAKE: 184 calories, 8 g protein, 8 g carbohydrates, 16 g total fat, 4 g saturated fat, 4 g fiber, 436 mg sodium

LEMON-POPPY SEED PANCAKES

PREP TIME: 15 MINUTES | **TOTAL TIME:** 25 MINUTES

Makes 4 servings (3 pancakes per serving)

If you've become bored with plain Wheat-Free Pancakes, there are numerous delicious variations you can make to liven up breakfast. Here's one such variation, a lemon–poppy seed version that is wonderful topped with whipped cream and sliced strawberries.

The lemon stevia is optional. If you are a fan of lemon, as I am, you can increase the proportions of lemon juice and peel a bit.

3 large eggs, separated

4 tablespoons buttermilk

1 tablespoon lemon juice

1 tablespoon freshly grated lemon peel

2 teaspoons poppy seeds

¼ teaspoon lemon stevia or to desired sweetness (optional)

1½ cups blanched almond flour

½ teaspoon baking powder

¼ teaspoon baking soda

¼ teaspoon sea salt

In a large bowl, whisk together the egg yolks, buttermilk, lemon juice, lemon peel, poppy seeds, and stevia (if using).

Add the almond flour, baking powder, baking soda, and salt and mix until thoroughly combined.

In a small bowl, whisk the egg whites until slightly stiff. Fold into the batter.

Grease a skillet or griddle and heat over medium heat. For each pancake, scoop 2 heaping tablespoons of batter onto the skillet. Cook for 1 minute, or until bubbles form around the edges. Turn and cook for 1 minute, or until underside is lightly browned. Remove to a serving platter. Repeat with the remaining batter, regreasing the skillet if needed.

PER SERVING: 416 calories, 20 g protein, 16 g carbohydrates, 36 g total fat, 4 g saturated fat, 8 g fiber, 416 mg sodium

CREPES WITH RICOTTA AND STRAWBERRIES

PREP TIME: 15 MINUTES | TOTAL TIME: 45 MINUTES

Makes 8 servings

I used to think of crepes as something that barely touched my appetite, they were so light and airy. Wheat-free crepes, in contrast, while appearing light and airy, are wonderfully satisfying and filling due to the coconut flour and flaxseeds.

Unsweetened Greek yogurt can be substituted, if desired, for the ricotta. Also, the xylitol can be replaced with other sweeteners in a quantity equivalent to 1 to 2 teaspoons of sugar.

FILLING

- 1 cup ricotta
- 1 teaspoon xylitol or 1 drop liquid stevia or to desired sweetness
- 1 teaspoon lemon peel
- 2 cups strawberries, halved

CREPES

- ¼ cup coconut flour
- ¼ cup golden flaxseed meal
- ⅛ teaspoon sea salt
- 1½ cups almond or carton-variety coconut milk
- 4 eggs
- ¼ teaspoon vanilla extract

To make the filling: In a small bowl, combine the ricotta, xylitol or stevia, and lemon peel. Set aside.

To make the crepes: In a large bowl, combine the coconut flour, flaxseed meal, and salt. In a small bowl, whisk together the milk, eggs, and vanilla. Add the egg mixture to the flour mixture and stir until combined.

Coat a small nonstick skillet with oil and heat over medium heat. Measure ⅓ cup of the batter and pour into the pan, swirling the batter around so it coats the bottom of the pan. Cook for 3 minutes, or until the top of the crepe appears dry. Turn the crepe and cook for 1 minute, or until the underside is dry. Repeat with the remaining batter, stacking the crepes as they are cooked.

Top each crepe with 2 tablespoons of the ricotta filling and ¼ cup of the strawberries.

PER SERVING: 130 calories, 8 g protein, 9 g carbohydrates, 7 g total fat, 2.5 g saturated fat, 4 g fiber, 128 mg sodium

CHEESE AND EGG QUESADILLAS

PREP TIME: 10 MINUTES | TOTAL TIME: 25 MINUTES

Makes 2 servings

These simple and quick-to-prepare quesadillas are near the top of my list of Foods Kids Are Likely to Enjoy. They also work well as a unique breakfast, a portable lunch, or a quick dinner.

1 tablespoon butter

½ red bell pepper, finely chopped

2 scallions, finely chopped

4 eggs

¼ cup milk

½ cup shredded cheese such as Cheddar, Swiss, or horseradish, divided

4 Wheat Belly Tortillas (page 227)

In a large skillet over medium heat, melt the butter. Cook the pepper and scallions, stirring frequently, for 5 minutes, or until tender. In a small bowl, whisk the eggs and milk. Pour into the skillet and add ¼ cup of the cheese. Cook, stirring frequently, until the mixture is scrambled and the eggs are cooked through but still moist. Cover and set aside.

Grease a medium skillet and place over medium heat. Place 1 tortilla in the skillet and sprinkle with 1 tablespoon of the remaining cheese. Add half of the egg mixture, sprinkle with 1 tablespoon of cheese, and top with a second tortilla. Cook for 2 minutes, or until the cheese is melted. Turn over and cook for 1 minute. Repeat.

PER SERVING: 736 calories, 42 g protein, 27 g carbohydrates, 56 g total fat, 15 g saturated fat, 20 g fiber, 639 mg sodium

GRILLED CHEESE BREAKFAST BAKE

PREP TIME: 30 MINUTES | **TOTAL TIME:** 1 HOUR 15 MINUTES + STANDING TIME

Makes 6 servings

Here's a variation on grilled cheese sandwiches you can put together in a few minutes, provided you have Basic Bread (page 225) on hand. (For this reason, I like having a supply of this bread handy, stored in the refrigerator, for just such occasions.) This breakfast bake can also serve as a lunch bake, or even a light dinner bake.

14 slices (½" thick) Basic Bread (page 225)

2 cups shredded Fontina or Gruyère cheese, divided

2 cups loosely packed baby spinach

2 tomatoes, sliced into 8 slices

4 eggs

1½ cups half-and-half

½ teaspoon nutmeg

1 teaspoon sea salt

½ teaspoon ground black pepper

Preheat the oven to 375°F. Grease an 9" × 9" baking pan with butter.

Toast the bread in a toaster on medium setting. Line the bottom of the baking pan with 7 slices, cutting to fit.

Sprinkle with 1 cup of the cheese, then top with the spinach. Top with the tomatoes.

Rotate the pan 45 degrees and place the remaining 7 slices of bread crosswise to the first (so that the bread is not stacked like a sandwich). Sprinkle the remaining 1 cup cheese over the bread.

In a medium bowl, whisk the eggs and half-and-half until the yolks are broken up. Add the nutmeg, salt, and pepper, and whisk to combine. Pour over the bread, making sure to soak all of it.

Cover with foil and bake for 20 minutes. Remove the foil and bake for 25 minutes, or until the eggs are puffy and set and the cheese is browned. (If the cheese browns before the eggs set, replace the foil for the final minutes.) Let stand for 10 minutes before serving.

PER SERVING: 485 calories, 25 g protein, 17 g carbohydrates, 37 g total fat, 13 g saturated fat, 5 g fiber, 1,001 mg sodium

BROCCOLI AND MUSHROOM FRITTATA

PREP TIME: 30 MINUTES | TOTAL TIME: 1 HOUR 5 MINUTES

Makes 8 servings

Frittatas are a perfect fit in the Wheat Belly lifestyle: They are rich in fats and nutrition, with limitless possibilities for unique flavor combinations.

1 clove garlic, thinly sliced

1 teaspoon extra-virgin olive oil

8 ounces cremini mushrooms, sliced

2 cups broccoli florets

1 teaspoon sea salt

½ teaspoon ground black pepper

1 cup shredded sharp Cheddar cheese

2 cups half-and-half

6 eggs

2 tablespoons loosely packed fresh dill, chopped

Preheat the oven to 375°F. Grease a 9" pie plate.

In a small skillet, cook the garlic in the oil over medium-low heat for 3 minutes. Remove the garlic and set aside. Increase the heat to medium. Cook the mushrooms, stirring frequently, for 8 minutes, or until golden.

Meanwhile, place a steamer basket in a large pot with 2" of water over medium-high heat. Steam the broccoli for 3 minutes, or until bright green and tender-crisp. Remove and roughly chop.

Add the broccoli to the skillet. Stir to coat. Sprinkle with salt and pepper. Remove from the heat, and add the reserved garlic.

Line the bottom of the pie plate with the vegetables. Top with the cheese.

In a bowl, whisk together the half-and-half and eggs. Add the dill and whisk to combine. Carefully pour over the cheese and vegetables.

Place the pie plate on a baking sheet and bake in the center of the oven for 35 minutes, or until a knife inserted in the center comes out clean.

PER SERVING: 168 calories, 8 g protein, 6 g carbohydrates, 13 g total fat, 8 g saturated fat, 1 g fiber, 299 mg sodium

GOOD-MORNING SOUFFLÉ

PREP TIME: 22 MINUTES | **TOTAL TIME:** 45 MINUTES

Makes 6 servings

The mere mention of "soufflé" sends many people running—but not this recipe, scaled down for people like me, who don't have formal training at Le Cordon Bleu.

Advance preparation is key. Don't make this during some hurried morning before work or school. Make it on the weekend and eat it, bit by bit, over the week or prepare it the night before.

To add variety to your soufflé, try adding up to ½ cup shredded cheese and either ½ cup vegetable puree or ⅓ cup finely diced cooked vegetables or crumbled cooked bacon to the base (before folding in the egg whites). Some ideas: butternut squash/ Gruyère/paprika; onion/roasted red pepper/rosemary/spinach; artichoke/red pepper/ Gruyère/thyme; red pepper/fennel/onion; or try blue cheese/walnuts by substituting finely ground walnuts for the Parmesan cheese.

4 tablespoons butter, melted and divided

2 tablespoons grated Parmesan cheese

4 eggs + 1 egg yolk

3 tablespoons garbanzo bean (chickpea) flour

1 cup milk, at room temperature

½ teaspoon fine sea salt

¼ teaspoon ground black pepper

¼ teaspoon nutmeg

Preheat the oven to 425°F. Brush six 6-ounce ramekins with 2 tablespoons melted butter, and dust with the cheese. Place on a baking sheet and set aside. Separate the eggs, placing the yolks in a medium bowl and the whites in a large bowl.

In a medium saucepan over medium heat, melt the remaining 2 tablespoons butter. Add the flour and cook, whisking constantly, for 1 to 2 minutes, or until blended and the mixture begins to bubble.

Gradually add the milk, whisking constantly until smooth. Cook, whisking constantly, for 5 minutes, or until the mixture begins to thicken. Do not let the mixture boil. Remove from the heat and add the salt, pepper, and nutmeg.

Whisking constantly, pour ⅓ cup of the milk mixture into the yolks. Then add the remaining milk mixture to the bowl and whisk thoroughly. If preparing the soufflé the night before serving it, cover the yolk mixture and the egg whites and refrigerate both overnight. Allow both to come to room temperature (enough to take the chill off) before proceeding.

With an electric mixer on high speed, beat the egg whites until soft peaks form. Fold one-third of the egg whites into the yolk mixture. Repeat.

Divide the mixture into the ramekins. Bake in the center of the oven for 17 to 18 minutes, or until puffed and golden. The centers should look set and firm, and a toothpick inserted into the center should come out clean.

Serve immediately.

PER SERVING: 167 calories, 7 g protein, 4 g carbohydrates, 13 g total fat, 7 g saturated fat, 0 g fiber, 353 mg sodium

SPINACH-TOMATO QUICHE

PREP TIME: 25 MINUTES | **TOTAL TIME:** 55 MINUTES

Makes 8 servings

This simple quiche uses a nonwheat crust. Nut meals work well, forming a crunchy layer that complements the softer filling ingredients. The duo of spinach and sun-dried tomatoes yields a wonderful combination of rich tastes and concentrated nutrition.

For easy variations, substitute cooked broccoli or asparagus for the spinach. You can also add chopped chicken, ham, sausage, or other meats.

For convenience, prepare the quiche ahead of time and refrigerate it until ready to serve. I'll occasionally make 2 at a time to save lots of prep time over a week of breakfasts, or even serve it for lunch or dinner. Quiche will keep in the refrigerator for several days. Just reheat briefly before serving.

1 **Basic Pie Crust (page 261), made with salted butter**

1 **tablespoon olive oil**

1 **large tomato, seeded and chopped**

4 **cups packed baby spinach**

1 **clove garlic, minced**

½ **cup grated Romano cheese or crumbled feta cheese**

4 **eggs**

1½ **cups heavy cream, half-and-half, or milk**

½ **teaspoon onion powder**

Preheat the oven to 350°F. Bake the pie crust in a 9" pie plate or tart pan for 15 minutes, or until firm to the touch. Remove to a rack.

Meanwhile, in a large skillet over medium heat, heat the oil. Cook the tomato, stirring occasionally, for 2 minutes, or until its juices begin to seep. Add the spinach and cook, stirring, for 2 minutes, or until the spinach begins to wilt. Add the garlic and cook for 1 minute. Spoon the filling into the baked pie crust. Sprinkle the cheese over the filling.

In a medium bowl, whisk together the eggs; cream, half-and-half, or milk; and onion powder. Pour over the cheese and vegetables.

Place the pie plate on a baking sheet and bake for 35 minutes, or until a knife inserted in the center comes out clean.

PER SERVING: 561 calories, 14 g protein, 12 g carbohydrates, 53 g total fat, 21 g saturated fat, 6 g fiber, 420 mg sodium

GREEN CHILE AND CHORIZO STRATA

PREP TIME: 15 MINUTES | **TOTAL TIME:** 1 HOUR 5 MINUTES + CHILLING TIME

Makes 9 servings

If you like hot and spicy foods, give this Green Chile and Chorizo Strata a try. You will never say that a wheat-free lifestyle is boring or tasteless!

The key to this breakfast casserole, or strata, is chorizo sausage, which is usually purchased already made with a mixture of paprika, ground red pepper, cumin, chile, and other spices, packing a delicious mixture of flavors.

2 links chorizo (about 7 ounces), casings removed

½ small onion, finely chopped

1 serrano chile pepper, seeded and finely chopped

4 eggs

2 cups milk

1 teaspoon sea salt

½ teaspoon ground black pepper

1 teaspoon cumin

2½ cups shredded Monterey Jack cheese, divided

½ loaf Basic Bread (page 225), cut into ½" cubes (about 4 cups)

Grease a 9" × 9" baking pan.

Heat a medium skillet over medium-high heat. Cook the chorizo, breaking with a wooden spoon, for 5 minutes. Reduce the heat to medium and add the onion and chile pepper. Cook, stirring occasionally, for 8 minutes, or until the chorizo is cooked through and the vegetables are softened. Transfer to a plate covered with a paper towel and set aside to cool slightly.

In a large bowl, whisk together the eggs, milk, salt, black pepper, and cumin. Stir in 2 cups of the cheese, the bread cubes, and the chorizo mixture until combined.

Pour into the baking pan. Cover and refrigerate for 8 hours or overnight.

To bake, preheat the oven to 375°F. Uncover the strata and top with the remaining ½ cup cheese. Bake for 35 minutes, or until puffed and a knife inserted into the center comes out clean.

PER SERVING: 215 calories, 12 g protein, 8 g carbohydrates, 16 g total fat, 5 g saturated fat, 2 g fiber, 528 mg sodium

GREEK FRITTATA

PREP TIME: 20 MINUTES | TOTAL TIME: 55 MINUTES

Makes 6 servings

In this modern collision of Greek and Italian, the rich tastes of kalamata olives, artichokes, sun-dried tomatoes, and fresh basil come together for a simple-to-prepare dish perfect for breakfast, lunch, dinner, or brunch. For convenience, prepare it on the weekend and store in the refrigerator to eat during the week.

8 eggs

2 tablespoons half-and-half or heavy cream

1 tablespoon extra-virgin olive oil

½ red onion, chopped

¼ cup pitted kalamata olives, chopped

½ cup artichoke hearts, finely chopped

¼ cup sun-dried tomatoes (soaked in oil), chopped

2 tablespoons chopped fresh basil

½ cup finely crumbled feta cheese

½ teaspoon ground black pepper

Preheat the oven to 350°F.

In a medium bowl, whisk the eggs and the half-and-half or cream. Set aside.

In an ovenproof skillet over medium heat, heat the oil. Cook the onion, stirring frequently, for 5 minutes, or until softened. Add the olives, artichokes, tomatoes, basil, cheese, and pepper. Cook for 5 minutes, or until the onion is browned.

Stir in the egg mixture. Cook for 3 minutes. Place in the oven and bake for 15 minutes, or until a knife inserted in the center comes out clean.

Using a spatula, release the frittata around the edges and bottom, and slide it onto a cutting board. Cool for 5 minutes, then cut into 6 wedges.

PER SERVING: 211 calories, 12 g protein, 5 g carbohydrates, 16 g total fat, 5 g saturated fat, 1 g fiber, 440 mg sodium

VARIATION

Add leftover chicken, pork, or steak, chopped into ½" pieces; trade the feta for grated Romano or Parmesan cheese; add ½ cup heavy cream for added richness.

ITALIAN SAUSAGE FRITTATA

PREP TIME: 20 MINUTES | TOTAL TIME: 1 HOUR

Makes 6 servings

Here's a simple variation on the frittata theme. The spiciness of the Italian sausage takes center stage in this recipe, so choose your favorite, preferably uncured. If serving this frittata for dinner, prepare some mashed cauliflower topped with ground black pepper, a pinch of salt, and butter as a side dish.

As with all frittata and quiche recipes, consider preparing ahead of time—on the weekend, for example—to store in the refrigerator and eat during the week.

8 eggs

1 cup ricotta cheese

3 tablespoons extra-virgin olive oil

12 ounces uncured Italian sausage, crumbled

½ large yellow onion, finely chopped

½ teaspoon sea salt

¼ teaspoon ground black pepper

1 cup coarsely chopped portobello mushrooms

2 cups packed fresh spinach, coarsely chopped

¼ cup grated Parmesan cheese

Preheat the oven to 350°F.

In a medium bowl, whisk together the eggs, ricotta, and 2 tablespoons of the oil. Set aside.

In a large ovenproof skillet over medium heat, heat the remaining 1 tablespoon oil. Cook the sausage and onion for 10 minutes, or until the sausage is cooked. Sprinkle with the salt and pepper.

Add the mushrooms and spinach and cook, stirring occasionally, for 2 minutes, or until the spinach wilts. Stir in the egg mixture until well blended. Cook for 3 minutes.

Sprinkle with the Parmesan. Transfer the skillet to the oven and bake for 20 minutes, or until a knife inserted in the center comes out clean.

Using a spatula, release the frittata around the edges and the bottom. Cool for 5 minutes, then slice and serve.

PER SERVING: 363 calories, 26 g protein, 9 g carbohydrates, 25 g total fat, 8 g saturated fat, 1 g fiber, 629 mg sodium

HOMEMADE TURKEY SAUSAGE PATTIES

PREP TIME: 10 MINUTES | **TOTAL TIME:** 25 MINUTES

Makes 6 patties (3" diameter)

Avoiding the sodium nitrite of cured, processed foods is sometimes tough, since most producers continue to use this oxidation-blocking agent in their sausages, pepperoni, ham, and other meat products. So why not make sausage patties yourself?

Because these are made starting with ground turkey (which can be easily substituted with ground beef, pork, or lamb), no curing goes into your own sausages.

2 tablespoons extra-virgin olive oil	2 teaspoons fennel seeds
1 medium yellow onion, finely chopped	2 teaspoons dried basil
2 cloves garlic, minced	1 teaspoon ground black pepper
1 pound ground turkey	2 teaspoons dried parsley
2 teaspoons dried oregano, crumbled	1 teaspoon sea salt

In a medium skillet over medium heat, heat the oil. Cook the onion and garlic for 5 minutes, or until the onion is browned and softened. Remove the skillet from the heat and cool for 10 minutes.

In a large bowl, combine the turkey and the onion mixture. Add the oregano, fennel, basil, pepper, parsley, and salt and blend by hand until thoroughly mixed.

Form patties to the desired width and thickness (3" wide by ½" to ¾" thick works well) by hand. Cook in the skillet over medium heat for 8 minutes, or until a thermometer inserted in the center registers 165°F and the meat is no longer pink.

PER SERVING: 172 calories, 14 g protein, 3 g carbohydrates, 11 g total fat, 3 g saturated fat, 1 g fiber, 288 mg sodium

CHEDDAR EGG MUFFINS

PREP TIME: 15 MINUTES | **TOTAL TIME:** 35 MINUTES

Makes 12

While a few minutes of preparation are required for these simple Cheddar egg muffins, you will be rewarded with breakfast for the next few days. These muffins are also popular with the kids.

After baking and cooling, store muffins in the refrigerator and heat briefly prior to serving.

8 ounces Turkey Sausage (opposite page)

2 cups broccoli, finely chopped

1 cup shredded Cheddar cheese

¼ cup sun-dried tomatoes (soaked in oil), finely chopped

1 teaspoon dried basil

½ teaspoon dried oregano

½ teaspoon onion powder

½ teaspoon sea salt

8 large eggs

1 tablespoon chives

Preheat the oven to 350°F. Grease a 12-cup muffin pan.

Cook the sausage according to the recipe directions.

In a large bowl, combine the sausage, broccoli, cheese, tomatoes, basil, oregano, onion powder, and salt.

In a medium bowl, whisk the eggs. Pour into the broccoli mixture and mix thoroughly. Divide the mixture evenly among the muffin cups. Top with the chives.

Bake for 30 minutes, or until a wooden pick inserted in the center of a muffin comes out clean.

PER SERVING: 127 calories, 10 g protein, 3 g carbohydrates, 9 g total fat, 3 g saturated fat, 1 g fiber, 224 mg sodium

BREAKFAST EGG BISCUITS

PREP TIME: 10 MINUTES | **TOTAL TIME:** 20 MINUTES

Makes 2

Think of this as a healthy alternative to a fast-food breakfast muffin. These Breakfast Egg Biscuits are easy to prepare beforehand. Alternatively, make only the biscuits ahead of time, then add the eggs, sausage, and cheese when you are ready to eat.

Rather than forming them by hand, using a whoopie pie pan or other shallow pan with 2½"- to 3"-wide wells really helps to generate the small but sturdy shape of a biscuit. Egg rings are also useful to get the fried eggs perfectly round and uniformly thick. A 3" round metal cookie cutter works perfectly.

2 **sausage patties or 2 slices Canadian bacon (preferably uncured)**

2 **medium eggs**

2 **Basic Biscuits (page 245), halved lengthwise**

2 **slices Cheddar cheese (1 ounce each)**

In a medium skillet, cook the sausage patties or Canadian bacon until cooked through. Remove to a plate and set aside. In the same skillet, break 1 egg into an egg ring, breaking the yolk. Cover and cook for 1 to 2 minutes, or until almost set. Use a knife to separate the egg from the ring and remove the ring. Turn the egg over and cook for 1 minute, or until set. Remove to a plate. Repeat with the remaining egg.

Place the bottom of 1 biscuit on a plate and top with 1 egg, 1 sausage patty or slice of Canadian bacon, and 1 slice of cheese. Cover with the biscuit top. Repeat to make a second sandwich.

PER SERVING: 512 calories, 34 g protein, 16 g carbohydrates, 37 g total fat, 9 g saturated fat, 7 g fiber, 1,139 mg sodium

SMOKED SALMON AND CREAM CHEESE SANDWICHES

PREP TIME: 10 MINUTES | **TOTAL TIME:** 10 MINUTES

Makes 2 servings

A match for any smoked salmon and cream cheese sandwich from the deli, this recipe can be whipped up in just a couple of minutes for a quick breakfast or toted to the office for lunch, provided you have a supply of Classic Scones handy.

As with all *Wheat Belly Cookbook* breads, scones, and muffins, think about preparing a supply in advance to save the time and effort when the impulse for a sandwich hits.

2 ounces cream cheese, softened

1 tablespoon finely chopped fresh herbs (dill, thyme, chives, parsley, basil, or rosemary)

Dash of ground black pepper

2 Classic Scones (page 248)

3 ounces sliced smoked salmon

¼ red onion, sliced

In a small bowl, mix the cheese, herbs, and pepper until smooth and well combined.

Cut each scone in half crosswise. Spread the bottoms with one-half of the cheese mixture. Top each with half of the salmon and half of the onion rings. Top with the scone tops.

PER SERVING: 347 calories, 18 g protein, 12 g carbohydrates, 28 g total fat, 9 g saturated fat, 6 g fiber, 801 mg sodium

GRAINLESS GRANOLA

PREP TIME: 5 MINUTES | **TOTAL TIME:** 25 MINUTES

Makes 8 servings (4 cups)

This recipe probably shouldn't be called granola, since there are no oats, wheat flour, or any of the usual suspects in it. But it is delicious and will please even the most die-hard wheat-consuming member of the family.

Use this granola as you would any other, as a snack eaten by hand, toted to your workplace in a portable container, or as a breakfast cereal in unsweetened almond milk, coconut milk (the thinner variety in the dairy section of the grocery store), or milk.

1 cup raw cashew pieces

1 cup raw pumpkin seeds

1 cup slivered almonds

2 tablespoons whole flaxseeds or chia seeds

1 cup unsweetened coconut flakes

2 teaspoons ground cinnamon

2 tablespoons extra-light olive oil, coconut oil, or walnut oil

¼ cup sugar-free hazelnut syrup (or sweetener equivalent to ½ cup sugar)

Preheat the oven to 350°F.

In a large bowl, combine the cashews, pumpkin seeds, almonds, flaxseeds or chia seeds, coconut, and cinnamon. Add the oil and syrup and mix together.

Spread the mixture on a baking sheet in a ½" thick layer. Bake for 20 minutes, stirring once, or until golden.

PER ½-CUP SERVING: 315 calories, 9 g protein, 11 g carbohydrates, 28 g total fat, 10 g saturated fat, 4 g fiber, 13 mg sodium

SUCCESS STORY

Gary Lost 55 Pounds

I was always the guy with the big—you might say voracious—appetite. Put me in front of an all-you-can-eat buffet and I'd eat till I was uncomfortable. It was as if an eating switch was turned on in my brain.

But I had a system for regulating my weight. Whenever I'd approach 250 pounds, I'd panic, go on a strict diet, hit the gym, and shed 25 pounds or so. It was a huge struggle, though—I'd fight constant hunger and exhaustion, and I couldn't sustain the regimen. Then, over the next year or so, I'd find myself pushing 250 again, and the cycle would start all over.

On Labor Day 2011, I stumbled across *Wheat Belly* just as I was finishing one of my

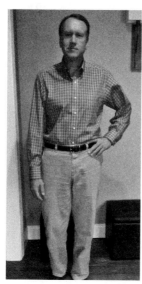

AFTER

25-pound weight-loss marathons. My knees and ankles hurt from exercising, and I felt pain with every step I took. I was hungry and discouraged.

But what I read as I paged through *Wheat Belly* seemed to make sense, and I decided to give it a try. The weight just started coming off. What was really remarkable, though, was that I wasn't the least bit hungry. It was as though I'd experienced a brain-chemistry makeover—my love affair with food seemed to be over at last.

My digestive system improved, too— I felt "light in the gut," without the typical bloat I'd always experienced after eating. My skin started improving, and my chronically dry, flaky elbows smoothed over. I no longer felt that afternoon fog and fatigue, and I slept so much better.

Since following *Wheat Belly,* I've lost 55 pounds, with virtually no effort—and no hunger. I didn't even go to the gym. I came to realize that working out is part of my overall health and well-being, not a weight-loss strategy.

It's such a satisfying plan—I eat as much as I want of lots of different foods, and I don't miss bread and pasta at all. The big payoff? At 175 pounds, I weigh now what I did in high school!

Wheat Belly has been a game changer for me—I only wish I'd known about this 20 years ago! At 47, I feel like I've regained my future.

SANDWICHES AND SALADS

OPEN-FACED BEEF AND ARUGULA SANDWICHES

PREP TIME: 15 MINUTES | TOTAL TIME: 15 MINUTES

Makes 4 servings

The combined taste of beef and horseradish is perfect for sandwiches, but incomplete without bread. Our Basic Focaccia comes to the rescue! You can save time by preparing the horseradish–sour cream sauce ahead of time.

¼ cup sour cream

2 tablespoons olive oil

1 tablespoon red wine vinegar or apple cider vinegar

1 tablespoon prepared horseradish

4 slices Basic Focaccia (page 228)

4 cups baby arugula

4 roasted red peppers, patted dry and cut into strips

12 ounces sliced cooked steak or roast beef

In a small bowl, whisk together the sour cream, oil, vinegar, and horseradish until blended.

On each of 4 lunch plates, place 1 slice of focaccia. Evenly divide the arugula, peppers, and steak or roast beef among the focaccia. Drizzle with the horseradish sauce.

PER SERVING: 427 calories, 28 g protein, 16 g carbohydrates, 29 g total fat, 5 g saturated fat, 6 g fiber, 630 mg sodium

CHICKEN SUN-DRIED TOMATO SANDWICHES

PREP TIME: 10 MINUTES | TOTAL TIME: 10 MINUTES

Makes 2 servings

Focaccia layered with chicken, turkey bacon, avocado, and sun-dried tomato makes a rich mix of flavors, with each bite exploding with the tastes of a deli sandwich—with none of the deli downside! For a simple variation, try either horseradish or wasabi mayonnaise in place of standard mayonnaise. Also try eliminating the chicken and adding more bacon, or replacing both the bacon and chicken with thinly sliced beef.

2 teaspoons mayonnaise

2 teaspoons olive oil

1 teaspoon white wine vinegar or apple cider vinegar

2 slices Basic Focaccia (page 228), sliced horizontally in half

1 cooked chicken breast, thinly sliced

1 medium avocado, peeled, pitted, and thinly sliced

¼ cup sun-dried tomatoes in olive oil

4 slices uncured turkey bacon, cooked

4 slices Swiss cheese

In a small bowl, stir together the mayonnaise, oil, and vinegar.

On 2 lunch plates, place the bottom halves of the bread. Arrange half of the chicken, avocado, tomatoes, bacon, and cheese on each slice of bread. Drizzle with the mayonnaise mixture and top with the remaining bread.

PER SERVING: 725 calories, 50 g protein, 21 g carbohydrates, 51 g total fat, 11 g saturated fat, 10 g fiber, 469 mg sodium

TURKEY BRIE SANDWICHES

PREP TIME: 10 MINUTES | TOTAL TIME: 10 MINUTES

Makes 2 servings

The key with this sandwich, as with many of the sandwiches in this cookbook, is to keep a small supply of focaccia bread on hand, ready to go for a quick lunch or dinner. If you'd like your cheese melted, microwave the sandwich for 20 seconds or bake it in the oven at 350°F for no more than 5 minutes.

Note that for this recipe to yield 2 servings, the full size of the focaccia is required, as described in the Basic Focaccia recipe on page 228.

2 slices Basic Focaccia (page 228), sliced horizontally in half

2 tablespoons mayonnaise

4 ounces sliced roasted turkey

1 medium tomato, thinly sliced

2 ounces Brie, thinly sliced

On 2 lunch plates, place the bottom halves of the bread. Spread with the mayonnaise. Arrange half of the turkey, tomato, and cheese slices (or spread on top if softened) on each slice of bread. Top with the remaining bread.

PER SERVING: 508 calories, 32 g protein, 14 g carbohydrates, 37 g total fat, 9 g saturated fat, 5 g fiber, 593 mg sodium

REUBEN SANDWICHES

PREP TIME: 15 MINUTES | TOTAL TIME: 15 MINUTES

Makes 2 servings

I thought I'd died and gone to heaven when I had a Reuben sandwich again! The Basic Focaccia serves as the bread for this sandwich. If you'd like less of the spiciness of the rosemary in this Reuben Sandwich, make the bread with less or no rosemary. In place of Thousand Island, you might also try horseradish mayonnaise or Dijon mustard. Note that the full size of the focaccia is required for this recipe.

4   **thin (¼–½") slices Rye Bread (page 226)**

6   **ounces sliced corned beef**

¼   **cup sauerkraut**

3   **tablespoons Thousand Island dressing**

2   **slices Swiss cheese**

On 2 lunch plates, place 1 slice of bread. Arrange half the corned beef, sauerkraut, Thousand Island dressing, and cheese on each bread slice. Top with the remaining bread and cut in half.

PER SERVING: 487 calories, 31 g protein, 14 g carbohydrates, 34 g total fat, 10 g saturated fat, 5 g fiber, 1,470 mg sodium

WASABI HAM AND SWISS SANDWICHES

PREP TIME: 10 MINUTES | TOTAL TIME: 10 MINUTES

Makes 4 servings

This variation on the traditional ham and Swiss sandwich tosses in the wonderfully electrifying taste of wasabi horseradish. Of course, if you are not into wasabi or anything horseradish, good old-fashioned mustard or mayonnaise works just fine, too.

8 slices Basic Bread (page 225)

¾ pound sliced ham

4 slices Swiss cheese

8 slices cucumber, diagonally cut

8 thin slices tomato

2 tablespoons Wasabi Cream Sauce (page 219)

Place 4 slices of the bread on a work surface. Top evenly with the ham, cheese, cucumber, and tomato slices. Spread the wasabi sauce on the remaining bread slices. Place on top of the tomatoes.

PER SERVING: 495 calories, 34 g protein, 18 g carbohydrates, 33 g total fat, 9 g saturated fat, 6 g fiber, 1,644 mg sodium

GRILLED CHICKEN PESTO SANDWICHES

PREP TIME: 15 MINUTES | **TOTAL TIME:** 15 MINUTES

Makes 4 servings

I'll use any excuse to spread some fresh basil pesto on a sandwich. Given the ingredients in this sandwich—lettuce, onion, lean chicken, healthy oil, and nuts—you can't get much healthier! Feel free to use deli chicken, turkey, or other meats for variety.

2 tablespoons extra-virgin olive oil

1 medium yellow onion, sliced

1 jar (12 ounces) sliced roasted red peppers

8 slices Basic Bread (page 225)

2 grilled boneless, skinless chicken breasts, sliced lengthwise

4 leaves romaine or other lettuce

4 tablespoons fresh basil pesto

In a large skillet over medium-high heat, heat the oil. Cook the onion and peppers for 5 minutes, or until lightly browned. Remove from the heat.

Place 4 slices of the bread on a work surface. Top evenly with the chicken, onion and pepper mixture, and lettuce.

Spread 1 tablespoon pesto on each of the remaining 4 slices of bread, then place on top of each sandwich.

PER SERVING: 567 calories, 31 g protein, 22 g carbohydrates, 41 g total fat, 7 g saturated fat, 7 g fiber, 899 mg sodium

AVOCADO BLT SANDWICHES

PREP TIME: 15 MINUTES | TOTAL TIME: 15 MINUTES

Makes 4 servings

Unlike wheat-based BLT sandwiches that leave you hungry, this smaller version (given the usually smaller nonwheat bread slices) will leave you positively stuffed! For variety, instead of spreading the bread with plain mayonnaise, try an olive tapenade, basil pesto, or wasabi mayonnaise. Or add sprouts, sun-dried tomatoes, or thinly sliced dill pickles.

8 slices Basic Bread (page 225), toasted

4 tablespoons mayonnaise, divided

8 slices uncured bacon, cooked

1 medium tomato, thinly sliced

1 avocado, halved, pitted, peeled, and thinly sliced

1 cup salad greens or lettuce

On each of 4 lunch plates, place 1 slice of bread. Spread each bread slice with ½ tablespoon of the mayonnaise. Place 2 slices of bacon, 2 slices of tomato, 2 slices of avocado, and a handful of greens or lettuce on the bread. Spread each of the remaining 4 bread slices with ½ tablespoon of mayonnaise and top each sandwich.

PER SERVING: 551 calories, 28 g protein, 19 g carbohydrates, 44 g total fat, 7 g saturated fat, 8 g fiber, 696 mg sodium

GRILLED CHEESE SANDWICHES

PREP TIME: 10 MINUTES | TOTAL TIME: 10 MINUTES

Makes 4 servings

Nothing says comfort food like grilled cheese—until, of course, you suffer all the discomfort of having consumed something made of wheat! So here it is again, all comfort with no discomfort.

Slice the bread more thinly to get the cheese melted without burning the bread. Try adding slices of tomato, red onion, fresh basil, or avocado for a change of pace. I like changing the cheese from the traditional Cheddar to Swiss or Gruyère for a slightly different spin.

8 **teaspoons butter**

8 **thin slices Basic Bread (page 225)**

8 **thin slices Cheddar cheese**

Spread 1 teaspoon butter on each of 4 slices of bread. Place in a large nonstick skillet, buttered side down. Top each with 2 slices of cheese and a slice of bread. Spread each top slice with 1 teaspoon butter.

Cook over medium heat for 7 minutes, turning once or until the bread is browned and the cheese melted.

PER SERVING: 544 calories, 25 g protein, 15 g carbohydrates, 44 g total fat, 17 g saturated fat, 5 g fiber, 933 mg sodium

SALMON SALAD SANDWICHES

PREP TIME: 15 MINUTES | **TOTAL TIME:** 15 MINUTES

Makes 4 servings

If you tire of tuna salad sandwiches, this simple variation replaces the tuna with salmon. Despite the relatively high cost of fresh wild salmon, canned wild salmon is usually surprisingly affordable yet provides all the wonderful health benefits of fish.

1 can (14.75 ounces) wild salmon
¼ cup mayonnaise
¼ yellow onion, finely chopped
1 rib celery, finely chopped
1 tablespoon chopped chives
½ teaspoon ground black pepper

1 teaspoon rice vinegar
Dash of sea salt
8 slices Basic Bread (page 225)
8 slices cucumber, cut diagonally
½ cup alfalfa or broccoli sprouts

In a medium bowl, combine the salmon, mayonnaise, onion, celery, chives, pepper, vinegar, and salt and mix together thoroughly.

Place 4 slices of the bread on a work surface and spread the salmon mixture evenly on each. Top each with 2 slices of cucumber. Divide the sprouts among the sandwiches. Top with another slice of bread.

PER SERVING: 536 calories, 41 g protein, 16 g carbohydrates, 37 g total fat, 6 g saturated fat, 6 g fiber, 1,039 mg sodium

NUT BUTTER AND STRAWBERRY SANDWICH

PREP TIME: 5 MINUTES | **TOTAL TIME:** 5 MINUTES

Makes 1 serving

Who doesn't miss a peanut butter and jelly sandwich? Portable, sweet, and delicious, this sandwich was a true childhood favorite for most of us. Minus the wheat bread and the sugar-laden jelly, how could we possibly enjoy it again without booby-trapping our health? Here's how!

Our Basic Bread provides a wheat-free, ultra-low-carbohydrate bread, while whole strawberries provide the familiar taste of strawberry jam. Swap out the strawberries for thinly sliced bananas, pears, apricots, or apples for other unique tastes.

2 slices Basic Bread (page 225)

2 tablespoons nut or seed butter, such as peanut, almond, cashew, hazelnut, or sunflower seed

½ cup whole strawberries, sliced

On a lunch plate, place 1 slice of bread. Spread with the nut or seed butter. Top with the strawberries and remaining bread slice.

PER SERVING: 537 calories, 20 g protein, 23 g carbohydrates, 43 g total fat, 6 g saturated fat, 8 g fiber, 739 mg sodium

GOAT CHEESE APRICOT FINGER SANDWICHES

PREP TIME: 15 MINUTES | TOTAL TIME: 15 MINUTES

Makes 12 servings

You don't have to have the ladies over to enjoy these delicious sandwiches. Sure, they're great to serve to friends, but they also make an excellent lunch, or even breakfast with coffee. Make up a bunch ahead of time for a quick meal or snack. Kids love them, too.

12 very thin slices Walnut Raisin Bread (page 243)

1 ounce goat cheese, at room temperature

4 tablespoons apricot butter (or other unsweetened fruit butter)

Place 6 slices of the bread on a work surface. Evenly spread the goat cheese on the bread and top with the fruit butter. Top with the remaining bread slices and cut in half.

PER SERVING: 95 calories, 4 g protein, 6 g carbohydrates, 7 g total fat, 1.5 g saturated fat, 2 g fiber, 163 mg sodium

STEAK AND VEGGIE FAJITA

PREP TIME: 15 MINUTES | TOTAL TIME: 15 MINUTES

Makes 1 serving

Here's a great way to use leftover steak. Or try substituting roast beef, pork, turkey, or chicken for the steak. For extra flavor, add some chopped fresh cilantro or a side dish of guacamole.

1 Flaxseed Wrap (page 231)

1 tablespoon coconut or olive oil

1 small onion, cut into wedges

1 cup frozen mixed peppers, thawed

1 clove garlic, minced

4 ounces cooked, sliced top round steak

⅓ cup prepared salsa

2 tablespoons shredded Cheddar or Monterey Jack cheese

Place the wrap on a plate. Set aside.

In a small skillet over medium heat, heat the oil. Cook the onion for 5 minutes, or until tender. Add the peppers and garlic and cook for 3 minutes, or until heated through. Place on half of the wrap.

Heat the steak in the same skillet for 2 minutes, or just until heated through. Place on top of the pepper mixture.

Top with the salsa and cheese. Fold the wrap.

PER SERVING: 786 calories, 53 g protein, 26 g carbohydrates, 52 g total fat, 30 g saturated fat, 10 g fiber, 967 mg sodium

MEDITERRANEAN TUNA SALAD WRAPS

PREP TIME: 20 MINUTES | **TOTAL TIME:** 20 MINUTES

Makes 4 servings

One way around having wheat flour in your life is to put other foods to work in wrapping your food for portability. Here's an easy breadless sandwich using large lettuce leaves as the "bread."

For variety, substitute canned salmon for the tuna, use green rather than kalamata olives, add sliced avocado, or add some sprouts.

2 tablespoons mayonnaise

2 tablespoons olive oil

1 tablespoon lemon juice

1 teaspoon Dijon mustard

2 cans (6 ounces each) water-packed tuna, drained

1 tomato, seeded and chopped

2 tablespoons chopped kalamata olives

2 scallions, thinly sliced

8 large leaves lettuce, such as Boston or leaf

In a medium bowl, combine the mayonnaise, oil, lemon juice, and mustard. Stir in the tuna, tomato, olives, and scallions. Arrange the lettuce on a work surface with the rib ends closest to you. Divide the tuna salad among the lettuce leaves and roll to enclose. Place 2 wraps on each of 4 plates and serve.

PER SERVING: 230 calories, 17 g protein, 4 g carbohydrates, 16 g total fat, 2 g saturated fat, 1 g fiber, 554 mg sodium

GINGER CHICKEN LETTUCE CUPS

PREP TIME: 15 MINUTES | **TOTAL TIME:** 25 MINUTES

Makes 2 servings

I love having these at Chinese restaurants, but they are generally served with a sweetened soy sauce that, to us wheat-free folk, can be excessively sweet. Here's an unsweetened version that is likely to be more palatable to those of us with heightened sensitivity to sweetness. Serve these alongside a stir-fry with shirataki noodles or some sushi.

1 tablespoon coconut oil

1 small onion, chopped

2 carrots, shredded

1 clove garlic, minced

1 tablespoon fresh ginger

½ cup water chestnuts, drained and chopped

1 cup diced cooked skinless dark meat chicken

2 tablespoons chicken broth or water

1 tablespoon gluten-free soy sauce

2 tablespoons rice wine vinegar

2 scallions, thinly sliced

4 leaves Bibb lettuce, washed

In a large skillet over medium-low heat, heat the oil. Cook the onion for 5 minutes, or until tender. Add the carrots, garlic, ginger, and water chestnuts and cook for 1 minute.

Add the chicken, broth or water, soy sauce, and vinegar and cook for 3 minutes, or until heated through. Remove from the heat and stir in the scallions.

Divide the chicken mixture equally among the lettuce leaves. Place 2 lettuce cups on each of 2 plates and serve.

PER SERVING: 279 calories, 22 g protein, 17 g carbohydrates, 14 g total fat, 8 g saturated fat, 4 g fiber, 683 mg sodium

WHEAT BELLY PIZZA

PREP TIME: 20 MINUTES | **TOTAL TIME:** 30 MINUTES

Makes 8 servings

Use the wheat-free Pizza Crust from page 233 and you convert a food awful for health into a healthy one that will keep you and your spouse full and the kids—even teenagers—happy!

For variety, use feta or provolone cheese instead of mozzarella; add fresh basil; try diced ham and Cheddar cheese; or use ground hamburger or turkey in place of the sausage.

¼ cup extra-virgin olive oil, divided

1 pound bulk or loose sausage

1 medium onion, chopped

2 cloves garlic, minced

1 recipe Pizza Crust II (page 233)

2 cups sugar-free pizza or marinara sauce

8 ounces fresh mozzarella, thinly sliced

½ red or green bell pepper, chopped

1 teaspoon dried oregano

2 tablespoons grated Parmesan or Romano cheese

Preheat the oven to 350°F.

In a skillet over medium heat, heat 2 tablespoons of the oil. Cook the sausage, onion, and garlic for 10 minutes, or until the sausage is cooked through and the onion is tender. Remove from the heat and drain if necessary.

Place the pizza crust on a baking sheet. Top with the sauce, mozzarella, sausage mixture, bell pepper, oregano, and Parmesan or Romano. Drizzle the remaining 2 tablespoons oil over the top.

Bake for 10 minutes, or until browned and the cheese melts.

PER SERVING: 491 calories, 23 g protein, 17 g carbohydrates, 38 g total fat, 9 g saturated fat, 6 g fiber, 664 mg sodium

MINI PIZZAS

PREP TIME: 30 MINUTES | TOTAL TIME: 1 HOUR 45 MINUTES

Makes 6 servings

Individual pizzas make a great lunch or light meal and are a favorite for the little ones. For super-fast pizzas, place a Flaxseed Wrap (page 231) or Wheat Belly Tortilla (page 227) on a baking sheet and top with your favorite toppings.

¾ cup warm water (100–110°F)

1¼ teaspoons active dry yeast

1 cup almond meal/flour

1 cup garbanzo bean (chickpea) flour

½ cup ground golden flaxseeds

1 teaspoon sea salt

2 tablespoons olive oil

1½ cups sugar-free pizza or marinara sauce

TOPPINGS (OPTIONAL)

1 cup ricotta cheese

1 cup shredded mozzarella cheese

8 ounces thinly sliced fresh mozzarella cheese

4 ounces thinly sliced pepperoni

Thinly sliced and sautéed bell pepper and onion

Thinly sliced and sautéed yellow squash and zucchini

Quartered grape tomatoes

2 tablespoons chopped fresh herbs

In a small bowl, whisk together the water and yeast until the yeast dissolves. Let stand for 10 minutes.

In a medium bowl, whisk together the almond meal/flour, garbanzo flour, flax-seeds, and salt. Add the oil and the yeast mixture and stir for 5 minutes, or until all of the ingredients are evenly distributed and a loose ball of dough forms. Cover with plastic wrap and let stand in a warm place for 1 hour. Divide into 6 equal pieces.

Preheat the oven to 350°F. Line 2 baking sheets with parchment paper.

Place a piece of parchment paper on the work surface. Place 1 piece of dough on a piece of parchment paper and top with a second sheet of parchment paper. Flatten with a rolling pin into a circle about 4". Place the dough on the baking sheet. Carefully remove the top layer of parchment paper. Use a spoon or your hands to form a crust edge. Repeat with the remaining pieces of dough.

Bake for 20 minutes, or until lightly browned. Remove from the oven and top each with ¼ cup pizza or marinara sauce and desired toppings. Bake for 10 minutes or until heated through.

PER SERVING (WITHOUT TOPPINGS): 317 calories, 11 g protein, 24 g carbohydrates, 21 g total fat, 2 g saturated fat, 10 g fiber, 545 mg sodium

PESTO CHICKEN PIZZA

PREP TIME: 20 MINUTES | TOTAL TIME: 30 MINUTES

Makes 8 servings

Minus the wheat flour, pizza crust becomes the platform for an endless range of healthy variations. Here's one of those variations: a delicious pizza combining the rich flavors of basil pesto with artichokes and goat cheese.

1 recipe Pizza Crust I (page 232)

⅓ cup prepared pesto

1 cup cooked chicken, cut into small strips

1 roasted red pepper, cut into small strips

½ cup water-packed canned artichoke hearts, rinsed and drained, patted dry and quartered

½ cup (3 ounces) crumbled goat cheese

Preheat the oven to 450°F.

Prepare the pizza crust and place on a baking sheet.

Evenly spread the pesto over the crust. Arrange the chicken, pepper strips, and artichokes over the pesto. Top with the cheese.

Bake for 10 minutes, or until heated through and the crust is crisp.

PER SERVING: 413 calories, 22 g protein, 10 g carbohydrates, 34 g total fat, 8 g saturated fat, 4 g fiber, 370 mg sodium

CAESAR SALAD WITH WHEAT-FREE CROUTONS

PREP TIME: 15 MINUTES | TOTAL TIME: 15 MINUTES

Makes 4 servings

Caesar salad isn't Caesar salad without big, crunchy croutons. When you order a Caesar salad without croutons at a restaurant, you invariably get funny looks and a generally unsatisfying salad. Fortunately, croutons return in all their olive oil–toasted glory using our Basic Bread!

4 slices Basic Bread (page 225), cut into ¾" cubes

2 tablespoons olive oil

¼ teaspoon sea salt

¼ teaspoon ground black pepper

⅓ cup mayonnaise

¼ cup grated Parmesan cheese

3 tablespoons lemon juice

2 cloves garlic, minced

1 head romaine lettuce (1 pound), torn into bite-size pieces

1 pound boneless, skinless chicken breasts, roasted or grilled

Preheat the oven to 450°F.

In a medium bowl, toss the bread cubes with the oil, salt, and pepper. Transfer to a baking sheet and spread evenly. Bake for 10 minutes, turning once, or until lightly browned. Place on a plate and set aside.

In a large bowl, whisk together the mayonnaise, cheese, lemon juice, and garlic. Add the lettuce and toss until coated.

Shred the chicken or cut diagonally into strips. Top the lettuce with the chicken and croutons.

PER SERVING: 534 calories, 36 g protein, 14 g carbohydrates, 38 g total fat, 7 g saturated fat, 6 g fiber, 785 mg sodium

CHIPOTLE STEAK SALAD

PREP TIME: 25 MINUTES | TOTAL TIME: 25 MINUTES

Makes 4 servings

The combination of steak and onions—plenty of onions!—comes together in this salad, along with the peppery taste of jalapeño. This salad easily serves as a main course or can be used as a hefty salad alongside some fajitas (using Flaxseed Wraps, page 231) or tortilla soup.

2 white or yellow onions, cut into wedges

1 red onion, cut into wedges

1 tablespoon olive oil

1 teaspoon gluten-free chipotle seasoning

½ teaspoon sea salt

1 pound lean top round or flank steak

2 ounces goat cheese, crumbled

¼ cup sour cream

1 tablespoon white wine vinegar

½ teaspoon Worcestershire sauce

6 cups mixed greens

4 plum tomatoes, seeded and chopped

Coat the grill racks or a broiler pan with cooking spray. Preheat the grill or broiler.

In a large bowl, combine the onions and 1 tablespoon of the oil.

Rub the seasoning and salt on the steak.

Grill or broil the steak for 10 minutes, turning once, or until a thermometer inserted in the center registers 145°F for medium-rare. Remove to a cutting board and let rest for 10 minutes before cutting across the grain into thin slices.

Place the onions in a grill basket or broiler pan. Grill or broil for 15 minutes, turning occasionally, or until browned.

Meanwhile, in a large bowl, whisk together the cheese, sour cream, vinegar, and Worcestershire sauce. Add the greens and tomatoes and toss well to coat. Divide among 4 serving bowls and top each with one-quarter of the sliced steak and the onions.

PER SERVING: 274 calories, 30 g protein, 14 g carbohydrates, 10 g total fat, 4 g saturated fat, 4 g fiber, 398 mg sodium

ORIENTAL CHICKEN SALAD

PREP TIME: 20 MINUTES | **TOTAL TIME:** 30 MINUTES

Makes 4 servings

This recipe was one of the dishes, I believe, that won my kids over to the wheat-free lifestyle, since they realized that eating foods without wheat could be every bit as tasty as eating those with wheat. With flavors of ginger and wasabi mingled together with the softness of rice vinegar, this Oriental Chicken Salad, while a great side salad, can also serve as the main course. Wasabi powder is optional (since it can be tough to find), but it adds some unexpected zing to the chicken.

2 large eggs

½ cup finely ground golden flaxseeds

2 tablespoons coconut flour

1 teaspoon onion powder

½ teaspoon wasabi powder (optional)

1 teaspoon ground ginger

4 boneless, skinless chicken breast halves, sliced lengthwise into 1" strips

4 cups mixed greens

¼ cup sliced almonds

½ cup Asian Dipping Sauce (page 214)

Preheat the oven to 400°F.

In a shallow bowl, whisk the eggs.

In another shallow bowl, combine the flaxseeds, coconut flour, onion powder, wasabi powder (if using), and ginger and mix together.

Dip each chicken strip in the eggs to coat and then roll in the flaxseed mixture. Place each strip on a baking sheet. Bake for 20 minutes, turning once, or until no longer pink and the juices run clear.

Divide the greens among 4 plates, sprinkle with the almonds, and drizzle with the vinaigrette. Top with the chicken strips.

PER SERVING: 344 calories, 36 g protein, 14 g carbohydrates, 17 g total fat, 2 g saturated fat, 8 g fiber, 1,277 mg sodium

PANZANELLA

PREP TIME: 25 MINUTES | TOTAL TIME: 55 MINUTES

Makes 4 servings

Panzanella is an Italian bread salad. Here, the Basic Focaccia, tossed with olives, tomatoes, and basil, adds its own great flavor to the dish.

3 cups cubed Basic Focaccia (page 228)

⅓ cup olive oil

3 tablespoons white balsamic vinegar

¼ teaspoon sea salt

1 large red tomato, seeded and cut into 1" chunks

1 large yellow bell pepper, cut into 1" chunks

1 small English cucumber, quartered lengthwise and thinly sliced crosswise

1 small red onion, halved and thinly sliced

¼ cup basil leaves, cut into thin strips

6 pitted kalamata olives, chopped

Preheat the oven to 350°F.

On a baking sheet, arrange the bread cubes. Bake for 10 minutes, or until toasted.

In a large bowl, whisk together the oil, vinegar, and salt. Add the tomato, pepper, cucumber, onion, basil, and olives, and toss well. Add the focaccia cubes and toss to coat. Allow to stand at room temperature for 30 minutes before serving.

PER SERVING: 385 calories, 8 g protein, 16 g carbohydrates, 35 g total fat, 4 g saturated fat, 5 g fiber, 426 mg sodium

MOCK POTATO AND SNAP BEAN SALAD

PREP TIME: 20 MINUTES | **TOTAL TIME:** 20 MINUTES

Makes 4 servings

Cauliflower works well as a substitute for potatoes in this flavorful salad, which is a perfect replacement for potato or pasta salad at a barbecue. To serve it as a main dish salad, add 1 pound cooked chicken, turkey, steak, or sausage.

1 head cauliflower, broken into florets

½ pound green beans, trimmed and cut in half

¼ cup mayonnaise

3 tablespoons prepared pesto

1 plum tomato, halved, seeded, and cut into thin strips

2 scallions, sliced

In a large saucepan over high heat, bring 2" of water to a boil. Place a steamer basket in the pan and add the cauliflower. Reduce the heat to medium, cover, and cook for 10 minutes, or until slightly tender. Add the green beans, cover, and cook for 4 minutes, or until the cauliflower is tender and the beans are tender-crisp.

Meanwhile, in a large bowl, stir together the mayonnaise and pesto. Add the cauliflower and green beans and toss to coat well. Stir in the tomato and scallions.

PER SERVING: 221 calories, 5 g protein, 13 g carbohydrates, 18 g total fat, 2 g saturated fat, 5 g fiber, 188 mg sodium

THAI NOODLE SALAD WITH PEANUT SAUCE

PREP TIME: 25 MINUTES | TOTAL TIME: 25 MINUTES

Makes 2 servings

Many Thai dishes are off the list in our wheat-free world, since noodles made from wheat flour usually serve as the centerpiece. Here is a way to have a peanutty Thai salad again using shirataki noodles.

This is the basic salad. For variety, add fresh cilantro, grated fresh ginger, or toasted sesame seeds, or top it with boiled or barbecued shrimp.

1 tablespoon natural creamy peanut butter	1 package (8 ounces) shirataki noodles, rinsed and drained
1 tablespoon rice wine vinegar	1 carrot, cut into matchsticks
2 teaspoons gluten-free soy sauce	½ cucumber, halved, seeded, and cut into matchsticks
2 teaspoons toasted sesame oil	2 tablespoons chopped peanuts
½ teaspoon ground ginger	

In a large bowl, whisk together the peanut butter, vinegar, soy sauce, sesame oil, and ginger. Set aside.

Bring a large pot of water to a boil over high heat. Cook the noodles and carrot for 1 minute. Drain, reserving ⅓ cup of the water. Rinse the noodles and carrot under cold water. Drain well.

Whisk the reserved water into the peanut mixture until smooth. Add the noodles, carrot, and cucumber, tossing to coat well. Top with the peanuts.

PER SERVING: 171 calories, 5 g protein, 11 g carbohydrates, 13 g total fat, 2 g saturated fat, 2 g fiber, 392 mg sodium

SUCCESS STORY

Kaylana: Psoriasis, memory problems, stuttering—gone!

In my neighborhood, everyone knew me for the breads and pastries I was always whipping up. It sure seemed healthier to do my own baking than to buy breads from the store, but this style of eating began to take its toll—and not in the ways you might expect.

My husband and I live in Latvia, where I homeschool my little ones. I began to notice that Samuel, my youngest, was having difficulty with language development. At 4½, he still couldn't remember his numbers, and a simple reading program was agony. He had no memory of things he'd learned just seconds before, and a year later things hadn't improved much at all.

We puzzled over what the problem could be. We knew he wasn't disabled—he had great motor skills and could ride a two-wheeler when he was only 3 years old. He had great people skills, too, showing more care and sympathy toward others than most kids his age. But when it came to his lessons, nothing seemed to work.

Around this time, we both developed psoriasis on our hands, and Samuel began to develop a stutter. He'd desperately want to tell me something but couldn't get the words out. As he slowly drifted into a shell, my heart broke to pieces.

Then I got a letter from my sister-in-law with some very surprising news: She and her family were all going on a wheat fast. If I was the queen of pastries, she was the ruler of all things wheat—she even ground her own wheat daily. So I was in shock and disbelief—until I started doing some research. I learned that wheat—all the wonderful, homemade goodies I was baking—was poisoning my family.

That was it. We immediately went on a wheat-free diet, and within 3 days I noticed a huge difference. Samuel's stuttering vanished, and he began flying through his lessons. Our skin problems have disappeared, too. And I've discovered amazing new wheat-free recipes, like nutrient-rich almond pancakes.

It's been a miraculous turnaround for my family, and we plan to stay on this road for a long, long time.

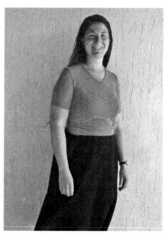

AFTER

APPETIZERS

ARTICHOKE AND SPINACH DIP

PREP TIME: 15 MINUTES | TOTAL TIME: 35 MINUTES

Makes 8 servings

This simple Artichoke and Spinach Dip is the perfect accompaniment to sliced raw vegetables or Flaxseed Crackers (page 241). I've even used it as a sandwich spread— heavenly on a ham and Swiss sandwich between 2 slices of Wheat Belly Basic Bread.

2 packages (8 ounces each) Neufchâtel cheese, at room temperature

⅓ cup sour cream

¼ cup mayonnaise

3 cloves garlic, halved

2 teaspoons Dijon mustard

½ cup grated Parmesan cheese, divided

2 jars (6 ounces each) marinated artichoke hearts, drained and finely chopped

1 package (10 ounces) frozen chopped spinach, thawed and squeezed dry

Assorted vegetables such as celery sticks, carrot sticks, and sliced bell peppers

Preheat the oven to 375°F. Coat a 1½- or 2-quart baking dish with cooking spray.

In a blender or food processor, combine the Neufchâtel, sour cream, mayonnaise, garlic, mustard, and ¼ cup of the Parmesan. Blend or process until smooth.

In a medium bowl, combine the artichoke hearts and spinach. Add the cheese mixture and toss to coat. Pour into the baking dish. Top with the remaining ¼ cup Parmesan. Bake for 20 minutes, or until bubbling hot.

Serve with the vegetables.

PER SERVING: 293 calories, 9 g protein, 6 g carbohydrates, 26 g total fat, 11 g saturated fat, 1 g fiber, 459 mg sodium

ALMOND RED PEPPER DIP

PREP TIME: 10 MINUTES | TOTAL TIME: 10 MINUTES

Makes 8 servings

Finely ground nut meals are surprisingly friendly bases for dips. This peppery dip calls for toasted almonds, but I've used walnuts successfully, too.

1 jar (10–12 ounces) roasted red peppers, drained well

⅓ cup sliced almonds, toasted

⅓ cup finely grated Parmesan cheese

1 tablespoon balsamic vinegar

1 clove garlic

Pinch of ground red pepper

⅛ teaspoon sea salt

⅛ teaspoon ground black pepper

Endive leaves and jicama sticks

In a food processor, combine the peppers, almonds, cheese, vinegar, garlic, and ground red pepper. Pulse until smooth. Transfer to a serving bowl, add the salt and black pepper, and stir to combine.

Serve with the vegetables.

PER SERVING: 45 calories, 2 g protein, 2 g carbohydrates, 3 g total fat, 1 g saturated fat, 1 g fiber, 151 mg sodium

CHEESE FONDUE

PREP TIME: 10 MINUTES | TOTAL TIME: 20 MINUTES

Makes 12 servings

Dust off the fondue pot! In the Wheat Belly style of life and eating, we don't shy away from fatty but wheat-free foods like cheeses. This fondue is a celebration of cheeses that you can combine with a wide variety of dipping foods.

2 cups shredded Gruyère cheese (8 ounces)

2 cups shredded Swiss cheese (8 ounces)

1 tablespoon arrowroot

½ teaspoon dry mustard

1 clove garlic, halved

1 cup chicken broth

3 ounces cream cheese, cut into chunks

In a medium bowl, toss the Gruyère and Swiss with the arrowroot and mustard until coated.

Rub the garlic halves all around the inside of the top of a double boiler, then discard.

Add the broth to the double boiler and place over simmering water. Gradually add the cheese mixture, stirring until the cheeses are melted. Stir in the cream cheese just until melted. Remove from the heat. Keep warm in a fondue pot or bowl.

PER SERVING: 178 calories, 11 g protein, 2 g carbohydrates, 14 g total fat, 8 g saturated fat, 0 g fiber, 204 mg sodium

BUFFALO CHICKEN WITH BLUE CHEESE SAUCE

PREP TIME: 10 MINUTES | TOTAL TIME: 55 MINUTES

Makes 6 servings

Know those chicken wings you like? Well, they probably contain wheat flour and/or high-fructose corn syrup in the sauce, converting a healthy food into a dish with health booby traps. Here's how to make a wheat-free, high-fructose corn syrup–free version with none of those worries.

2 pounds chicken drummettes	2 tablespoons mayonnaise
1 teaspoon chili powder	¼ cup crumbled blue cheese
½ teaspoon sea salt	2 tablespoons butter
¼ teaspoon ground black pepper	¼ cup hot-pepper sauce
¼ teaspoon ground red pepper	Celery sticks (optional)
½ cup plain Greek yogurt	

Preheat the oven to 400°F.

In a large bowl, toss the chicken with the chili powder, salt, black pepper, and ground red pepper. Arrange on a baking sheet. Roast for 45 minutes, or until browned and cooked through.

Meanwhile, in a small bowl, combine the yogurt, mayonnaise, and blue cheese. Cover and chill until ready to serve.

In a small skillet over medium-low heat, melt the butter. Add the hot-pepper sauce, reduce the heat to low, and keep warm.

Place the cooked drummettes in a large bowl. Toss with the pepper sauce mixture. Serve with the blue cheese sauce and celery sticks, if desired.

PER SERVING: 445 calories, 30 g protein, 1 g carbohydrates, 35 g total fat, 12 g saturated fat, 0 g fiber, 695 mg sodium

TERIYAKI MEATBALLS

PREP TIME: 20 MINUTES | TOTAL TIME: 40 MINUTES

Makes 10 servings

Teriyaki Meatballs serve as a great standalone appetizer, a side dish alongside some vegetables, or a topper to a vegetable stir-fry that includes shiitake mushrooms and a side of cauliflower "rice." Beef or pork works equally well in place of the turkey.

⅓ cup wheat-free soy sauce

2 tablespoons mirin (sweet Japanese rice wine) or medium-dry sherry

3 tablespoons rice vinegar

2½ tablespoons minced fresh ginger, divided

2 tablespoons xylitol or 8 drops liquid stevia or to desired sweetness

1 teaspoon dark sesame oil

1 pound lean ground turkey

¼ cup ground flaxseeds

1 egg

1 clove garlic, minced

¼ teaspoon sea salt

In a medium saucepan, combine the soy sauce, mirin or sherry, vinegar, 1½ tablespoons of the ginger, and the xylitol or stevia and heat over medium heat. Simmer for 10 minutes, or until reduced to about ½ cup. Stir in the sesame oil.

Meanwhile, preheat the oven to 400°F. Coat a broiler pan with cooking spray.

In a large bowl, combine the turkey, flaxseeds, egg, garlic, salt, and the remaining 1 tablespoon ginger. Shape into approximately twenty 2" meatballs and place on the pan.

Bake for 15 minutes, turning once, or until no longer pink. Transfer to the saucepan with the sauce. Cover and cook for 5 minutes, or until the flavors are blended.

PER SERVING: 107 calories, 10 g protein, 3 g carbohydrates, 6 g total fat, 1 g saturated fat, 1 g fiber, 620 mg sodium

WASABI CUCUMBERS

PREP TIME: 15 MINUTES | TOTAL TIME: 15 MINUTES

Makes 4 servings

The unique horseradishy heat of wasabi combines with the tastes of smoky salmon and cool cucumber in this simple but tantalizing appetizer.

⅓ cup cream cheese

2 tablespoons wasabi paste (without added sugar)

1 large cucumber, cut into 24 slices

2 ounces smoked salmon, cut into 24 strips

In a small bowl, stir together the cheese and wasabi. Arrange the cucumber slices on a platter and top each with a spoonful of cheese mixture. Garnish each with a small twist of salmon.

PER SERVING: 149 calories, 10 g protein, 8 g carbohydrates, 9 g total fat, 4 g saturated fat, 0 g fiber, 220 mg sodium

GOAT CHEESE AND OLIVE STUFFED DATES

PREP TIME: 10 MINUTES | TOTAL TIME: 10 MINUTES

Makes 8 servings

When a somewhat sweeter appetizer is needed alongside, say, your Mozzarella Sticks (page 150) and Barbecue Bacon Shrimp (page 151), these stuffed dates will do the job. Be sure to use Deglet Noor dates because they are the lowest in carbohydrates.

2 ounces soft goat cheese, at room temperature

2 tablespoons finely chopped pitted kalamata olives

½ teaspoon orange peel

16 large pitted Deglet Noor dates

In a small bowl, stir together the goat cheese, olives, and orange peel until combined. Stuff into the dates.

PER SERVING: 80 calories, 2 g protein, 13 g carbohydrates, 3 g total fat, 1 g saturated fat, 2 g fiber, 107 mg sodium

PEPPER AND ALMOND GOAT CHEESE

PREP TIME: 10 MINUTES | TOTAL TIME: 10 MINUTES

Makes 5 servings

This is one of my favorite appetizers, as it combines the earthy flavors of fresh basil and olive oil and the creamy mouth feel of goat cheese. If you serve this to friends or family, save a few pieces for breakfast!

1 package (5 ounces) soft goat cheese

1 roasted red pepper, drained, patted dry, and cut into thin strips

¼ cup fresh basil leaves, cut into thin strips

1 tablespoon extra-virgin olive oil

1 tablespoon balsamic vinegar

2 tablespoons sliced almonds, toasted

Slice the goat cheese into 10 thin slices. Place on a serving plate. Sprinkle with the red pepper, basil, oil, vinegar, and almonds.

PER SERVING: 118 calories, 6 g protein, 0 g carbohydrates, 10 g total fat, 5 g saturated fat, 1 g fiber, 111 mg sodium

MOZZARELLA STICKS

PREP TIME: 5 MINUTES | TOTAL TIME: 45 MINUTES

Makes 6 servings

These yummy Mozzarella Sticks are similar to those served in many Italian restaurants. While they are perfect as an appetizer, they are also great for kids to eat for lunch or a snack. Look for marinara sauces that do not have added sucrose or high-fructose corn syrup.

2 tablespoons arrowroot	½ teaspoon dried basil, crushed
2 eggs	12 sticks string cheese, unwrapped
¾ cup golden flaxseed meal	6 tablespoons coconut oil
¼ cup grated Parmesan or Romano cheese	1 cup sugar-free marinara sauce, warmed

In a shallow bowl or plate, place the arrowroot. In a shallow bowl, beat the eggs until blended. In another shallow bowl or on a plate, combine the flaxseed meal, Parmesan or Romano, and basil.

Roll 1 string cheese stick in the arrowroot until coated. Dip into the eggs and reroll in the arrowroot. Dip into the eggs again and roll in the flaxseed mixture, turning to coat well. (Be sure to coat the ends well.) Place on a baking sheet. Repeat with the remaining cheese sticks. Cover and place in the freezer for 30 minutes.

In a large skillet over medium-high heat, heat ½ inch of coconut oil. Cook 3 to 6 cheese sticks in the oil for 1 minute, turning once, or until golden brown. Repeat with the remaining cheese sticks.

Serve with the marinara sauce.

PER SERVING: 427 calories, 24 g protein, 14 g carbohydrates, 34 g total fat, 20 g saturated fat, 6 g fiber, 729 mg sodium

BARBECUE BACON SHRIMP

PREP TIME: 10 MINUTES | TOTAL TIME: 20 MINUTES

Makes 8 servings

Minus the breading on shrimp, minus the ubiquitous high-fructose corn syrup and sugar in barbecue sauce, minus the nitrites of cured meats, these Barbecue Bacon Shrimp are converted into a healthy, problem-free appetizer. To make this recipe as hassle-free as possible, keep a supply of the Kansas City–Style Barbecue Sauce (page 215) on hand, premade for such occasions.

 1 **pound large shrimp, peeled and deveined**

 ¼ **cup Kansas City–Style Barbecue Sauce (page 215)**

 ½ **pound nitrite-free bacon, each slice halved**

Preheat the broiler to low.

Brush the shrimp with the sauce and wrap each with 1 piece of bacon. Secure with a wooden pick. Place on a broiler pan and broil 4 to 6" from the heat for 6 minutes, turning once, or until the bacon is crisp and the shrimp are opaque.

PER SERVING: 171 calories, 23 g protein, 2 g carbohydrates, 10 g total fat, 5 g saturated fat, 0 g fiber, 847 mg sodium

SUCCESS STORY

Marilyn W.: Indigestion and bloating— disappeared

I'd never really been sick, but when I think about it, it had been a long, long time since I'd really been well, either. On the outside, I probably looked okay—I'm fashionable, attractive woman with a high-powered job—but I hated the bloated belly that I'd always struggled to lose.

So when a friend told me about *Wheat Belly,* I grabbed my e-reader and down-loaded the book that very same day. I had a gut sense that I had a wheat intolerance, even though I'd tested negative for celiac disease 5 years earlier. But at age 62, I'd been carrying more than 40 excess pounds and feeling bloated, achy, exhausted, and hypoglycemic for a decade—and every single diet I'd attempted was sabotaged within a couple of weeks by my intense food cravings.

Today is only the 6th day of my wheat-free life, but already the change has been amazing. A couple of days ago, a friend remarked, "You look great! Have you been exercising?" I think what he noticed was the loss of bloat and my improved skin tone and coloring. I told

him about the book and going wheat free.

If full health feels like a 10, I think I must have muddled along at a 4 for decades. After less than a week, I've returned to a 7, and I'm still climbing. My body confirms that wheat was poisonous for me. I no longer feel like a doughboy—or doughgirl—which is the perfect analogy for wheat belly. Just last week I was suffering chronic pain from indigestion. Today that's completely disappeared. I can feel myself healing at a very deep level, and I feel wonderful in ways I'd long since forgotten—no more aches or bloating, no more cravings, hardly any hunger. In their place, I have energy I hadn't felt in years.

Giving up the wheat? Easy. I had no withdrawal symptoms, and in just a few days I've shed the bloat and probably lots of the fat. And I'm on the road to better health, a big plus when you come from a family in which diabetes is common.

For me, *Wheat Belly* is a life-changing, health-giving book, and I talk about it to anyone who'll listen. I plan to follow this way of eating forever.

SOUPS AND STEWS

CREAM OF BROCCOLI SOUP

PREP TIME: 15 MINUTES | **TOTAL TIME:** 50 MINUTES

Makes 4 servings

Sure, there's comfort food in this wheat-free lifestyle! Here's a wheat-free, dairy-free version of Cream of Broccoli Soup. The use of coconut milk and coconut flour, rather than the usual wheat flour, cornstarch, or evaporated milk, slashes carbohydrate and sugar content but makes no sacrifice in taste.

1 pound broccoli

1 tablespoon butter or coconut oil

1 leek, sliced (white part only)

1 rib celery, sliced

4 cups chicken broth

2 cups carton-variety coconut milk, divided

1½ tablespoons coconut flour

1 teaspoon chopped fresh thyme or ½ teaspoon dried

Cut the broccoli into florets and set aside. Trim and discard the tough, fibrous skin from the stems. Coarsely chop the stems and set aside.

In a medium saucepan over medium-low heat, heat the butter or oil. Cook the leek and celery, stirring occasionally, for 8 minutes, or until the leek is soft. Add the broccoli stems and broth. Bring to a boil, then reduce the heat to low, cover, and simmer for 15 minutes. Add the broccoli florets and simmer for 10 minutes.

Transfer the mixture to a blender or food processor. Puree until smooth. Return to the saucepan and increase the heat to medium.

Meanwhile, in a small bowl, whisk together ¼ cup of the coconut milk and the coconut flour until smooth. Slowly add to the broccoli mixture, stirring constantly. Stir in the remaining 1¾ cups coconut milk and the thyme. Cook, stirring, for 3 minutes, or until thickened.

PER SERVING: 135 calories, 8 g protein, 14 g carbohydrates, 6 g total fat, 5 g saturated fat, 4 g fiber, 628 mg sodium

CREAM OF TOMATO SOUP

PREP TIME: 10 MINUTES | TOTAL TIME: 50 MINUTES

Makes 4 servings

If wheat infiltrates everything from Twizzlers to tomato soup, can we still have a nice bowl of tomato soup without it? Yes—if you make it yourself! Here's how to restore this traditional and tasty lunch or dinner dish to your life. Top this soup with croutons made with any leftover Basic Bread (page 225).

1 tablespoon extra-virgin olive oil

1 small onion, chopped

2 cups vegetable or chicken broth

1 can (14 ounces) diced tomatoes

2 tablespoons tomato paste

1 teaspoon dried basil, crushed

1 cup half-and-half or canned coconut milk

¼ cup fresh basil, chopped

In a large saucepan over medium-high heat, heat the oil. Cook the onion, stirring occasionally, for 5 minutes, or until soft. Add the broth, tomatoes (with juice), tomato paste, and dried basil. Bring to a boil. Reduce the heat to low, cover, and simmer for 20 minutes, or until slightly thickened. Let cool for 10 minutes.

Transfer the mixture in batches to a blender or food processor. Puree until smooth. Return to the saucepan. Add the half-and-half or coconut milk. Cook, stirring, for 3 minutes, or until heated and thickened. Serve garnished with the fresh basil.

PER SERVING: 153 calories, 3 g protein, 12 g carbohydrates, 10 g total fat, 5 g saturated fat, 2 g fiber, 577 mg sodium

SHRIMP BISQUE

Makes 4 servings

This Shrimp Bisque is perfect to accompany a salad of mixed greens with creamy avocado dressing as lunch, or as the starting dish of a more elaborate holiday meal. Serve it as is or with sour cream.

2 tablespoons butter or extra-virgin olive oil

1 medium onion, chopped

¾ pound peeled and deveined medium shrimp

1 cup tomato puree

1 tablespoon minced fresh parsley

2 teaspoons minced fresh dill

1 teaspoon lemon juice

2 cups chicken or vegetable broth

1½ cups half-and-half or canned coconut milk

Dash of ground red pepper

Fresh chives, finely chopped, for garnish

In a medium saucepan over medium heat, heat the butter or oil. Cook the onion for 5 minutes, or until soft.

Add the shrimp, tomato puree, parsley, dill, lemon juice, and broth. Simmer for 10 minutes. Add the half-and-half or coconut milk and the pepper and heat through. Serve garnished with the chives.

PER SERVING: 302 calories, 23 g protein, 13 g carbohydrates, 18 g total fat, 10 g saturated fat, 2 g fiber, 732 mg sodium

BUTTERNUT SQUASH BISQUE

PREP TIME: 10 MINUTES | TOTAL TIME: 40 MINUTES

Makes 4 to 8 servings

Here's an old favorite to accompany your Wheat Belly Pizza (page 131) or Meat Loaf (page 173) or to serve with some Walnut Raisin Bread (page 243).

Given the higher carbohydrate content of this soup, it is better served as a side dish, rather than as the primary dish in a meal for adults. Kids, of course, can go to town on this soup.

If you'd like, sprinkle ground nutmeg and finely chopped chives on top before serving.

1 large butternut squash	½ teaspoon ground red pepper
2 tablespoons butter or coconut oil + 2 tablespoons butter (optional)	½ teaspoon ground cumin
	2¼ cups chicken broth
2 medium onions, chopped	¼ teaspoon sea salt
1 medium red bell pepper, chopped	¼ teaspoon ground black pepper
2 cloves garlic, minced	¼ cup whole plain yogurt or sour cream

Pierce the squash several times with a sharp knife; place it on a paper towel in the microwave oven. Microwave on high power for 5 minutes. Halve the squash lengthwise and remove and discard the seeds; microwave on high power for 5 minutes. Set aside to cool slightly.

In a large pot over medium-high heat, heat 2 tablespoons of the butter or oil. Cook the onions, bell pepper, and garlic, stirring occasionally, for 5 minutes.

Scoop the squash flesh from its shell and cut into chunks; add the squash chunks, ground red pepper, cumin, and broth to the soup. Bring to a boil. Reduce the heat to medium-low. If desired, add 2 tablespoons of butter for a richer taste. Cover and simmer for 15 minutes.

Transfer the soup to a blender or food processor. Puree until smooth. Return the soup to the saucepan. Stir in the salt and black pepper. Heat through. Garnish each serving with yogurt or sour cream.

PER SERVING: 123 calories, 3 g protein, 23 g carbohydrates, 3 g total fat, 2 g saturated fat, 4 g fiber, 262 mg sodium

AFRICAN CHICKEN SOUP

PREP TIME: 20 MINUTES | TOTAL TIME: 1 HOUR

Makes 4 servings

The warm scents of coriander, cilantro, and cumin greet you in this soup thickened with peanut butter. For variety, try adding 2 tablespoons of tomato paste along with the peanut butter, adding 2 to 3 cups of raw spinach during the last 5 minutes of simmering, or topping the soup with finely chopped scallions.

2 tablespoons olive or coconut oil, divided

12 ounces boneless, skinless chicken breasts, cut into 1½" pieces

3 carrots, sliced

1 onion, chopped

1 red bell pepper, coarsely chopped

5 cloves garlic, minced

1 tablespoon ground cumin

2 teaspoons ground coriander

3 cups chicken broth

¼ cup natural smooth peanut butter

3 tablespoons chopped cilantro

In a large pot over medium-high heat, heat 1 tablespoon of the oil. Cook the chicken, turning occasionally, for 5 minutes, or until no longer pink and the juices run clear. Transfer to a plate and set aside.

In the same pot, heat the remaining 1 tablespoon oil and cook the carrots, onion, and pepper for 5 minutes, stirring often, or until lightly browned. Add the garlic, cumin, and coriander and cook for 1 minute.

Add the broth and bring to a boil. Reduce the heat to medium-low, cover, and simmer for 10 minutes, or until the vegetables are tender. In a small bowl, combine the peanut butter and ¼ cup of the hot broth. Stir until smooth. Stir the peanut butter mixture into the soup.

Add the reserved chicken and simmer for 5 minutes, or until the chicken is heated through. Remove from the heat and stir in the cilantro.

PER SERVING: 321 calories, 26 g protein, 15 g carbohydrates, 18 g total fat, 3 g saturated fat, 4 g fiber, 613 mg sodium

CREAMY CHICKEN AND WILD RICE SOUP

PREP TIME: 10 MINUTES | **TOTAL TIME:** 50 MINUTES

Makes 6 servings

Here's yet another traditional comfort food re-created minus unhealthy ingredients. I like serving this soup as the main dish alongside a light sandwich made with Basic Focaccia (page 228). It also serves as an excellent starter for a larger dinner.

This is a good example of how to use nonwheat grains safely and effectively. We use small portions—in this case ½ cup for the entire recipe to serve six—of the least processed form, in this case wild rice. This soup thereby remains a healthy soup packed with nutrition but with limited potential to overstimulate insulin.

6 cups chicken broth

½ cup wild rice

1 pound boneless, skinless chicken breasts, cubed

2 medium carrots, chopped

1 small onion, chopped

2 teaspoons lemon-pepper seasoning

½ teaspoon sea salt

2 stalks broccoli, cut into small florets (2 cups)

2 cups half-and-half

In a large pot over medium-high heat, combine the broth and rice. Cover and bring to a boil. Reduce the heat to medium-low and cook for 20 minutes.

Add the chicken, carrots, onion, lemon-pepper seasoning, and salt. Cook for 15 minutes. Add the broccoli and cook for 5 minutes, or until the broccoli and rice are tender.

Gradually stir in the half-and-half. Cook, stirring, for 5 minutes, or until heated through.

PER SERVING: 300 calories, 27 g protein, 21 g carbohydrates, 13 g total fat, 7 g saturated fat, 3 g fiber, 455 mg sodium

THAI CHICKEN CURRY SOUP

PREP TIME: 15 MINUTES | TOTAL TIME: 35 MINUTES

Makes 4 servings

With this flavorful variation on chicken soup, you will impress your family that you can do anything a Thai restaurant can do. Serve this soup alongside a salad of fresh greens, watercress, and shredded carrots, topped with Asian Dipping Suace (page 214).

2 tablespoons olive or coconut oil, divided

¾ pound boneless, skinless chicken thighs, cut into strips

3 ribs celery, sliced

3 cloves garlic, chopped

1 onion, chopped

1 red bell pepper, chopped

1 tablespoon minced fresh ginger

3 cups chicken broth

1 can (13.6 ounces) coconut milk

1 tablespoon green curry paste

2 tablespoons Thai fish sauce or gluten-free soy sauce

¼ cup fresh cilantro, chopped

In a large pot over medium-high heat, heat 1 tablespoon of the oil. Cook the chicken, stirring, for 8 minutes, or until browned. Remove to a plate and keep warm.

In the same pot, heat the remaining 1 tablespoon oil. Cook the celery, garlic, onion, pepper, and ginger, stirring occasionally, for 3 minutes. Add the broth, coconut milk, curry paste, fish sauce or soy sauce, and the reserved chicken. Bring to a boil over high heat. Reduce the heat to low and simmer, stirring occasionally, for 4 minutes, or until the chicken is no longer pink and the vegetables are tender-crisp. Sprinkle with the cilantro.

PER SERVING: 424 calories, 20 g protein, 11 g carbohydrates, 35 g total fat, 22 g saturated fat, 3 g fiber, 657 mg sodium

CHICKEN AND DUMPLINGS

PREP TIME: 10 MINUTES | TOTAL TIME: 1 HOUR 5 MINUTES

Makes 8 servings

If wheat can do it, we can do it just as well without. And in this recipe, dumplings are back! Just as you would ordinarily make dumplings using wheat flour, we use almond meal. The end result is every bit as good. I like putting a teaspoon of dried rosemary in my biscuit dough for a bit of added flavor.

2 tablespoons butter or coconut oil, divided

8 boneless, skinless chicken thighs

2 onions, chopped

2 carrots, sliced

2 ribs celery, sliced

3 cups chicken broth

1 teaspoon dried thyme

1 recipe Basic Biscuits (page 245)

½ cup sour cream or canned coconut milk

Preheat the oven to 350°F.

In a Dutch oven over medium-high heat, heat 1 tablespoon of the butter or oil. Cook the chicken, turning occasionally, for 5 minutes, or until golden on all sides. Remove to a plate and set aside.

Heat the remaining 1 tablespoon butter or oil. Cook the onions, carrots, and celery, stirring occasionally, for 5 minutes, or until the onions start to soften. Add the broth, thyme, the remaining ⅛ teaspoon salt, and the reserved chicken. Increase the heat to high. Bring to a boil. Bake, uncovered, for 20 minutes.

Meanwhile, prepare the biscuits. Remove the Dutch oven from the oven and stir in the sour cream or coconut milk. Increase the oven temperature to 400°F.

Dollop 8 biscuits onto the chicken mixture. Bake uncovered for 15 minutes. Cover and bake for 15 minutes, or until a thermometer inserted in the thickest portion of the chicken registers 170°F.

PER SERVING: 342 calories, 23 g protein, 15 g carbohydrates, 23 g total fat, 6 g saturated fat, 7 g fiber, 810 mg sodium

TURKEY CHILI

PREP TIME: 20 MINUTES | **TOTAL TIME:** 1 HOUR 30 MINUTES

Makes 4 servings

Here is a beanless chili recipe that, minus the beans and other unhealthy stuff like wheat flour, cornstarch, and sugars, won't mess with blood sugar or insulin. And it's also delicious!

Serve it with sour cream, if desired. This chili also serves as a great topping for shirataki noodles.

1 tablespoon olive or coconut oil	1 teaspoon sea salt
1 pound ground turkey breast	1 can (28 ounces) diced tomatoes
2 red or yellow bell peppers, chopped	1 can (14 ounces) chicken broth
2 carrots, chopped	1 can (8 ounces) tomato puree
1 large onion, chopped	1 chipotle chile pepper in adobo sauce, minced (optional)
4 large cloves garlic, minced	
2 tablespoons ancho chili powder	2 zucchini, chopped
1 tablespoon ground cumin	½ cup sour cream (optional)
1 teaspoon dried oregano	

In a large pot over medium-high heat, heat the oil. Cook the turkey, bell peppers, carrots, and onion, stirring frequently, for 8 minutes, or until the turkey is no longer pink. Add the garlic, chili powder, cumin, oregano, and salt. Cook, stirring constantly, for 1 minute.

Add the diced tomatoes (with juice), chicken broth, tomato puree, and chile pepper (if using). Bring to a boil. Reduce the heat to low, cover, and simmer, stirring occasionally, for 30 minutes.

Stir in the zucchini. Return to a simmer. Cover and simmer for 30 minutes, stirring occasionally, or until the flavors are blended and the vegetables are tender. Top each serving with sour cream, if using.

PER SERVING: 357 calories, 26 g protein, 31 g carbohydrates, 14 g total fat, 3 g saturated fat, 7 g fiber, 842 mg sodium

CHEESEBURGER SOUP

PREP TIME: 10 MINUTES | TOTAL TIME: 50 MINUTES

Makes 4 servings

Yell "cheeseburger soup!" and the kids will come running. You won't tell them, of course, that they are actually eating healthy foods like cauliflower, onions, herbs, beef, and cheese.

4 cups chicken broth, divided	½ teaspoon sea salt
½ head cauliflower, cut into florets	¼ teaspoon paprika
1 tablespoon butter or coconut oil	⅛ teaspoon ground black pepper
1 small onion, chopped	1 tablespoon coconut flour
½ pound ground beef	½ cup shredded sharp Cheddar cheese
1 tablespoon minced fresh parsley	

In a large saucepan, combine 3¾ cups of the broth and the cauliflower. Cover and bring to a boil over high heat. Reduce the heat to medium-low. Cook for 15 to 20 minutes, or until the cauliflower is tender when pierced with a fork.

Meanwhile, in a medium skillet over medium-high heat, heat the butter or oil. Cook the onion, stirring occasionally, for 5 minutes, or until golden. Crumble in the beef. Cook, stirring occasionally, for 8 minutes, or until no longer pink. Stir in the parsley, salt, paprika, and pepper. Remove from the heat and set aside.

Transfer the cauliflower mixture to a food processor or blender and puree until smooth. Return to the saucepan. In a small bowl, whisk the coconut flour with the remaining ¼ cup broth until smooth. Gradually add to the cauliflower mixture and cook, whisking constantly, over medium heat for 3 minutes, or until slightly thickened. Whisk in the cheese just until it melts. Remove the pan from the heat. Stir in the reserved beef mixture.

PER SERVING: 292 calories, 19 g protein, 9 g carbohydrates, 21 g total fat, 10 g saturated fat, 2 g fiber, 533 mg sodium

ASIAN BEEF AND VEGGIE BOWL

PREP TIME: 45 MINUTES | TOTAL TIME: 1 HOUR 10 MINUTES

Makes 4 servings

Shirataki noodles shine in Asian dishes. Here's an Asian stir-fry with beef, veggies, and ginger that will make a satisfying dinner alongside a few pieces of fresh sushi or Fried "Rice" (page 204).

3 tablespoons gluten-free soy sauce

1 tablespoon rice wine vinegar

¼ teaspoon red-pepper flakes

12 ounces trimmed boneless beef top round, cut across the grain into thin slices, slices cut into 1" pieces

2 stalks broccoli, cut into small florets, stems halved lengthwise and very thinly sliced crosswise (about 5 cups)

⅓ cup chicken broth

1 teaspoon arrowroot or coconut flour

2 tablespoons coconut oil, divided

2 tablespoons thin matchstick strips peeled fresh ginger

3 cloves garlic, thinly sliced

1 large red bell pepper, cut into thin strips

2 tablespoons unsalted cashews

2 packages (7 or 8 ounces each) shirataki noodles, rinsed and drained

In a medium bowl, combine the soy sauce, vinegar, and red-pepper flakes. Add the beef and toss to coat. Let stand at room temperature for 30 minutes.

Meanwhile, place a steamer basket in a large pot with 4" of water. Bring to a boil over high heat. Place the broccoli in the basket, cover, and steam for 6 minutes, or until tender-crisp. Remove the broccoli from the steamer and rinse briefly under cold running water. Set aside. Reduce the heat to low and cover the pot to keep the water warm.

Drain the beef, reserving the marinade. In a cup, whisk the broth and arrowroot or coconut flour. Set aside.

In a large, deep nonstick skillet or wok over medium-high heat, heat 1 tablespoon of the oil until hot but not smoking. Cook the ginger and garlic, stirring constantly, for 30 seconds, or just until fragrant; do not brown. Add half the drained beef strips and cook, stirring constantly, for 2 minutes, or just until no longer pink; transfer to a clean plate. Repeat with the remaining beef strips.

Add the remaining 1 tablespoon oil to the skillet. Cook the bell pepper for 2 minutes, stirring constantly, until just tender-crisp. Return the beef and any juices, the reserved marinade, and the steamed broccoli to the skillet. Toss to mix. Cook, stirring constantly, for 2 minutes, or until heated through. Stir the arrowroot mixture again; add to the skillet and cook, stirring, until the mixture boils and thickens. Remove from the heat and sprinkle with the cashews.

Meanwhile, bring the reserved pot of water to a boil. Cook the noodles for 1 to 2 minutes, or until heated through. Drain and pat dry with a towel. Divide the noodles and stir-fry among 4 plates.

PER SERVING: 254 calories, 24 g protein, 12 g carbohydrates, 13 g total fat, 8 g saturated fat, 3 g fiber, 589 mg sodium

BEEF STEW

PREP TIME: 10 MINUTES | TOTAL TIME: 1 HOUR 40 MINUTES

Makes 4 servings

You'd make your grandmother proud by whipping up this old-fashioned Beef Stew. Except this beef stew has no wheat flour or other unhealthy ingredients to thicken it, nor will it make you fat or diabetic, like many other modern dishes.

Enjoy this Beef Stew with Grilled Cheese Sandwiches (page 124) or Basic Biscuits (page 245) to mop up the gravy.

2 tablespoons extra-virgin olive oil	¾ teaspoon sea salt
1½ pounds trimmed beef chuck, cut into 1" chunks	¼ teaspoon ground black pepper
	1¾ cups beef broth, divided
1 large onion, coarsely chopped	2 pounds peeled butternut squash, cut into 3" chunks
1 rib celery, thinly sliced	
1 carrot, sliced	2 tablespoons lemon juice
1 teaspoon dried thyme	2 teaspoons coconut flour

In a Dutch oven over medium heat, heat the oil. Cook the beef, working in batches if necessary, for 5 minutes, or until browned all over. Using a slotted spoon, transfer the beef to a bowl and set aside.

Add the onion, celery, and carrot to the pot and cook, stirring occasionally, for 5 minutes, or until the onion is tender.

Stir in the thyme, salt, and pepper. Return the reserved beef to the pot. Add 1½ cups of the broth and bring to a boil. Reduce the heat, cover, and simmer for 45 minutes.

Stir in the squash and lemon juice. Cover and simmer for 30 minutes, or until the meat and squash are tender.

In a small bowl, whisk the coconut flour with the remaining ¼ cup broth. Add to the pot and cook, stirring constantly, for 3 minutes, or until the sauce thickens.

PER SERVING: 421 calories, 38 g protein, 34 g carbohydrates, 16 g total fat, 4 g saturated fat, 6 g fiber, 625 mg sodium

BEEF BURGUNDY WITH FETTUCCINE

PREP TIME: 25 MINUTES | **TOTAL TIME:** 2 HOURS 55 MINUTES

Makes 8 servings

While we sacrifice the wheat, you can instead indulge in some of the other ingredients, most notably the red wine.

1½ pounds beef stew meat

¼ teaspoon sea salt

¼ teaspoon ground black pepper

2 tablespoons extra-virgin olive oil, divided

1 pound mushrooms, quartered

½ pound pearl onions

3 cloves garlic, minced

2 cups Burgundy wine or beef broth

5 cups beef broth, divided

¼ cup tomato paste

1 bay leaf, crushed

1 bag (8 ounces) baby carrots, halved

1 cup frozen peas, thawed

1½ tablespoons coconut flour

3 packages (7 or 8 ounces each) shirataki fettuccine

¼ cup chopped parsley

On a work surface, season the beef evenly with the salt and pepper.

In a large saucepan over medium-high heat, heat 1 tablespoon of the oil. Cook the beef, working in batches if necessary and stirring frequently, for 5 minutes, or until browned. Remove to a plate and set aside.

Add the remaining 1 tablespoon oil to the pan. Cook the mushrooms, onions, and garlic, stirring often, for 10 minutes, or until lightly browned.

Add the wine or 2 cups broth, 4¾ cups of the broth, the tomato paste, bay leaf, and reserved beef. Bring to a boil. Reduce the heat to low, cover, and simmer for 1½ hours.

Add the carrots and simmer, covered, for 40 minutes, or until the beef and vegetables are tender. Add the peas and cook for 5 minutes. In a small bowl, whisk the coconut flour with the remaining ¼ cup broth. Add to the stew and cook, stirring constantly, for 3 minutes, or until thickened.

Meanwhile, prepare the fettuccine according to package directions. Serve the beef burgundy over the fettuccine, sprinkled with the parsley.

PER SERVING: 270 calories, 23 g protein, 17 g carbohydrates, 10 g total fat, 3 g saturated fat, 6 g fiber, 569 mg sodium

SALSA PORK STEW WITH ORZO

PREP TIME: 15 MINUTES | TOTAL TIME: 2 HOURS 25 MINUTES

Makes 6 servings

Don't panic: I haven't lost my wheat-free resolve with this recipe that includes orzo! To make this delicious Salsa Pork Stew, you will need shirataki orzo, i.e., shirataki noodles cut in an orzo shape. (The Miracle Noodle company makes this variety.) If unavailable, substitute another shirataki noodle variety or Faux Rice (page 203).

2 pounds boneless pork shoulder, cut into 1" cubes

½ teaspoon sea salt

½ teaspoon ground black pepper

Dash of ground red pepper

1 tablespoon olive or coconut oil

1 medium onion, chopped

1 large green bell pepper, chopped

1 jalapeño chile pepper, seeded and finely chopped

1 bottle (15 ounces) green salsa

1 cup chicken broth

1 package (7 or 8 ounces) shirataki orzo, rinsed and drained

2 limes, quartered

1 medium avocado, pitted and sliced

1 cup sour cream

Season the pork with the salt, black pepper, and ground red pepper. In a large pot over high heat, heat the oil. Working in batches, cook the pork, turning occasionally, until seared on all sides. (Don't overcrowd the pork or it will steam, not brown.) Transfer the pork to a plate and set aside.

Add the onion, bell pepper, and chile pepper to the pot. Cook, stirring occasionally, for 4 minutes, or until starting to brown. Add the salsa and broth, stirring to loosen any brown bits. Return the reserved pork to the pot. Reduce the heat to medium-low. Cover and simmer for 2 hours, or until the pork is fork-tender.

Bring a saucepan of water to a boil. Add the orzo and cook for 1 minute. Drain and pat dry. Serve with the stew. Garnish with the limes, avocado, and sour cream.

PER SERVING: 393 calories, 31 g protein, 15 g carbohydrates, 24 g total fat, 9 g saturated fat, 5 g fiber, 719 mg sodium

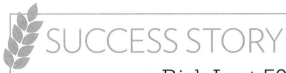

Rick Lost 50 Pounds

I was knocked off my couch and into action by a number and a little piece of white paper. The number was 220/110, and on the paper was scrawled a prescription for high blood pressure medication. All those years of moving very little and eating a lot had brought me there, and I didn't like it very much.

As I adjusted to the medicine, I started looking for an exercise program that would help me get my weight down, and I found ways to lower my blood pressure by reducing grains and sugar but not eliminating them. Little by little, I began to feel better as I dropped 25 pounds, but I started to plateau, and I really wanted to get off those drugs.

In the fall of 2011, a good friend told me about *Wheat Belly* and his success with it. I started right in, and by the new year I was completely wheat free and feeling great. Eating was easy, the cravings were gone, and even fasting was a breeze.

The first thing I noticed was that my joints, especially my hips, knees, hands, and shoulders, had stopped aching, and I had so much more energy. Commuting to my job in New York City, I started taking the stairs—two at a time—instead of the long, slow escalators as I emerged from the subway. And when I got to the top of the hundred-step staircase? I wasn't even out of breath! My wife noticed that I wasn't snoring anymore, and I was falling out of my clothes as my waist size dropped from 44 to 35—and counting.

Those first 25 pounds I lost before *Wheat Belly* took 14 months to disappear. But the next 25—after eliminating wheat— were gone in only 4.

Best of all, that scary number that shocked me into action isn't scary anymore. My blood pressure is down, and I'm off the medication. Because of *Wheat Belly*, I don't need to pollute my body with chemicals. All this time, the answer has been right in front of me: Lose the wheat, lose the weight!

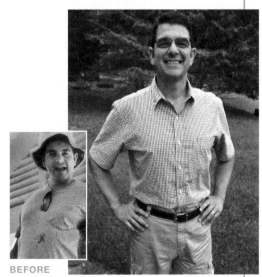

BEFORE

AFTER

MAIN DISHES

BRAISED POT ROAST WITH VEGETABLES

PREP TIME: 15 MINUTES | **TOTAL TIME:** 2 HOURS 40 MINUTES

Makes 6 servings

This traditional pot roast is a perfect demonstration of how you can eat like a king, yet maintain your wheat-free lifestyle. Coconut flour is a wonderful thickener for gravies and sauces and does not raise blood sugar or result in any other adverse health effects, such as those generated by using wheat flour or cornstarch. And it's not just about nutrition: In this recipe, coconut flour yields a delicious sauce that, I believe, tastes *better* than that made with traditional thickeners.

1½ pounds boneless beef chuck roast

¾ teaspoon dried oregano

½ teaspoon dried thyme

½ teaspoon sea salt

¼ teaspoon ground black pepper

1 can (15½ ounces) beef broth

½ cup red wine or beef broth

1 teaspoon gluten-free soy sauce

2 teaspoons extra-virgin olive oil

1 bay leaf

¾ pound white turnips, peeled and cut into eighths

2 cups frozen pearl onions, thawed

2 cups baby carrots

2 tablespoons coconut flour

¼ cup water

Preheat the oven to 400°F.

On a work surface, season the beef with the oregano, thyme, salt, and pepper. In a bowl, combine the broth, wine or broth, and soy sauce. Set aside.

In an ovenproof pot or Dutch oven over medium-high heat, heat the oil. Cook the beef for 2 minutes per side, or until browned. Remove from the heat and stir in the reserved broth mixture and bay leaf. Cover and bake for 1½ hours. Add the turnips, onions, and carrots. Cover and return to the oven. Bake for 45 to 55 minutes, or until the meat and vegetables are tender.

With a slotted spoon, transfer the beef and vegetables to a serving platter. Set the pot over medium-high heat. In a small bowl, whisk the coconut flour and water. Gradually add to the pan gravy and cook, whisking constantly, for 4 minutes, or until thickened. Remove the bay leaf and pour the sauce over the beef and vegetables.

PER SERVING: 238 calories, 28 g protein, 13 g carbohydrates, 6 g total fat, 2 g saturated fat, 4 g fiber, 584 mg sodium

PEPPERED STEAK

PREP TIME: 15 MINUTES | TOTAL TIME: 15 MINUTES

Makes 4 servings

If you've been misled down the low-fat pathway and have been avoiding beef, then it's time to get reacquainted with steak! This peppered steak goes perfectly alongside some steamed green beans or asparagus. If you're craving potatoes with it, consider mashing some cauliflower instead. Remember: If your budget permits, try to purchase pasture-fed cuts of beef.

2 beef round sirloin tip center steaks, 1" thick

2 teaspoons coarsely ground black pepper

¼ teaspoon sea salt

2 tablespoons olive or coconut oil

¼ cup beef broth

1 tablespoon tomato paste

1 tablespoon balsamic vinegar

2 teaspoons chopped parsley or thyme

On a work surface, cut each steak in half to make 4 steaks total. Press the pepper and salt evenly onto the steaks.

In a large skillet over medium heat, heat the oil until sizzling. Cook the steaks for 6 minutes, turning once, or until a thermometer inserted in the center registers 145°F for medium-rare. Transfer to a platter.

Meanwhile, in a small bowl, whisk the broth, tomato paste, and vinegar. Pour the broth mixture into the skillet. Cook for 2 minutes, stirring to loosen any browned bits, or until boiling. Add the parsley or thyme. Serve the sauce over the steaks.

PER SERVING: 183 calories, 19 g protein, 2 g carbohydrates, 11 g total fat, 2 g saturated fat, 0 g fiber, 264 mg sodium

MEAT LOAF

PREP TIME: 10 MINUTES | **TOTAL TIME:** 1 HOUR 45 MINUTES

Makes 8 servings

This Meat Loaf is an example of just how easy it can be to convert traditional wheat-containing dishes to healthier wheat-free versions: All the taste and textures are preserved, with none of the health destruction and weight gain. After dinner, save leftovers for meat loaf sandwiches served on Basic Bread (page 225).

2 tablespoons olive or coconut oil	2 large eggs
1 small onion, finely chopped	½ cup tomato juice
1 carrot, finely chopped	2 tablespoons chopped parsley
1 rib celery, finely chopped	1 teaspoon sea salt
2 cloves garlic, minced	½ teaspoon ground black pepper
2 pounds ground beef	4 strips bacon, cut in half
¼ cup ground flaxseeds	

Preheat the oven to 350°F. Lightly oil a rimmed baking sheet.

In a large skillet over medium heat, heat the oil. Cook the onion, carrot, celery, and garlic, stirring occasionally, for 5 minutes, or until tender. Transfer to a large bowl and let cool to room temperature.

Add the beef, flaxseeds, eggs, tomato juice, parsley, salt, and pepper to the bowl. Mix thoroughly.

With your hands, transfer the mixture to the baking sheet and shape into a log about 9" × 5". Lay the bacon strips lengthwise over the top and sides. Press to adhere. Bake for 1 hour 15 minutes, or until a thermometer inserted in the center registers 160°F and the meat is no longer pink. Let rest for 10 minutes before slicing.

PER SERVING: 416 calories, 24 g protein, 4 g carbohydrates, 34 g total fat, 11 g saturated fat, 2 g fiber, 536 mg sodium

SPAGHETTI BOLOGNESE

PREP TIME: 25 MINUTES | TOTAL TIME: 1 HOUR 35 MINUTES

Makes 4 servings

Good old-fashioned spaghetti fits nicely into our wheat-free lifestyle when we use shirataki noodles. Remember the sleepiness and fogginess that usually occur after a plate of wheat flour–based spaghetti? Well, that's all gone when you replace pasta with shirataki, a virtual zero-carbohydrate substitute.

If you prefer meatballs, don't add the meat to the mixture. Instead, add ¼ cup ground golden flaxseeds, ¼ cup grated Parmesan cheese, and 1 egg to the meat, mix well, and form into balls. Cook in 1 to 2 tablespoons olive or coconut oil in a skillet over medium heat until cooked through.

2 tablespoons extra-virgin olive oil	1 cup crushed tomatoes
1 rib celery, finely chopped	1 cup beef broth
1 small carrot, finely chopped	2 tablespoons tomato paste
1 small onion, finely chopped	1 teaspoon dried oregano
2 cloves garlic, minced	2 tablespoons chopped basil or parsley (optional)
½ pound ground beef chuck	
¼ pound ground pork	3 packages (7 or 8 ounces each) shirataki spaghetti, rinsed and drained
¼ pound ground veal or turkey breast	
¾ cup dry red wine or beef broth	

In a saucepan over medium-low heat, heat the oil. Cook the celery, carrot, onion, and garlic for 6 minutes, or until the celery and onion are soft. Add the beef, pork, and veal or turkey. Increase the heat to medium-high and cook, stirring to break up the meat, for 5 minutes, or until the meat is no longer pink. Add the wine or broth and reduce the heat to medium. Simmer for 15 minutes.

Stir in the tomatoes, 1 cup broth, tomato paste, and oregano. Partially cover and cook for 40 minutes, or until thick. Sprinkle with the basil or parsley, if using.

Meanwhile, bring a large pot of water to a boil. Add the spaghetti and cook according to package directions. Toss with the sauce.

PER SERVING: 351 calories, 25 g protein, 16 g carbohydrates, 18 g total fat, 5 g saturated fat, 6 g fiber, 240 mg sodium

TACO PIE

PREP TIME: 10 MINUTES | TOTAL TIME: 55 MINUTES

Makes 6 servings

Here's a Mexican-style dish that, minus the wheat and cornmeal, becomes healthy. There's no cornmeal or taco in this Taco Pie—just don't tell that to the kids!

Serve this Taco Pie with salsa or pico de gallo and some sour cream.

1 tablespoon olive or coconut oil	2 tablespoons ground golden flaxseeds
1 onion, chopped	2 pickled jalapeño chile peppers, minced
1 green bell pepper, chopped	
1 pound ground beef sirloin	1½ cups shredded sharp Cheddar cheese, divided
1½ teaspoons ground cumin	
½ teaspoon sea salt	1 recipe prepared Wheat Belly Tortillas (page 227)
1 tomato, chopped	
⅓ cup chopped fresh cilantro	

Preheat the oven to 350°F. Coat a 9" deep-dish pie pan with cooking spray. Line the pie pan with 2 tortillas.

In a skillet over medium heat, heat the oil. Cook the onion and bell pepper for 2 to 3 minutes, or until golden. Crumble the beef into the pan. Add the cumin and salt. Cook, stirring occasionally, for 5 minutes, or until the beef is no longer pink. Turn off the heat. Stir in the tomato, cilantro, flaxseeds, and chile peppers. Place in the pie pan. Sprinkle with ½ cup of the cheese.

Top with the remaining 2 tortillas. Sprinkle with the remaining 1 cup cheese.

Bake for 30 minutes, or until the crust is golden. Let stand for 5 minutes before cutting into wedges.

PER SERVING: 402 calories, 29 g protein, 12 g carbohydrates, 27 g total fat, 9 g saturated fat, 8 g fiber, 585 mg sodium

BALSAMIC GLAZED PORK TENDERLOIN

PREP TIME: 5 MINUTES | TOTAL TIME: 50 MINUTES

Makes 4 servings

Tenderloin yields small medallions from the tenderest part of the pig, livened up in this recipe with a balsamic vinegar and Dijon mustard glaze.

I like serving this pork tenderloin alongside a green salad topped with slices of roasted or grilled portobello mushrooms.

1 pound pork tenderloin	2 tablespoons coconut oil, extra-virgin olive oil, or butter
1 teaspoon ground cardamom	¼ cup beef broth
½ teaspoon ground black pepper	1 tablespoon balsamic vinegar
¼ teaspoon sea salt	2 tablespoons Dijon mustard

Preheat the oven to 350°F.

On a work surface, rub the tenderloin evenly with the cardamom, pepper, and salt. In a heatproof baking pan or ovenproof skillet over medium-high heat, heat the oil. Cook the tenderloin, turning occasionally, for 8 minutes, or until browned on all sides.

Place in the oven. Roast for 20 minutes, or until a thermometer inserted in the center registers 160°F and the juices run clear. Remove from the oven and transfer the pork to a cutting board. Let stand for 10 minutes.

Place the skillet over medium-high heat. Add the broth and vinegar. Bring to a boil, stirring to remove any browned bits. Cook until the mixture is reduced by about half. Whisk in the mustard. Slice the pork and drizzle with the sauce.

PER SERVING: 239 calories, 24 g protein, 3 g carbohydrates, 14 g total fat, 8 g saturated fat, 0 g fiber, 423 mg sodium

PECAN-BREADED PORK CHOPS

PREP TIME: 10 MINUTES I TOTAL TIME: 25 MINUTES

Makes 4 servings

Ground pecans replace wheat flour in this old favorite you likely had many times growing up. For Italian flavor, add 1 teaspoon dried oregano, 1 teaspoon dried basil, and 1 tablespoon grated Parmesan cheese to the flaxseed mixture and serve with tomato sauce.

2 tablespoons ground golden flaxseeds

½ teaspoon sea salt

½ teaspoon smoked paprika

1 large egg

1 teaspoon gluten-free soy sauce

½ cup ground pecans

4 boneless pork loin chops, ¾" thick

2 tablespoons olive or coconut oil

On a plate, combine the flaxseeds, salt, and paprika. In a wide shallow bowl, whisk the egg and soy sauce. Place the pecans on a plate.

Dip each chop into the flax mixture, then in the egg mixture, and then into the pecans to coat.

In a large skillet over medium-high heat, heat the oil. Cook the pork chops for 8 minutes, turning once, or until a thermometer inserted sideways in a chop registers 160°F and the juices run clear.

PER SERVING: 452 calories, 22 g protein, 3 g carbohydrates, 40 g total fat, 10 g saturated fat, 2 g fiber, 454 mg sodium

SLOW-COOKER COQ AU VIN

PREP TIME: 10 MINUTES | TOTAL TIME: 5 HOURS 10 MINUTES

Makes 6 servings

The use of a slow cooker for this surprisingly simple coq au vin eliminates several steps: no more need for reductions of this or that. Just pop the ingredients in the slow cooker and you're off!

The combination of Provençal herbs and red wine makes this traditional French dish a perennial winner. While coq au vin is traditionally made with French Burgundy wine, any dry red wine will do, such as a Chianti, Zinfandel, or Pinot Noir.

½ cup tomato paste

2 tablespoons coconut flour

1 cup dry red wine or chicken broth

1½ teaspoons herbes de Provence

1½ teaspoons sea salt

1½ teaspoons ground black pepper

3 pounds boneless, skinless chicken thighs

½ pound frozen pearl onions, thawed

8 ounces button mushrooms

6 slices bacon, coarsely chopped

2 large cloves garlic, minced

Coat a 5- to 6-quart slow-cooker with cooking spray. In the pot, whisk the tomato paste with the coconut flour until the flour dissolves. Whisk in the wine or broth, herbs, salt, and pepper until smooth. Add the chicken, onions, mushrooms, bacon, and garlic. Stir to coat the chicken with the sauce.

Cover and cook on high for 2½ to 3 hours or on low for 5 to 6 hours.

PER SERVING: 447 calories, 46 g protein, 11 g carbohydrates, 20 g total fat, 6 g saturated fat, 3 g fiber, 661 mg sodium

BRUSCHETTA CHICKEN OVER ANGEL HAIR PASTA

PREP TIME: 10 MINUTES | TOTAL TIME: 1 HOUR 25 MINUTES

Makes 4 servings

The tomatoes, basil, and garlic of the bruschetta make this chicken a flavorful dish appropriate for just about any occasion. Choose vine-ripened red tomatoes, ideally heirloom varieties such as Beefsteak or Gardener's Delight.

We use the angel hair variety of shirataki noodles in place of wheat flour–based noodles.

1 pound boneless, skinless chicken breast

¼ cup balsamic vinegar

6 ripe tomatoes, chopped

½ cup fresh basil, thinly sliced, + extra basil for garnish

2 tablespoons extra-virgin olive oil

2 cloves garlic, minced

½ teaspoon sea salt

3 packages (7 or 8 ounces each) angel hair shirataki, rinsed and drained

¼ cup shaved Parmesan cheese

In a resealable plastic storage bag, combine the chicken and vinegar. Knead to coat the chicken thoroughly. Refrigerate for 1 hour.

Meanwhile, in a large bowl, combine the tomatoes, basil, oil, garlic, and salt. Cover and let stand at room temperature for 1 hour.

Bring a large pot of water to a boil over high heat. Coat a grill rack or broiler rack with cooking spray. Preheat the grill or broiler. Grill or broil the chicken for 7 minutes, turning once, or until a thermometer inserted in the thickest portion registers 165°F and the juices run clear. Remove and let stand for 5 minutes.

Cook the angel hair in the boiling water for 1 minute, or until heated through. Drain and pat dry. Divide among 4 plates. Cut the chicken diagonally into thin slices. Place atop the angel hair. Top with the tomato mixture and the cheese.

PER SERVING: 190 calories, 15 g protein, 16 g carbohydrates, 10 g total fat, 2 g saturated fat, 8 g fiber, 407 mg sodium

CREAMY PARMESAN CHICKEN

PREP TIME: 10 MINUTES | TOTAL TIME: 40 MINUTES

Makes 4 servings

This chicken oozes with creamy cheese, made even creamier with the use of coconut milk.

This basic recipe can be jazzed up a bit by adding some chopped sun-dried tomatoes or chopped fresh parsley. Serve it alongside freshly sliced tomatoes, steamed broccoli, or wild rice.

4 **boneless, skinless chicken breast halves**

6 **scallions, white and light green parts, thinly sliced**

1 **can (13.6 ounces) coconut milk**

1 **cup shredded Gouda, Swiss, or Colby cheese**

½ **cup grated Parmesan cheese, divided**

Preheat the oven to 375°F. Coat a 9" × 9" baking dish with cooking spray. Place the chicken in the dish. Sprinkle with the scallions.

In a medium bowl, combine the coconut milk, Gouda, Swiss, or Colby, and ¼ cup of the Parmesan. Pour over the chicken mixture. Sprinkle with the remaining ¼ cup Parmesan.

Bake for 30 minutes, or until bubbling and a thermometer inserted in the thickest portion registers 165°F and the juices run clear. Let stand for 5 minutes before serving.

PER SERVING: 476 calories, 38 g protein, 5 g carbohydrates, 34 g total fat, 26 g saturated fat, 2 g fiber, 538 mg sodium

CHICKEN NUGGETS

PREP TIME: 10 MINUTES | TOTAL TIME: 30 MINUTES

Makes 4 servings

Nothing fried here, Mom! And no wacky artificial, don't-know-what-that-is ingredients, either. Likewise, the chicken in these chicken nuggets is as good as the chicken you choose.

1 pound boneless, skinless chicken breasts	½ cup grated Parmesan cheese
2 eggs	½ teaspoon onion powder
2 tablespoons butter, melted	¼ teaspoon garlic powder
½ cup ground golden flaxseeds	¼ teaspoon sea salt
	¼ teaspoon ground black pepper

Preheat the oven to 375°F. Line a rimmed baking sheet with parchment paper. Slice the chicken into 1½ to 2" pieces.

In a small bowl, whisk the eggs and butter.

In a shallow bowl, combine the flaxseeds, cheese, onion powder, garlic powder, salt, and pepper.

Coat each piece of chicken in the egg mixture and then roll in the flaxseed mixture. Place on the baking pan.

Bake for 20 minutes, turning once, or until no longer pink and the juices run clear.

PER SERVING: 274 calories, 22 g protein, 5 g carbohydrates, 19 g total fat, 7 g saturated fat, 4 g fiber, 380 mg sodium

HERBED CHICKEN

PREP TIME: 5 MINUTES | TOTAL TIME: 15 MINUTES

Makes 4 servings

Simple and elegant to serve for dinner, herbed chicken will be as varied as the herbs you choose. In this version, we use thyme, dill, or sage, brightened with lemon peel.

If you'd like, shake some grated Parmesan or Romano cheese over the top just before serving.

1 tablespoon coconut flour	½ cup chicken broth
1 tablespoon chopped fresh thyme, dill, or sage or 1 teaspoon dried	Grated peel of 1 lemon
1 pound chicken cutlets	2 tablespoons chopped fresh parsley
3 tablespoons extra-virgin olive oil	⅛ teaspoon sea salt
	⅛ teaspoon ground black pepper

On a plate or in a shallow bowl, combine the coconut flour and thyme, dill, or sage. Place the chicken slices in the flour mixture to coat.

In a large skillet over medium-high heat, heat the oil until hot. Cook the chicken for 4 minutes, turning once. Remove to a plate.

Add the broth and lemon peel to the pan. Bring to a boil. Add the chicken, parsley, salt, and pepper. Cook for 5 minutes, or until the chicken is no longer pink and the juices run clear.

PER SERVING: 235 calories, 25 g protein, 2 g carbohydrates, 14 g total fat, 2 g saturated fat, 1 g fiber, 289 mg sodium

CHICKEN POT PIE

PREP TIME: 15 MINUTES | TOTAL TIME: 1 HOUR 20 MINUTES

Makes 4 servings

You thought you'd never again eat TV dinners or watch reruns of the *Addams Family*, and you thought you'd never eat chicken pot pie again, didn't you? Well, here you go! Rather than a biscuit crust, we use cauliflower to create a light, creamy topping.

2 pounds cauliflower florets (1 medium head)

½ cup shredded Cheddar cheese

4 tablespoons butter, divided

¾ teaspoon sea salt, divided

2 carrots, thinly sliced

2 cups broccoli florets, cut into small pieces

1 package (10 ounces) sliced mushrooms

12 ounces chicken tenders, cut into cubes

½ cup sour cream

¼ teaspoon ground black pepper

Preheat the oven to 375°F.

Place the cauliflower in a steamer basket set in a pot of boiling water over medium heat. Cover and cook for 15 minutes, or until very tender. Place in a large bowl with the cheese, 2 tablespoons of the butter, and ¼ teaspoon of the salt. Mash until smooth and set aside.

Meanwhile, in a large ovenproof skillet over medium-high heat, heat 1 tablespoon of the butter. Cook the carrots, broccoli, and mushrooms, stirring frequently, for 5 minutes, or until tender-crisp. Remove to a plate and set aside.

Return the skillet to the heat. Add the remaining 1 tablespoon butter. Cook the chicken, stirring, for 5 minutes, or until no longer pink.

Stir in the sour cream, pepper, the remaining ½ teaspoon salt, and the reserved vegetables.

Cover with the mashed cauliflower. Bake for 35 minutes, or until heated through.

PER SERVING: 400 calories, 32 g protein, 21 g carbohydrates, 24 g total fat, 15 g saturated fat, 8 g fiber, 579 mg sodium

INDIAN CHICKEN CURRY

PREP TIME: 10 MINUTES | TOTAL TIME: 30 MINUTES

Makes 6 servings

Indian Chicken Curry fits so easily in our wheat-free lifestyle that I provide a recipe for one version here. In this version, I add cilantro and a bit of white wine for an added dimension to the dominant flavors of curry and paprika.

If you are minding your carbs, serve this dish with finely chopped cauliflower as "rice." If carbs aren't as much of a concern, such as when you're cooking for children or friends, serve the curry with basmati or jasmine rice. A salad of spring greens, sliced red onions, and golden raisins is a nice accompaniment. This chicken curry can also be used as the filling in Flaxseed Wraps (see page 231) with added sliced tomatoes and spinach.

3 tablespoons olive oil	½ teaspoon sea salt
1 medium yellow onion, finely chopped	2 tablespoons tomato paste
2 cloves garlic, minced	½ cup coconut milk
1 pound boneless, skinless chicken breasts, cut into 1" cubes	½ teaspoon ground red pepper
2 tablespoons curry powder	3 tablespoons cilantro, finely chopped
1 teaspoon paprika	¼ cup water
1 teaspoon grated fresh ginger	¼ cup white wine

In a large skillet over medium heat, heat the oil. Cook the onion, garlic, and chicken for 5 minutes, or until the chicken and onion are lightly browned.

Add the curry powder, paprika, ginger, salt, tomato paste, coconut milk, red pepper, cilantro, and water. Reduce the heat to low, cover, and cook, stirring occasionally, for 10 minutes, or until the chicken is cooked through. Add the wine and cook, covered, for 2 to 3 minutes.

PER SERVING: 213 calories, 17 g protein, 5 g carbohydrates, 13 g total fat, 5 g saturated fat, 2 g fiber, 333 mg sodium

ALMOND-CRUSTED CHICKEN

PREP TIME: 10 MINUTES | TOTAL TIME: 30 MINUTES

Makes 4 servings

It's easy to "bread" meats without bread crumbs! This is my favorite method because the combination of ground almonds and ground golden flaxseeds provides a fine breading texture that sticks fairly well to the meat. The same mixture can be used to bread pork chops, beef or turkey burgers, or fish. For variety, add herbs and spices, such as dried basil or rosemary, to your breading. Onion and/or garlic powder can also be added.

2 tablespoons extra-virgin olive oil

1 tablespoon Dijon mustard

¼ teaspoon sea salt

¼ teaspoon ground black pepper

1 cup chopped almonds

½ cup ground golden flaxseeds

2 boneless, skinless chicken breasts

Preheat the oven to 375°F. Coat a baking sheet with cooking spray.

In a shallow bowl, combine the oil, mustard, salt, and pepper. On a plate, combine the almonds and flaxseeds.

Place the chicken breasts between 2 sheets of waxed paper and pound with a meat mallet to ½" thickness. Dip the chicken in the mustard mixture, spreading with a spatula to coat evenly. Dip into the nut mixture, pressing lightly to coat on both sides. Place the chicken on the baking sheet.

Bake for 20 minutes, or until a thermometer inserted in the thickest portion registers 165°F and the juices run clear.

PER SERVING: 354 calories, 22 g protein, 11 g carbohydrates, 27 g total fat, 2 g saturated fat, 8 g fiber, 257 mg sodium

"FRIED" PARMESAN-CRUSTED CHICKEN

PREP TIME: 10 MINUTES | **TOTAL TIME:** 45 MINUTES

Makes 4 servings

Who doesn't love fried chicken? This "fried" chicken is easy to whip up in minutes and will serve you well with the kids.

Make the "breading" as bland or spicy as you or your family desires by reducing or loading up on the oregano and paprika. For added spiciness, add some hot-pepper sauce to the egg mixture or ground red pepper or chipotle pepper to the dry "bread" crumb mixture.

It's best to reheat any leftovers in the oven or toaster oven, rather than the microwave, because the "breading" has a tendency to get soggy when stored.

2 eggs	1 teaspoon dried oregano
2 tablespoons extra-virgin olive oil	¼ teaspoon paprika
1 cup ground flaxseeds	½ teaspoon sea salt
½ cup grated Parmesan cheese	2 pounds chicken drumsticks
1 teaspoon onion powder	

Preheat the oven to 375°F. Coat a large baking pan with cooking spray.

In a shallow bowl, whisk the eggs and oil until blended.

In another shallow bowl, combine the flaxseeds, Parmesan, onion powder, oregano, paprika, and salt and mix thoroughly.

Dip each drumstick into the egg mixture to coat and then roll in the flax mixture, shaking or tapping off any excess. Place in the baking pan, leaving space between each drumstick.

Bake for 35 minutes, or until a thermometer inserted in the thickest portion registers 170°F and the juices run clear.

PER SERVING: 516 calories, 43 g protein, 10 g carbohydrates, 35 g total fat, 7 g saturated fat, 9 g fiber, 610 mg sodium

GRILLED SALMON WITH HORSERADISH SAUCE

PREP TIME: 5 MINUTES | TOTAL TIME: 15 MINUTES

Makes 4 servings

If you love horseradish as much as I do, you'll love this quick and simple salmon recipe. Serve it with a salad or a steamed green vegetable, and you have a perfect heart-healthy meal!

4 salmon fillets (5 ounces each)	1 tablespoon stone-ground mustard
¼ teaspoon sea salt	1 teaspoon grated lemon peel
½ cup mayonnaise	½ teaspoon ground black pepper
1 tablespoon prepared horseradish	

Coat a nonstick grill pan or large nonstick skillet with cooking spray and heat over medium-high heat. Sprinkle the salmon with the salt. Cook the salmon for 8 minutes, turning once, or until lightly browned and just opaque.

Meanwhile, in a medium bowl, whisk the mayonnaise, horseradish, mustard, lemon peel, and pepper until blended.

Top the salmon evenly with the sauce.

PER SERVING: 404 calories, 28 g protein, 1 g carbohydrates, 31 g total fat, 4 g saturated fat, 0 g fiber, 383 mg sodium

COD WITH ROMESCO SAUCE

PREP TIME: 5 MINUTES | TOTAL TIME: 15 MINUTES

Makes 4 servings

Traditional Spanish romesco sauce, rich with the flavors of peppers and tomatoes, livens up cod and other fish.

2 tablespoons olive oil	½ teaspoon sea salt
4 skinless cod fillets (5 ounces each)	¼ teaspoon ground black pepper
2 teaspoons chopped fresh chives	½ cup Romesco Sauce (page 216)

In a large nonstick skillet over medium-high heat, heat the oil. Sprinkle the cod with the chives, salt, and pepper. Cook for 8 minutes, turning once, or until the fish flakes easily. Remove to a plate.

Add the Romesco Sauce to the skillet, reduce the heat to medium, and bring to a boil. Cook, stirring, for 1 minute, or until heated through. Drizzle over the cod.

PER SERVING: 234 calories, 27 g protein, 3 g carbohydrates, 12 g total fat, 2 g saturated fat, 1 g fiber, 359 mg sodium

FETA SPINACH SWORDFISH

PREP TIME: 15 MINUTES I TOTAL TIME: 35 MINUTES

Makes 2 servings

Vegetable meets sheep meets fish in this collision of disparate flavors and textures. The unique saltiness of the feta cheese nicely complements the rich flavor of fresh spinach alongside the neutral and wonderfully nonfishy swordfish.

For variety, try grilling or pan roasting the swordfish. This recipe is also delicious using whitefish, mahi mahi, or salmon in place of the swordfish.

3 tablespoons extra-virgin olive oil

8 ounces button or portobello mushrooms, sliced

2 cloves garlic, minced

⅛ teaspoon sea salt

½ teaspoon ground black pepper

3 cups fresh spinach

1 can (14.5 ounces) diced tomatoes, drained

2 swordfish fillets (5 ounces each)

½ cup feta cheese, crumbled

Preheat the oven to 350°F. Coat a baking pan with cooking spray.

In a large skillet over medium heat, heat the oil. Cook the mushrooms, garlic, salt, and pepper for 5 minutes, or until the mushrooms are softened. Add the spinach and tomatoes and cook, covered, for 10 minutes, stirring occasionally, or until the spinach is wilted and the flavors are blended.

Meanwhile, place the swordfish fillets in the baking pan and bake for 15 minutes. Turn the oven to broil and broil for 5 minutes, or until the fish is just opaque.

Divide the mushroom mixture between 2 plates and sprinkle the feta over the top. Lay the swordfish alongside.

PER SERVING: 515 calories, 38 g protein, 15 g carbohydrates, 35 g total fat, 10 g saturated fat, 3 g fiber, 1,022 mg sodium

FISH AND VEGGIE CHIPS

PREP TIME: 10 MINUTES | TOTAL TIME: 40 MINUTES

Makes 4 servings

The kids will get their fries while also getting some veggies with this fun and easy recipe. We use turnips, an underappreciated but versatile root vegetable, in this recipe to make the fries. If your turnips come with their turnip greens, serve this recipe with the greens sautéed in butter.

3 turnips, peeled and cut into thick sticks

2 tablespoons extra-virgin olive oil

1 teaspoon sea salt, divided

1 teaspoon ground black pepper, divided

1 large egg

1 cup ground golden flaxseeds

1 teaspoon dried thyme

1½ pounds catfish (or other white fish) fillets

1 lemon, cut into wedges

Hot-pepper sauce

Preheat the oven to 425°F. Line a large baking pan with foil. Place the turnip sticks on the pan. Drizzle with the oil and season with ½ teaspoon of the salt and ½ teaspoon of the pepper. Toss to coat evenly and then spread out on the pan. Bake for 15 minutes.

Meanwhile, in a shallow bowl, whisk the egg and the remaining ½ teaspoon salt and ½ teaspoon pepper. On a plate, combine the flaxseeds and thyme. Dip the fish in the egg mixture and then into the flax mixture to coat.

When the fries have baked for 15 minutes, remove the pan and push the fries to one side. Place the fish on the pan. Bake for 12 minutes (with the fries), or until the fish flakes easily. Serve with the lemon wedges and hot-pepper sauce.

PER SERVING: 467 calories, 35 g protein, 16 g carbohydrates, 31 g total fat, 4 g saturated fat, 11 g fiber, 759 mg sodium

FETTUCCINE ALFREDO

PREP TIME: 5 MINUTES   I   **TOTAL TIME:** 15 MINUTES

Makes 4 servings

Remember: Don't be afraid of fat! Cheese, butter, and heavy cream shine in this Fettuccine Alfredo, minus the *truly* unhealthy ingredient, wheat. Surely the kids will eat their broccoli when it's served along with this pasta dish.

3 packages (7 or 8 ounces each) shirataki fettuccine, rinsed and drained

4 tablespoons butter

1 clove garlic, minced

¾ cup heavy cream

¾ cup grated Parmesan cheese

¼ cup grated Pecorino Romano cheese

¼ teaspoon sea salt

¼ teaspoon ground black pepper

   Pinch of ground red pepper

1 tablespoon minced fresh parsley (optional)

Set a large pot of water over high heat.

Cook the fettuccine according to package directions. Drain.

In the same pot over low heat, cook the butter and garlic for 2 minutes, or just until the garlic is fragrant. Add the cream, Parmesan, Pecorino Romano, salt, black pepper, and red pepper. Cook for 2 minutes, or until heated through. Add the fettuccine and toss to coat well.

Sprinkle with the parsley, if using.

PER SERVING: 350 calories, 9 g protein, 8 g carbohydrates, 34 g total fat, 22 g saturated fat, 5 g fiber, 590 mg sodium

EGGPLANT PARMESAN

PREP TIME: 15 MINUTES I TOTAL TIME: 1 HOUR 15 MINUTES

Makes 6 servings

The trick to making Eggplant Parmesan without frying, using eggplant coated with wheat-free "bread crumbs," is to bake the eggplant separately coated in the bread-crumb equivalent until it is nearly done and *then* add the tomato sauce and other ingredients. This keeps the "breading" from getting soggy and shapeless.

2 large eggs

1 cup ground golden flaxseeds

½ teaspoon ground black pepper

2 medium eggplants, peeled and cut into ¼" slices (2 pounds)

2 tablespoons extra-virgin olive oil

3 cans (8 ounces each) tomato sauce

½ cup refrigerated basil pesto

1 cup shredded provolone cheese

½ cup grated Parmesan cheese

Preheat the oven to 400°F. Coat 2 large baking sheets with cooking spray. Grease a 9" × 9" baking dish.

Beat the eggs in a shallow dish. On a plate, combine the flaxseeds and pepper. Dip the eggplant slices into the egg and then into the flaxseed mixture, pressing to coat. Shake off any excess.

Arrange the eggplant slices on the baking sheets. Drizzle with the oil. Bake for 40 minutes, or until golden and tender, turning once and reversing the pans from the top to the bottom oven rack.

Meanwhile, in a medium bowl, combine the tomato sauce and pesto. Spread ¼ cup of the sauce on the bottom of the baking dish. Arrange half of the eggplant slices on top. Spoon on half of the remaining sauce and sprinkle with half of the provolone and Parmesan. Top with the remaining eggplant slices. Spoon on the remaining sauce and sprinkle with the remaining provolone and Parmesan.

Bake for 20 minutes, or until heated through and the cheese is golden.

PER SERVING: 408 calories, 19 g protein, 24 g carbohydrates, 29 g total fat, 7 g saturated fat, 13 g fiber, 1,066 mg sodium

NO-MACARONI 'N CHEESE

PREP TIME: 20 MINUTES | TOTAL TIME: 1 HOUR

Makes 6 servings

This recipe transforms the incredibly unhealthy stuff that comes out of a box into a dish that is healthy and has the same irresistible salty, cheesy taste that everyone loves.

5 tablespoons butter, divided

1 small onion, minced

1 clove garlic, minced

2 tablespoons coconut flour

1 can (13.6 ounces) coconut milk

½ teaspoon dry mustard

¼ teaspoon sea salt

2 cups shredded extra-sharp Cheddar cheese

1 large head cauliflower, broken into florets and cut into bite-size pieces

¼ cup grated Parmesan cheese

2 tablespoons ground golden flaxseeds

Preheat the oven to 350°F. Grease a 2-quart baking dish.

In a medium saucepan over medium-high heat, melt 3 tablespoons butter. Cook the onion, stirring, for 5 minutes, or until lightly browned. Add the garlic and cook for 1 minute. Stir in the coconut flour and cook, stirring constantly, for 3 minutes or until lightly browned. Stir in the coconut milk, mustard, and salt. Bring to a boil, stirring constantly. Remove from the heat and stir in the Cheddar and cauliflower until blended. Pour into the baking dish.

In a small bowl, combine the Parmesan, flaxseeds, and the remaining 2 tablespoons butter. Sprinkle over the casserole. Bake for 30 minutes, or until bubbling and lightly browned.

PER SERVING: 323 calories, 11 g protein, 11 g carbohydrates, 27 g total fat, 20 g saturated fat, 4 g fiber, 409 mg sodium

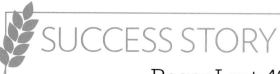

SUCCESS STORY

Roger Lost 40 Pounds

When I looked in the mirror, I hardly recognized the face that looked back at me. I was only 49, but my hair was graying, my skin was wrinkling and losing its healthy glow, and store clerks were asking me for my senior citizen discount card. I couldn't concentrate, and I had a hard time following conversations or even finding my way on familiar roads. Even my prescription glasses were failing me—reading became more and more difficult, and I had to drop out of my doctoral program.

I was 230 pounds and more than 50 inches in my midsection, and I was hungry almost all the time. Something had to change.

That happened on March 1, 2012, when I started to read *Wheat Belly.* A few weeks after I embarked on this new road, my life took a turn for the better. My hair began to grow in darker, and those wrinkles and dark circles around my eyes disappeared. It was amazing how many ways my life changed when I stopped eating wheat—I had no idea about the pancreatic hell I was causing my body by consuming all that man-made garbage. My anxiety while driving? Gone. Eyesight? Better, even without glasses. The constant ringing in my ears? Completely quiet! Aches and pains in my joints? They've almost entirely stopped. Even the itching and flaking of my skin have improved.

Best of all, I've finally experienced relief from the constant bowel problems that plagued me since my early teens and the anxiety and depression that made it almost impossible to think, read, and reason, let alone hold a job. Since losing the wheat, my depression has lifted.

The loss of wheat has been a wonderful gain in my life, as I begin to see my body as something to live in rather than a house of pain. As I lose weight, I'm losing inches around my middle, too, and I'm optimistic that I'll reach my 200-pound goal and stay there for good.

SIDE DISHES

BROCCOLI WITH CHEESE SAUCE

PREP TIME: 10 MINUTES | **TOTAL TIME:** 10 MINUTES

Makes 4 servings

Remember: We're no longer terrified of the fat content of cheese in this new Wheat Belly lifestyle. So have that rich, creamy cheese sauce on top of your broccoli or other vegetables without a moment of guilt or regret! For variety, replace the broccoli with other vegetables such as asparagus, Brussels sprouts, or green beans. Or vary the cheese, replacing the Cheddar with Swiss or Gruyère, for instance.

1 large bunch broccoli, cut into florets

1 tablespoon butter

1 teaspoon coconut flour

1¼ cups milk

½ teaspoon ground mustard

1½ cups shredded sharp Cheddar cheese

Place a steamer basket in a large pot with 2" of water. Bring to a boil over high heat. Place the broccoli in the basket and steam for 5 minutes, or until tender-crisp.

Meanwhile, in a small saucepan over medium heat, melt the butter. Stir in the coconut flour until smooth. Gradually add the milk and cook, whisking constantly, until the sauce thickens.

Add the mustard and cheese and stir until melted.

Place the broccoli in a serving bowl and top with the cheese sauce.

PER SERVING: 297 calories, 16 g protein, 17 g carbohydrates, 20 g total fat, 12 g saturated fat, 5 g fiber, 373 mg sodium

CAULIFLOWER MUSHROOM DRESSING

PREP TIME: 15 MINUTES | **TOTAL TIME:** 1 HOUR

Makes 8 servings

There's no need to abandon stuffing or dressing at the holidays with this wheat-free alternative! This dressing is heavier than the usual bread-based dressing or stuffing. Because it contains meat, it should not be stuffed into the turkey to cook, as this will not ensure a sufficiently high temperature.

While this dressing works best as a two-step process—stove top to oven—if pressed for time, you could just cook it on the stove top a bit longer.

1 head cauliflower, cut into florets

2 tablespoons olive oil

½ pound loose pork sausage

4 ounces mushrooms, sliced

3 ribs celery, chopped

1 small onion, finely chopped

2 cloves garlic, minced

2 cups shredded mild Cheddar cheese

2 eggs, lightly beaten

1 teaspoon ground sage

1 teaspoon ground thyme

½ teaspoon sea salt

¼ teaspoon ground black pepper

2 tablespoons ground golden flaxseeds

Preheat the oven to 350°F. Grease a 2½-quart baking dish.

Place a steamer basket in a large pot with 2" of water. Bring to a boil over high heat. Add the cauliflower to the basket and steam for 5 minutes, or until tender-crisp.

Meanwhile, in a large skillet over medium heat, heat the oil. Cook the sausage, mushrooms, celery, onion, and garlic for 10 minutes, stirring, or until the sausage is cooked and the vegetables are softened. Remove from the heat. Stir in the cauliflower, cheese, eggs, thyme, salt, and black pepper.

Place in the baking dish and sprinkle with flaxseeds. Bake for 20 minutes, or until heated through and the cheese is melted.

PER SERVING: 271 calories, 14 g protein, 7 g carbohydrates, 21 g total fat, 9 g saturated fat, 3 g fiber, 550 mg sodium

OLIVE OIL AND BALSAMIC ROASTED VEGETABLES

PREP TIME: 10 MINUTES | TOTAL TIME: 40 MINUTES

Makes 6 servings

This mix of healthy vegetables, fresh basil, garlic, and olive oil can serve as a simple, healthy side dish or even a main course. It also makes a wonderful filling tucked between Basic Focaccia (page 228).

Optionally, consider topping the roasted vegetables with shredded mozzarella cheese or grated Parmesan or Romano cheese during the last few minutes of baking.

1 medium eggplant, cut into ½" cubes (1 pound)

1 green bell pepper, sliced

1 red bell pepper, sliced

1 yellow onion, quartered and sliced

2 cloves garlic, minced

¼ cup fresh basil, chopped

¼ cup extra-virgin olive oil

2 tablespoons balsamic vinegar

Preheat the oven to 350°F.

In a large baking pan, combine the eggplant, green and red bell peppers, onion, garlic, and basil and mix. Drizzle the oil and vinegar over the vegetables. Toss to coat well.

Roast, turning occasionally, for 30 minutes, or until browned.

PER SERVING: 126 calories, 2 g protein, 10 g carbohydrates, 10 g total fat, 1 g saturated fat, 4 g fiber, 5 mg sodium

GREEN BEAN CASSEROLE

PREP TIME: 25 MINUTES | TOTAL TIME: 50 MINUTES

Makes 6 servings

Miss onion rings? In addition to the Wheat Belly Onion Rings recipe, here's another way to revisit these old favorites minus wheat while adding to your daily intake of healthy green vegetables.

Topped with onion rings, this Green Bean Casserole yields a side dish that stands proudly alongside baked fish, poultry, beef, or pork, or it can even serve as a main dish itself. It's also great for leftovers, warmed briefly in the microwave prior to serving.

4 tablespoons butter or coconut oil, divided

1 large yellow onion, cut into rings

¼ cup ground golden flaxseeds

1 yellow onion, chopped

4 ounces button mushrooms, sliced

1 bag (16 ounces) French-cut green beans, thawed

1 cup chicken broth

8 ounces cream cheese, cut into cubes

3 tablespoons grated Parmesan cheese

⅛ teaspoon ground red pepper

Preheat the oven to 350°F. Grease a 1½- to 2-quart shallow baking dish.

In a large skillet over medium-high heat, heat 2 tablespoons of the butter or oil. Add the onion rings and cook, stirring occasionally, for 10 minutes, or until lightly browned.

Place the flaxseeds on a large plate. Add the browned onion rings and toss with the flaxseeds to coat. Set aside.

In the same skillet over medium-high heat, heat the remaining 2 tablespoons butter or oil. Cook the chopped onion and mushrooms for 8 minutes, or until most of the liquid has absorbed. Add the green beans and broth and bring to a simmer. Stir in the cream cheese until melted. Stir in the Parmesan and red pepper. Pour into the baking dish. Arrange the onion rings over the top.

Bake for 25 minutes, or until hot and bubbling.

PER SERVING: 276 calories, 7 g protein, 13 g carbohydrates, 23 g total fat, 13 g saturated fat, 4 g fiber, 315 mg sodium

WHEAT BELLY ONION RINGS

PREP TIME: 10 MINUTES | **TOTAL TIME:** 25 MINUTES

Makes 4 servings

Satisfy the fussiest wheat-eater in your family with these Wheat Belly Onion Rings. Too many people fear that, minus wheat, they will be denied all the indulgent foods that populate the wheat world. Not so. Re-create conventional onion rings using healthy nonwheat ingredients, and you will no longer seem like the food tyrant of the house denying everyone their fun foods.

While great served by themselves as an appetizer or snack, Wheat Belly Onion Rings also serve as a useful side dish with steak, fish, poultry, or pork.

¾ cup coconut flour, divided

½ teaspoon smoked paprika

1 egg

1 tablespoon melted coconut oil or olive oil

1 cup ground golden flaxseeds

½ cup almond meal

2 large sweet onions, cut into ½"-thick slices and separated into rings

Preheat the oven to 450°F. Coat 2 baking sheets with cooking spray.

In a shallow bowl, combine ¼ cup of the coconut flour and the paprika. In another shallow bowl, beat the egg and oil until blended. On a large plate, combine the flaxseeds, the remaining ½ cup coconut flour, and the almond meal.

Dredge the onion rings in the coconut flour–paprika mixture, gently shaking off the excess. Dip in the egg mixture, letting the excess drip off. Dredge in the flaxseed mixture to coat. Place on the baking sheets and lightly coat with cooking spray.

Bake for 12 minutes, turning once, or until lightly browned.

PER SERVING: 400 calories, 15 g protein, 39 g carbohydrates, 24 g total fat, 5 g saturated fat, 21 g fiber, 36 mg sodium

BETTER THAN MASHED POTATOES

PREP TIME: 25 MINUTES | TOTAL TIME: 35 MINUTES

Makes 4 servings

While potatoes, of course, contain none of the Evil Grain, they have problems all their own, including the potential for causing extreme blood sugar rises. Many potatoes sold today are also genetically modified, introducing a whole new level of uncertainty.

So here is how to re-create the taste and feel of mashed potatoes that are every bit as good as—no, better than! —the dish made from potatoes, but with none of the worries.

1 large head cauliflower, cut into florets

2 ounces cream cheese

2 tablespoons butter

¼ teaspoon sea salt

Place a steamer basket in a large pot with 2" of water. Bring to a boil over high heat. Place the cauliflower in the basket and steam for 20 minutes, or until very soft.

Remove from the heat and drain. In a blender or food processor, combine the cauliflower, cream cheese, butter, and salt. Blend or process until smooth.

PER SERVING: 152 calories, 5 g protein, 11 g carbohydrates, 11 g total fat, 7 g saturated fat, 4 g fiber, 297 mg sodium

PISTACHIO QUINOA PILAF

PREP TIME: 15 MINUTES | TOTAL TIME: 25 MINUTES

Makes 8 servings

While I am no friend to carbohydrates or to nonwheat grains in general, an occasional serving of benign grains like quinoa or sorghum can fit into an otherwise wheat-free, healthy diet. The only caveat: Keep your portion sizes modest. This recipe yields 8 servings, each of which contains 15 grams "net" carbohydrate (total carbohydrate minus fiber) from the quinoa, a modest exposure.

Children should not be restricting carbohydrates as much as adults should, so this recipe may be one to serve the kids, too, without limiting portion size.

2 tablespoons butter or coconut oil

1 onion, finely chopped

1 small red bell pepper, finely chopped

1 small clove garlic, minced

1 carrot, shredded

1¼ cups chicken or vegetable broth

1 cup quinoa, rinsed and drained

¼ teaspoon sea salt

½ teaspoon orange peel

¼ cup pistachios, toasted

In a medium saucepan over medium-high heat, melt the butter or oil. Cook the onion and pepper for 5 minutes, or until the onion is lightly browned. Add the garlic and carrot and cook for 1 minute.

Stir in the broth and bring to a boil. Stir in the quinoa, cover, and reduce the heat to low. Simmer for 12 to 15 minutes, or until the broth is absorbed. Remove from the heat and stir in the salt, orange peel, and pistachios.

PER SERVING: 140 calories, 4 g protein, 18 g carbohydrates, 6 g total fat, 2 g saturated fat, 3 g fiber, 255 mg sodium

FAUX RICE

PREP TIME: 10 MINUTES | **TOTAL TIME:** 10 MINUTES

Makes 4 servings

Like potatoes, rice is not a wheat-containing problem food. But rice is not entirely without its own issues, especially the triggering of high blood sugar if consumed in high enough quantities. We can re-create "rice" quite nicely by using cauliflower to produce a ricelike food that does anything rice can do, just minus the carbohydrates.

There are several ways to create the ricelike pieces of cauliflower needed for this dish. One method is to cut the cauliflower into large pieces and shred it on a box grater using the largest holes. Another method is to use a food processor with a shredding disk attachment.

1 head cauliflower, broken into large pieces

1 tablespoon butter

¼ teaspoon sea salt

Using a food processor with a shredding disk attachment or the largest holes of a box grater, shred the cauliflower.

Place the shredded cauliflower in a microwaveable bowl. Cover and microwave on high power for 3 minutes, stirring once, or until desired doneness.

Toss with the butter and salt.

PER SERVING: 62 calories, 3 g protein, 7 g carbohydrates, 3 g total fat, 2 g saturated fat, 3 g fiber, 212 mg sodium

FRIED "RICE"

PREP TIME: 25 MINUTES | **TOTAL TIME:** 35 MINUTES

Makes 4 servings

If you'd like some fried rice along with your shirataki noodles, stir-fry, or other Asian dish, give this Fried "Rice" a try. Made with cauliflower but without, of course, any nasty wheat or carbohydrate-rich rice, it yields none of the unhealthy effects of the real thing.

For variety, add finely chopped and sautéed pork, chicken, turkey, or beef; cubed tofu (non-GMO); or sliced shiitake mushrooms.

1 small head cauliflower, cut into large pieces	4 scallions, sliced
1 egg	2 carrots, shredded
1 tablespoon water	2 cloves garlic, minced
2 tablespoons coconut oil or olive oil	1 tablespoon shredded fresh ginger
½ cup chicken, beef, or vegetable broth	1½ teaspoons tamari or gluten-free soy sauce
	1 teaspoon dark sesame oil

Using a food processor with a shredding disk attachment or the largest holes of a box grater, shred the cauliflower. Set aside.

In a small bowl, beat the egg and water with a fork until smooth. Set aside.

In a large skillet over medium-high heat, heat the oil. Cook the cauliflower, stirring, for 5 minutes, or until lightly browned. Add the broth and bring to a simmer. Cover and cook for 5 minutes, or until tender. Add the scallions, carrots, garlic, and ginger and cook, stirring, for 4 minutes, or until lightly browned. Stir in the tamari or soy sauce and the sesame oil. Push the mixture to the outside of the skillet.

Pour the egg mixture into the center of the skillet and cook, stirring, for 2 minutes, or until cooked through. Stir into the "rice" mixture.

PER SERVING: 131 calories, 4 g protein, 9 g carbohydrates, 10 g total fat, 7 g saturated fat, 3 g fiber, 259 mg sodium

CREAMED SPINACH

PREP TIME: 15 MINUTES I **TOTAL TIME:** 15 MINUTES

Makes 4 servings

There never was anything wheat in creamed spinach, but it wonderfully accompanies so many of the main dishes in the *Wheat Belly Cookbook* that I thought I had to include it!

2 tablespoons coconut oil or butter	10 ounces baby spinach
1 onion, finely chopped	3 ounces cream cheese
1 red bell pepper, finely chopped	½ cup shredded Swiss cheese, cut into small cubes
1 clove garlic, minced	⅛ teaspoon ground nutmeg
½ cup chicken broth	

In a skillet over medium heat, melt the oil or butter. Cook the onion and pepper, stirring often, for 5 minutes, or until tender. Add the garlic and cook, stirring, for 2 minutes, or until lightly browned.

Stir in the broth and spinach and cook, stirring often, for 4 minutes, or until wilted. Stir in the cream cheese, Swiss cheese, and nutmeg. Stir until the cheeses are melted and well blended.

PER SERVING: 235 calories, 7 g protein, 14 g carbohydrates, 18 g total fat, 12 g saturated fat, 4 g fiber, 280 mg sodium

SPAGHETTI SQUASH
WITH BROWN BUTTER AND SAGE

PREP TIME: 1 HOUR I TOTAL TIME: 1 HOUR 5 MINUTES

Makes 4 servings

This interesting spaghetti squash recipe can be used as a delicious side dish alongside turkey at a holiday dinner, or as a unique accompaniment to beef, chicken, or pork along with a steamed green vegetable.

Other ways to use spaghetti squash include using it as a replacement for pasta in any pasta recipe; combining it with a generous dollop of basil pesto and a few dashes of grated Romano cheese; or tossing it with extra-virgin olive oil, sun-dried tomatoes, and chopped fresh basil. Also see the recipe for Spaghetti Squash Latkes.

1 medium spaghetti squash
   (about 3 pounds)

4 tablespoons butter

3 tablespoons chopped fresh sage

1 clove garlic, minced

1 tablespoon lemon juice

Preheat the oven to 350°F.

Pierce the squash in several places with a small sharp knife or fork. Place on a baking sheet and roast, turning once, for 1 hour, or until tender.

About 10 minutes before the squash is ready, in a small skillet over medium heat, melt the butter. Continue cooking for 3 minutes, or until the butter begins to brown. (Be sure to keep a close watch over the butter so that it doesn't burn.) Add the sage and garlic and cook for 2 minutes, or just until crisp. Remove the pan from the heat and stir in the lemon juice.

Allow the squash to cool slightly. Cut in half lengthwise and scoop out and discard the seeds. With a fork, scrape the squash strands into a large bowl. Toss with the butter mixture.

PER SERVING: 172 calories, 2 g protein, 17 g carbohydrates, 12 g total fat, 8 g saturated fat, 4 g fiber, 126 mg sodium

SPAGHETTI SQUASH LATKES

PREP TIME: 40 MINUTES | **TOTAL TIME:** 40 MINUTES

Makes 8 servings

No wheat flour or potatoes figure in this reimagined latke recipe. The light flavor of spaghetti squash means these latkes will companionably accompany a wide variety of dishes, from casual foods like bratwurst to more serious main courses like steak or baked salmon.

2   large eggs

4   scallions, sliced

½   teaspoon sea salt

¼   teaspoon ground black pepper

2   tablespoons coconut flour

1   tablespoon ground golden flaxseeds

3   cups cooked spaghetti squash, drained and patted dry

6   tablespoons coconut oil, divided

Preheat the oven to 250°F. Grease a baking sheet.

In a large bowl, whisk together the eggs, scallions, salt, pepper, coconut flour, and flaxseeds. Stir in the squash.

In a large skillet over medium heat, heat 2 tablespoons of the oil. Working in batches, drop the squash mixture by ⅓ cupfuls onto the skillet. Cook for 8 minutes, turning once, or until golden brown. Place on the baking sheet and keep warm in the oven.

Repeat with the remaining squash mixture and oil.

PER SERVING: 139 calories, 3 g protein, 6 g carbohydrates, 12 g total fat, 10 g saturated fat, 2 g fiber, 127 mg sodium

ROMANO TOMATOES

PREP TIME: 10 MINUTES | TOTAL TIME: 25 MINUTES

Makes 4 servings

Here's yet another simple, straightforward recipe that helps you say goodbye to bread crumbs. In these Romano Tomatoes, ground golden flaxseeds substitute for the Evil Grain. I'd be shocked if anyone in the family can tell the difference!

6 plum tomatoes

¼ cup grated Romano cheese

3 tablespoons ground golden flaxseeds

½ teaspoon Italian seasoning

2 tablespoons olive oil

Preheat the oven to 400°F. Cut the tomatoes in half lengthwise. Cut a thin slice off the rounded side of each tomato half and place cut side up in a 13" × 9" baking dish.

In a small bowl, combine the cheese, flaxseeds, seasoning, and oil. Top the tomato halves evenly with the mixture.

Bake for 15 minutes, or until browned and the tomatoes are tender.

PER SERVING: 131 calories, 5 g protein, 5 g carbohydrates, 11 g total fat, 3 g saturated fat, 3 g fiber, 132 mg sodium

ZUCCHINI GRATIN

PREP TIME: 15 MINUTES | TOTAL TIME: 20 MINUTES

Makes 4 servings

Here's a replacement for your potatoes au gratin—no wheat bread crumbs or potatoes in sight! Serve this Zucchini Gratin as an accompaniment to baked chicken, beef, or pork main courses.

2 tablespoons butter or coconut oil

3 medium zucchini, cut into ¼" slices

1 onion, finely chopped

2 cloves garlic, minced

1 tablespoon chopped fresh thyme leaves or 1 teaspoon dried

½ cup heavy cream or canned coconut milk

1 tablespoon coconut flour

¼ teaspoon sea salt

½ cup shredded Romano cheese, divided

½ cup ground golden flaxseeds

Preheat the oven to 450°F. Grease a 2-quart baking dish.

In a large skillet over medium heat, melt the butter or oil. Cook the zucchini, onion, garlic, and thyme, stirring, for 5 minutes, or until tender-crisp.

Add the cream or coconut milk, coconut flour, and salt and cook for 5 minutes, or until thickened. Stir in ¼ cup of the cheese.

Place in the baking dish and sprinkle with the flaxseeds and the remaining ¼ cup cheese. Bake for 10 minutes, or until golden brown.

PER SERVING: 320 calories, 11 g protein, 15 g carbohydrates, 26 g total fat, 13 g saturated fat, 7 g fiber, 463 mg sodium

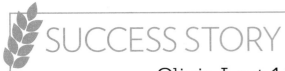

SUCCESS STORY

Olivia Lost 14 Pounds

Tucked away in my medicine chest above the bathroom sink, I kept a multitude of prescriptions: hydrochlorothiazide for high blood pressure, amoxicillin for acne, lorazepam for anxiety, albuterol for asthma, Effexor for depression. I had a host of allergies, irritable bowel syndrome, diarrhea, abdominal cramps, gas and bloating, swollen calves, heart palpitations, joint pain—you name it. I was only 41 but felt like 90.

That was 3 months ago. Today my medicine cabinet is empty, and I feel like a whole different person—all because of *Wheat Belly.*

When a friend told me about this book, I went straight to Amazon and clicked the "buy" button. Then I filled my pantry with gluten-free snacks and got started on my new life. It was pretty smooth sailing—I experienced some mild headaches the first few days, but by the time my first full week was over, I felt so different that I began to cry. They were tears of joy for how well I was feeling, mixed with a little sadness for all the years I'd felt so sick.

With my joint pain gone, I started exercising right away—I dropped about 5 pounds almost immediately, and the swelling in my legs disappeared. After 6 weeks I gave up my afternoon nap, and by week 9 my energy level exploded.

Now, after 3 months, I've lost 14 pounds. I'm no longer bloated, fatigued, or anxious—I can work, run errands, and shuttle the kids all day long, and everything seems so effortless. When I see cakes, rolls, and bread, most of the time they look no different to me than something inedible, like paper—no cravings! I feel too good now to ruin my health by eating wheat again.

Those gluten-free goodies I stashed before I went wheat free? Twelve weeks later, they're still in my pantry, unopened. I'd rather have other snacks, like no-bake cookies or a few squares of dark chocolate.

I had a dozen health issues that I never realized could be connected, and my doctors couldn't help me at all. But *Wheat Belly* totally changed my life.

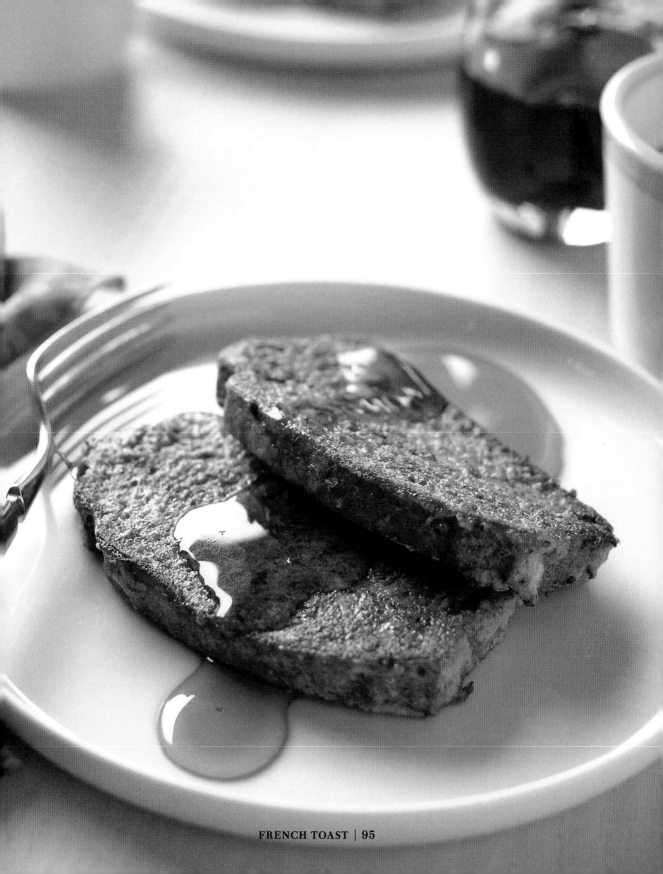

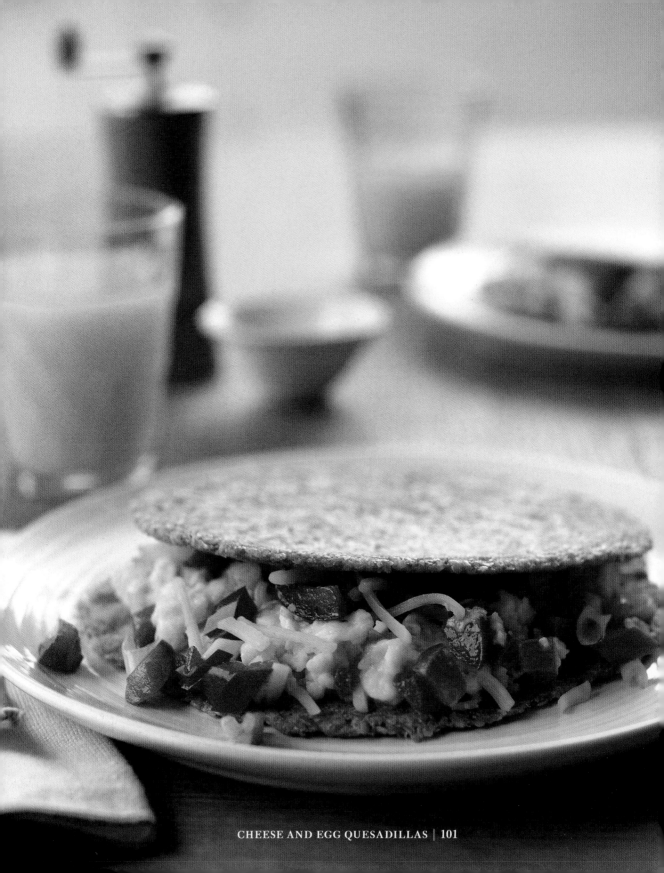

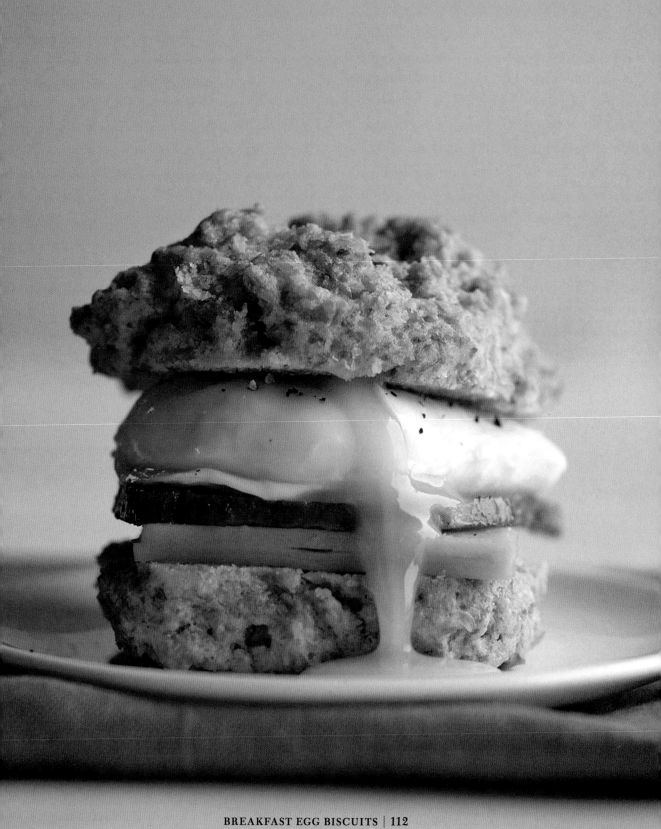

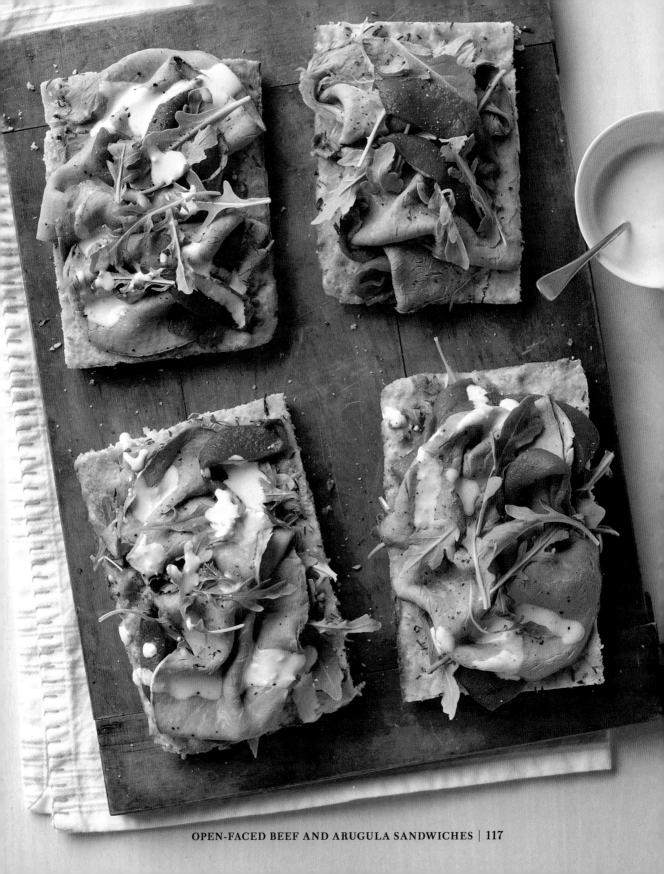

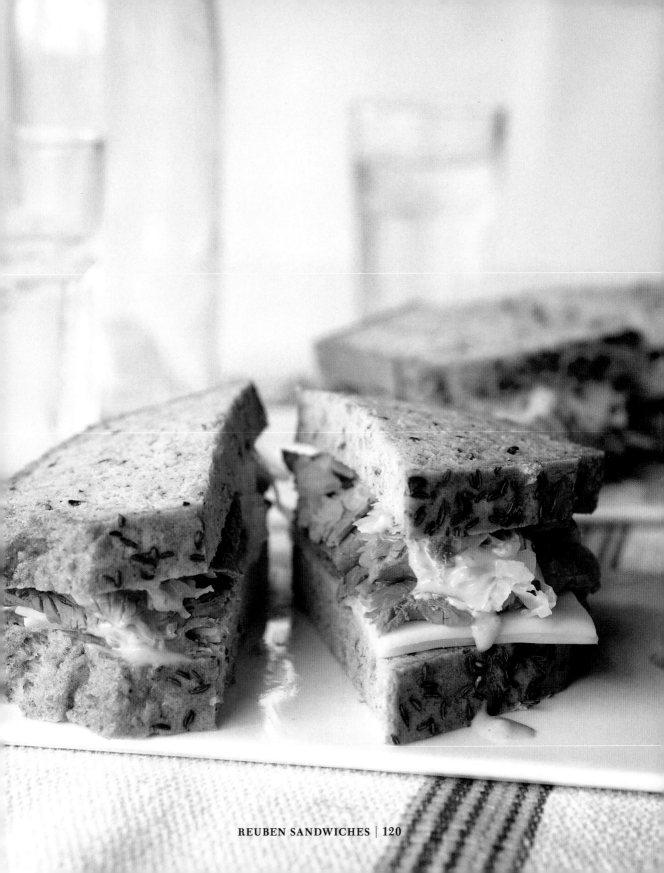

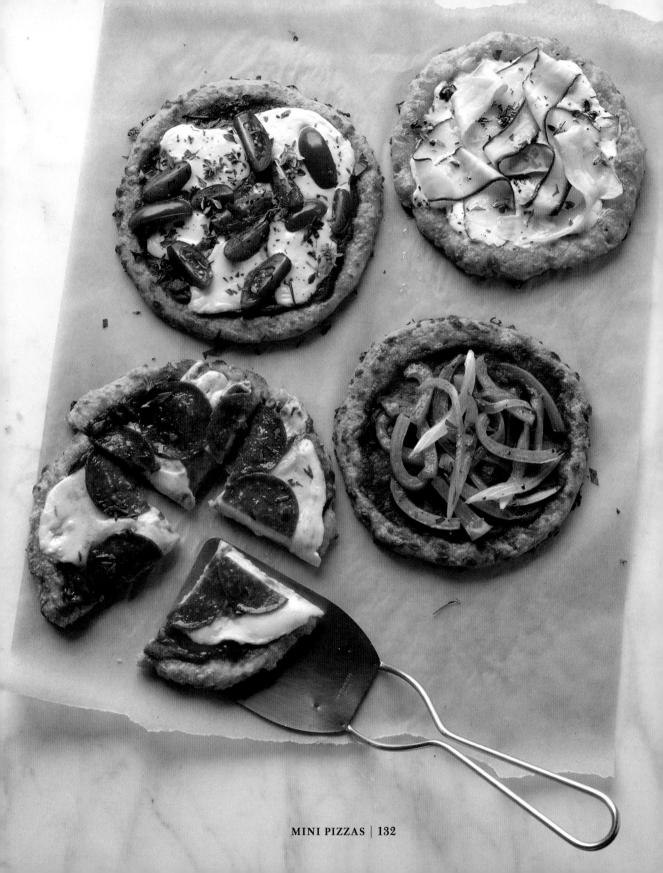

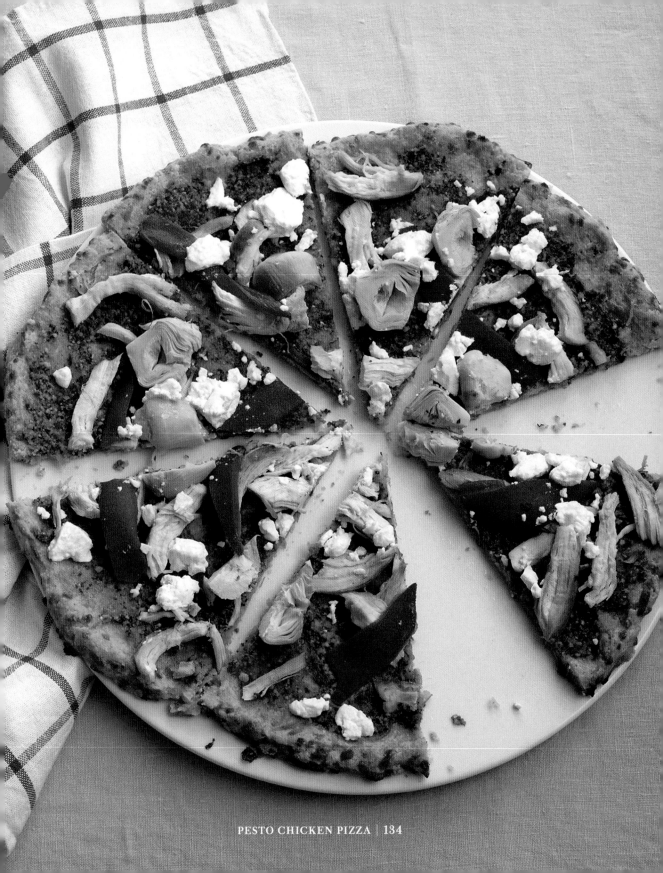

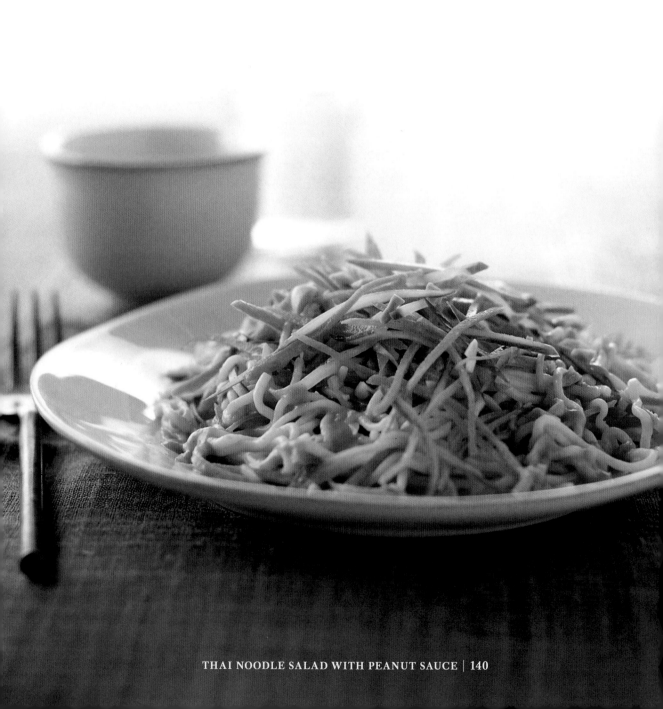

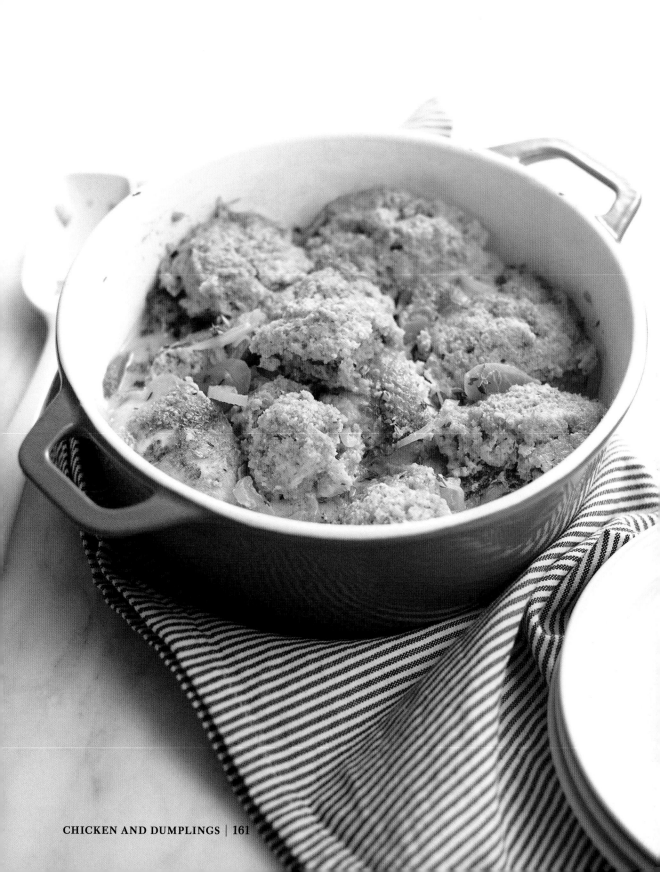

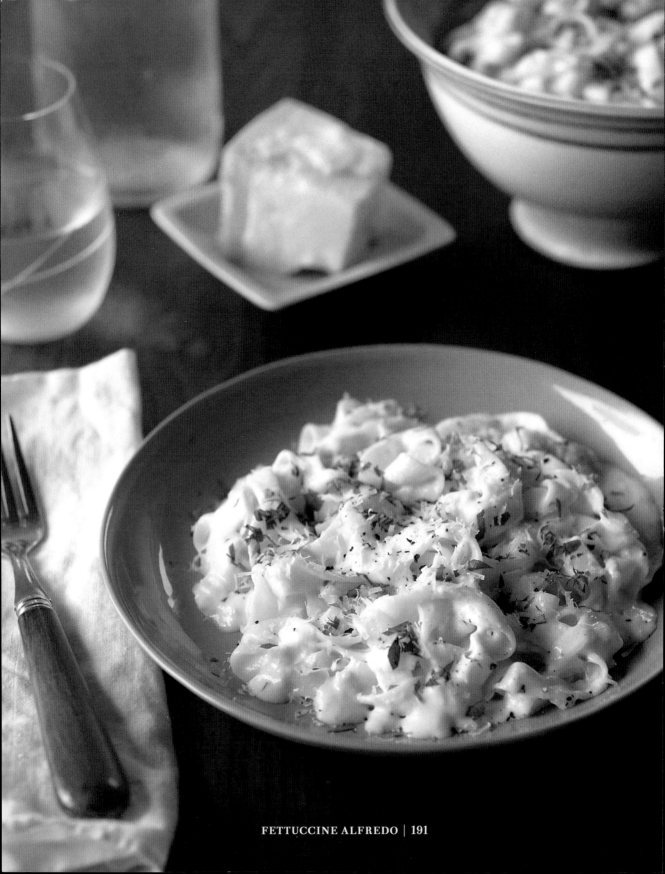

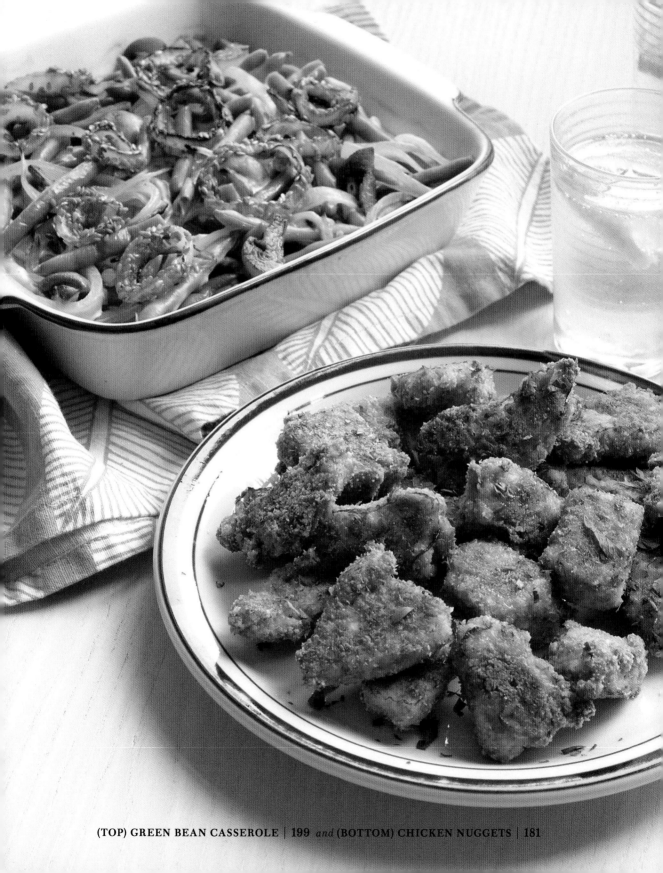

(TOP) GREEN BEAN CASSEROLE | 199 *and* (BOTTOM) CHICKEN NUGGETS | 181

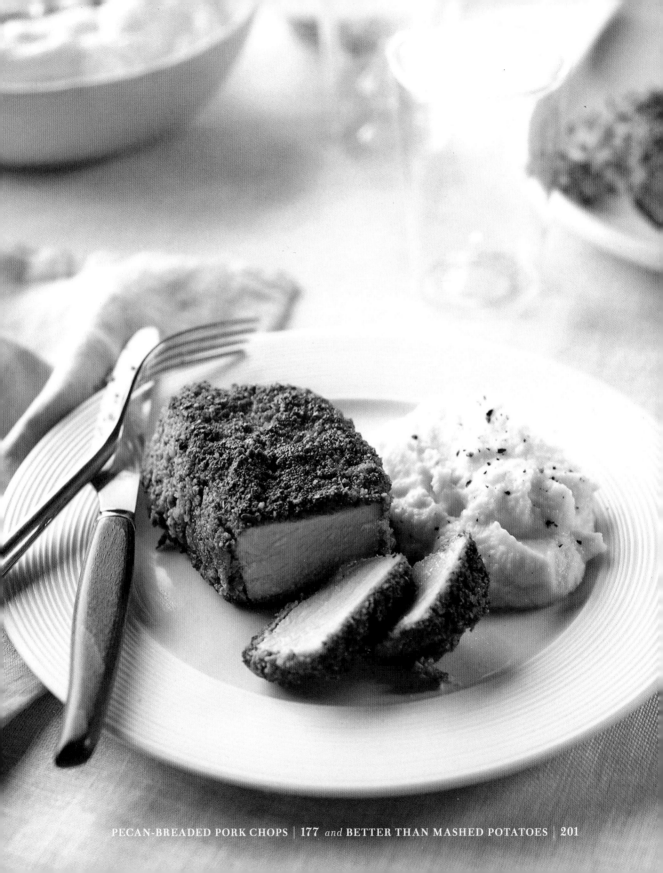

PECAN-BREADED PORK CHOPS | 177 *and* BETTER THAN MASHED POTATOES | 201

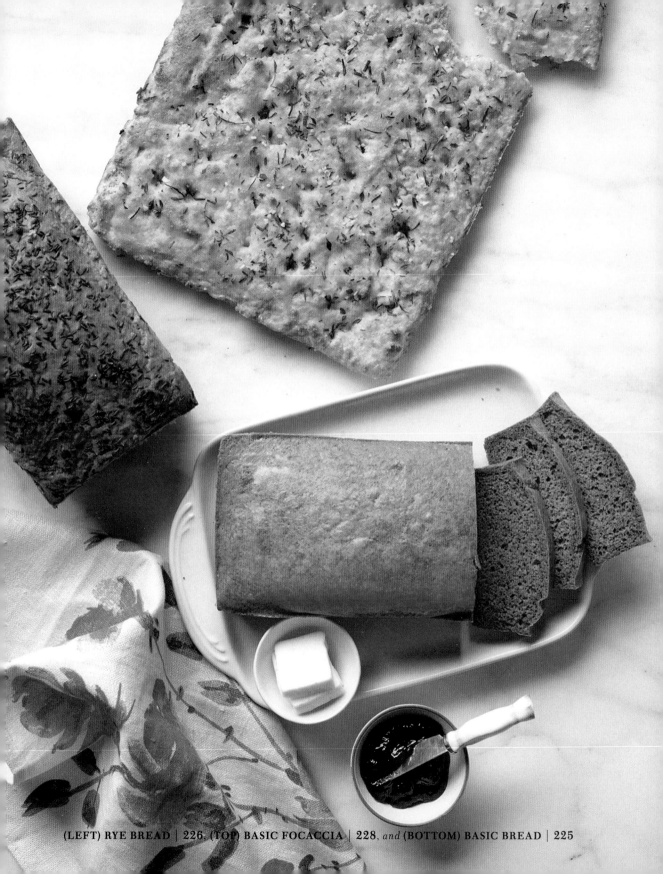

(LEFT) RYE BREAD | 226. (TOP) BASIC FOCACCIA | 228, *and* (BOTTOM) BASIC BREAD | 225

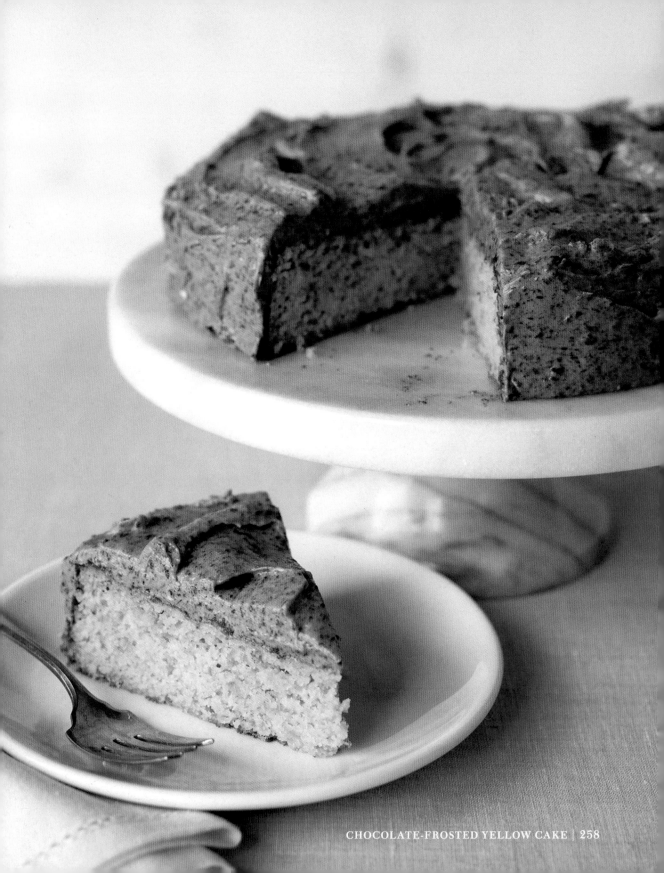

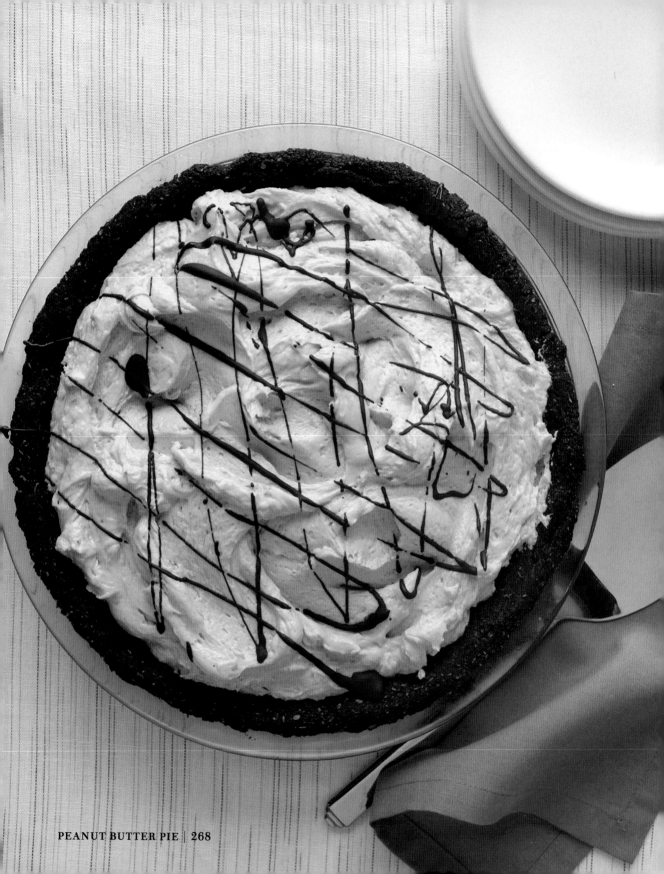

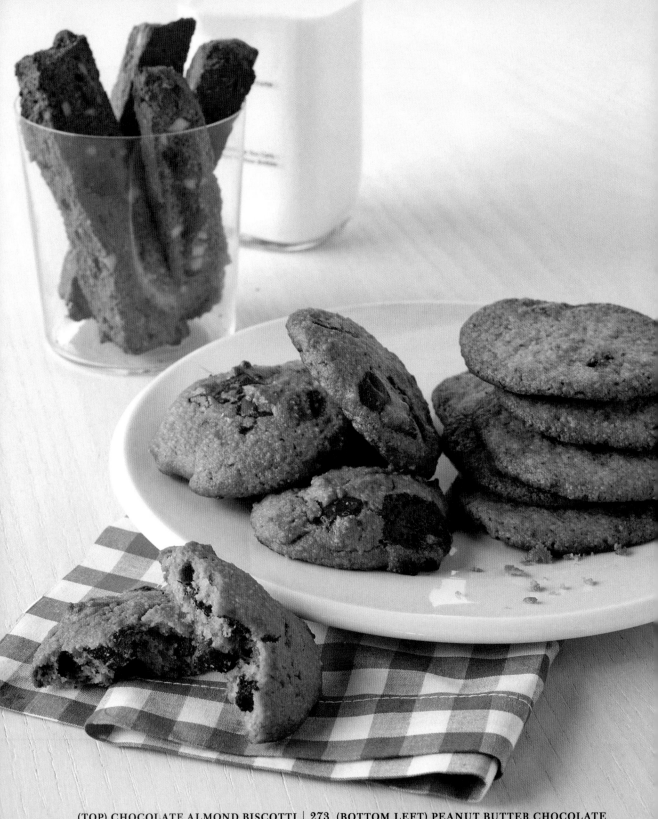

(TOP) CHOCOLATE ALMOND BISCOTTI | 273, (BOTTOM LEFT) PEANUT BUTTER CHOCOLATE
CHIP COOKIES | 277, *and* (BOTTOM RIGHT) CHOCOLATE CHIP COOKIES | 276

SAUCES AND SALAD DRESSINGS

WHITE SAUCE

PREP TIME: 10 MINUTES | TOTAL TIME: 10 MINUTES

Makes 16 servings (2 cups)

Béchamel, or white sauce, provides the basic starting sauce for many variations, including classic Cheddar cheese sauce, mustard sauce, Parmesan sauce, and even a mushroom sauce. Though white sauce is traditionally thickened with wheat flour, coconut flour is substituted in this version, a problem-free method that yields a delicious and versatile starting sauce.

The sauce can be used as is, poured over vegetables, chicken, or a meat- and vegetable-filled flaxseed wrap. Several variations are listed below.

2 tablespoons butter

1 small yellow onion, finely chopped

1 tablespoon coconut flour

2 cups whole milk

In a medium saucepan over medium heat, melt the butter. Cook the onion, stirring, for 5 minutes, or until golden brown. Stir in the coconut flour and cook, stirring constantly, for 1 minute. Slowly whisk in the milk and cook for 3 minutes, whisking constantly, or until thickened.

PER SERVING (2 TABLESPOONS): 35 calories, 1 g protein, 2 g carbohydrates, 2 g total fat, 2 g saturated fat, 0 g fiber, 24 mg sodium

VARIATIONS

Classic Cheese Sauce: Stir 3 cups shredded Cheddar cheese or a mix of your favorite cheeses into the finished sauce.

Mushroom Sauce: Cook 8 ounces mixed mushrooms and 1 teaspoon fresh thyme in 2 tablespoons butter for 6 minutes, or until the mushrooms release their juices and their liquid evaporates. Stir into the finished sauce.

Mustard Sauce: Stir 2 teaspoons Dijon mustard into the finished sauce.

WHEAT-FREE TURKEY GRAVY

PREP TIME: 10 MINUTES I TOTAL TIME: 10 MINUTES

Makes 8 servings

Thickness is obtained without wheat, cornstarch, or other carbohydrate-rich thickeners but with use of coconut flour and coconut milk. Many people worry that the use of coconut will allow a coconut flavor to show through. It should not, but if you have an especially sensitive palate and do sense a bit of the coconut, add a bit more onion and/or garlic powders. Other herbs and spices, of course, can be added, such as thyme, rosemary, or sage.

Because the quantity of drippings obtained will vary widely, depending on the size of your turkey, ingredient quantities are suggested and nutrition information is eliminated from this recipe. Rely on taste as you prepare your gravy to gauge ingredient quantity.

The same method can be applied to other meats besides turkey, provided you have sufficient drippings. At least 1 cup of drippings is generally required.

2¼ **cups turkey drippings**

1–3 **tablespoons coconut flour**

¼–½ **cup coconut milk**

½ **teaspoon onion powder**

¼ **teaspoon garlic powder**

½ **teaspoon sea salt**

In the roasting pan or a saucepan over low heat, heat the drippings. Meanwhile, in a small measuring cup or bowl, whisk together the flour and water. Pour in the coconut milk slowly, stirring, until the desired color is achieved. Slowly whisk the mixture into the drippings, and cook for 3 minutes, or until thickened.

Stir in the onion powder, garlic powder, and sea salt.

PER SERVING: 87 calories, 3 g protein, 2 g carbohydrates, 7 g total fat, 2 g saturated fat, 0 g fiber, 166 mg sodium

ASIAN DIPPING SAUCE

PREP TIME: 10 MINUTES | **TOTAL TIME:** 10 MINUTES

Makes 8 servings (1 cup)

This sauce is perfect for dipping cold vegetables or drizzling over steamed vegetables and Faux Rice (page 203). I love thinly slicing a fresh cucumber, bruising the slices with a flat object, such as a heavy spoon or a potato masher, and then soaking the cucumbers in the sauce for an hour in the refrigerator prior to serving.

The combined flavors of soy sauce, sesame, and ginger also provide an excellent marinade for chicken, pork, beef, or fish. Marinate for a minimum of 30 minutes, preferably 2 hours, prior to roasting or grilling.

½ cup gluten-free soy sauce

¼ cup water

2 tablespoons seasoned rice vinegar

2 tablespoons sesame oil

1 teaspoon grated fresh ginger

1 tablespoon xylitol or 2 drops liquid stevia or to desired sweetness

¼ teaspoon crushed red-pepper flakes (optional)

In a small bowl, whisk together the soy sauce, water, vinegar, oil, ginger, xylitol or stevia, and pepper flakes (if using).

PER SERVING (2 TABLESPOONS): 48 calories, 2 g protein, 3 g carbohydrates, 3 g total fat, 0 g saturated fat, 0 g fiber, 1,091 mg sodium

KANSAS CITY–STYLE BARBECUE SAUCE

PREP TIME: 5 MINUTES I TOTAL TIME: 25 MINUTES + COOLING TIME

Makes 32 servings (4 cups)

Who doesn't love the flavor of barbecue sauce brushed on ribs or used to slow-marinate pork chops? But what if you don't want a load of sugar, high-fructose corn syrup, and wheat flour or cornstarch with your sauce? Here is your solution.

This sauce is a variation on the popular Kansas City–style barbecue sauce based on a sweet mix of the flavors of tomato, vinegar, and spices. In addition to the traditional application to grilled meats, you can use this sauce in your Flaxseed Wraps (page 231) or quesadillas, as pizza sauce, as a dip for Chicken Nuggets (page 181), or on top of Meat Loaf (page 173).

2 cups sugar-free ketchup, or 1 can (6 ounces) tomato paste and 1 can (8 ounces) tomato sauce

1 cup apple cider vinegar

½ cup xylitol or ¼ teaspoon liquid stevia or to desired sweetness

¼ cup chili powder

2 tablespoons smoked paprika

2 tablespoons lemon juice

2 tablespoons gluten-free Worcestershire sauce

2 teaspoons garlic powder

2 teaspoons onion powder

In a heavy saucepan, combine the ketchup, vinegar, xylitol or stevia, chili powder, paprika, lemon juice, Worcestershire, garlic powder, and onion powder. Bring to a slow boil. Cook, stirring occasionally, for 20 minutes, or until thickened. Remove from the heat and cool completely.

Store in an air-tight container in the refrigerator for up to 2 weeks.

PER SERVING (2 TABLESPOONS): 19 calories, 0 g protein, 6 g carbohydrates, 0 g total fat, 0 g saturated fat, 0 g fiber, 71 mg sodium

ROMESCO SAUCE

PREP TIME: 10 MINUTES | TOTAL TIME: 15 MINUTES

Makes 16 servings (2 cups)

This traditional Spanish sauce, rich with the flavors of fire-roasted tomatoes and olive oil, is a perfect topping for fish, such as in Cod with Romesco Sauce (page 188).

Use the highest-quality olive oil for the best flavor.

2 tablespoons extra-virgin olive oil, divided

¾ cup slivered almonds

4 cloves garlic, coarsely chopped

¼ teaspoon red-pepper flakes

1 can (14.5 ounces) diced fire-roasted tomatoes

¼ cup chopped pimientos, drained

2 tablespoons ground golden flaxseeds

2 tablespoons red wine vinegar

½ teaspoon sea salt

In a small skillet over medium-high heat, heat 1 tablespoon of the oil. Cook the almonds, garlic, and pepper flakes, stirring, for 3 minutes, or until the almonds are lightly toasted. Transfer the almond mixture to a food processor along with the tomatoes, pimientos, flaxseeds, vinegar, salt, and the remaining 1 tablespoon oil. Process until well combined and smooth.

Store in an airtight container in the refrigerator for up to 2 weeks or in the freezer for up to 3 months.

PER SERVING (2 TABLESPOONS): 57 calories, 2 g protein, 3 g carbohydrates, 5 g total fat, 0.5 g saturated fat, 1 g fiber, 98 mg sodium

HOISIN SAUCE

PREP TIME: 5 MINUTES | **TOTAL TIME:** 5 MINUTES

Makes 8 servings (½ cup)

Traditional Chinese hoisin sauce is often made with wheat flour or other starch and is therefore off the Wheat Belly list of healthy foods. However, this tasty sauce, especially useful for topping Asian dishes, can be easily re-created without wheat.

In addition to its use as a topping for Asian dishes, try this Hoisin Sauce as a marinade for pork or beef, a unique sauce for barbecued ribs, or the sauce base for a stir-fry.

2 tablespoons gluten-free soy sauce

2 tablespoons fermented black bean paste or peanut butter

2 tablespoons tomato paste

2 tablespoons xylitol or 4 drops liquid stevia or to desired sweetness

1 tablespoon lemon juice

1 tablespoon sesame oil

½ teaspoon sriracha (Chinese hot sauce) or other hot sauce

¼ teaspoon garlic powder

¼ teaspoon onion powder

¼ teaspoon ground black pepper

In a medium bowl, whisk together the soy sauce, bean paste or peanut butter, tomato paste, xylitol or stevia, lemon juice, oil, sriracha, garlic powder, onion powder, and pepper. Store in an air-tight container in the refrigerator for up to 2 weeks.

PER SERVING (1 TABLESPOON): 34 calories, 1 g protein, 5 g carbohydrates, 2 g total fat, 0 g saturated fat, 0 g fiber, 332 mg sodium

THAI PEANUT SAUCE

PREP TIME: 10 MINUTES | TOTAL TIME: 10 MINUTES

Makes 8 servings (1 cup)

This delicious creamy, peanutty Thai sauce is perfect for dipping chicken satay or grilled shrimp or for tossing with shirataki noodles. Consider using it as the sauce on your next Flaxseed Wrap (page 231).

Optionally, top this sauce with chopped fresh cilantro.

½ cup natural peanut butter

¼ cup chicken broth

¼ cup canned coconut milk

3 tablespoons xylitol or 3 drops liquid stevia or to desired sweetness

2 tablespoons rice wine vinegar

1 tablespoon gluten-free soy sauce

1 tablespoon grated fresh ginger

In a small saucepan over medium heat, combine the peanut butter, broth, coconut milk, xylitol or stevia, vinegar, soy sauce, and ginger. Cook, stirring often, for 3 minutes, or until very smooth and thickened.

Store in an air-tight container in the refrigerator for up to 2 weeks, reheating as necessary.

PER SERVING (2 TABLESPOONS): 128 calories, 4 g protein, 9 g carbohydrates, 10 g total fat, 2 g saturated fat, 1 g fiber, 212 mg sodium

WASABI CREAM SAUCE

PREP TIME: 5 MINUTES | TOTAL TIME: 5 MINUTES

Makes 8 servings (1 cup)

If your life needs some excitement, try some wasabi!

Ideally, this sauce is prepared just before serving, as the wasabi tends to lose its characteristic horseradishy zing over time when mixed into the sauce. If leftover sauce is stored and loses its wasabi flavor, stir in some additional wasabi before serving.

This versatile sauce serves as an interesting spread for sandwiches, a dip for raw vegetables, or a salad dressing. It's also delicious brushed onto seafood before putting in the oven.

1	cup sour cream or mayonnaise	1	teaspoon grated fresh ginger
2	teaspoons wasabi powder	1	tablespoon chopped chives
2	teaspoons rice vinegar		Pinch of sea salt

In a medium bowl, stir together the sour cream or mayonnaise, wasabi powder, vinegar, ginger, chives, and salt until well blended.

Store in an air-tight container in the refrigerator for up to 1 week.

PER SERVING (2 TABLESPOONS): 48 calories, 1 g protein, 1 g carbohydrates, 5 g total fat, 3 g saturated fat, 0 g fiber, 56 mg sodium

RANCH DRESSING

PREP TIME: 5 MINUTES I TOTAL TIME: 5 MINUTES

Makes 16 servings (2 cups)

This Ranch Dressing recipe was included among the recipes in the first *Wheat Belly* book. Despite its simplicity, it proved so popular that I reproduce it here.

In addition to topping salads, this version of Ranch Dressing, enlivened with the tangy combination of vinegar and Parmesan cheese, is also great as a sauce on a Flaxseed Wrap (page 231) or a dip for raw veggies.

1 cup sour cream

½ cup mayonnaise

1 tablespoon distilled white vinegar

1 tablespoon water

½ cup grated Parmesan cheese

1 teaspoon garlic powder or finely minced garlic

1½ teaspoons onion powder

Pinch of sea salt

In a medium bowl, stir together the sour cream, mayonnaise, vinegar, and water. Stir in the Parmesan, garlic powder or garlic, onion powder, and salt. If desired, stir in 1 to 2 tablespoons additional water for a thinner consistency.

Store in an air-tight container in the refrigerator for up to 1 week.

PER SERVING (2 TABLESPOONS): 53 calories, 1 g protein, 2 g carbohydrates, 5 g total fat, 2 g saturated fat, 0 g fiber, 104 mg sodium

THOUSAND ISLAND DRESSING

PREP TIME: 5 MINUTES | TOTAL TIME: 5 MINUTES

Makes 16 servings (2 cups)

An old favorite, Thousand Island Dressing, as served in restaurants and even in fast-food outlets, is typically made with sugar and a variety of thickeners. But it is very easy to whip up on your own minus the unhealthy ingredients simply by using some common ones most people already keep around the house. If you lack the pickle relish, replace it with 1 table-spoon of finely chopped onion or whatever pickles you have on hand.

For added richness and thickness, a whole hard-cooked egg can be finely chopped and blended into the sauce.

Use this Thousand Island Dressing as the sauce in a Reuben Sandwich (page 120) or Flaxseed Wrap (page 231), or as a dip for raw veggies.

½ cup sour cream

½ cup mayonnaise

¼ cup sugar-free ketchup

1 tablespoon sugar-free pickle relish

½ teaspoon paprika

1 teaspoon lemon juice

In a medium bowl, stir together the sour cream, mayonnaise, ketchup, relish, paprika, and lemon juice.

Store in an air-tight container in the refrigerator for up to 1 week.

PER SERVING (2 TABLESPOONS): 63 calories, 0 g protein, 1 g carbohydrates, 7 g total fat, 2 g saturated fat, 0 g fiber, 65 mg sodium

CREAMY PESTO DRESSING

PREP TIME: 5 MINUTES | **TOTAL TIME:** 5 MINUTES

Makes 8 servings (1 cup)

Basil and Romano cheese are a heavenly combination in this Creamy Pesto Dressing. This dressing makes a great spread for sandwiches, as well as a dressing for green salads. Optionally, add a clove of minced garlic.

Turn this into blue cheese dressing by substituting crumbled blue cheese for the pesto.

¼ cup sour cream

¼ cup buttermilk

¼ cup basil pesto

2 tablespoons grated Romano cheese

1 teaspoon onion powder

½ teaspoon sea salt

In a medium bowl, stir together the sour cream, buttermilk, pesto, Romano, onion powder, and salt.

Store in an air-tight container in the refrigerator for up to 1 week.

PER SERVING (2 TABLESPOONS): 61 calories, 2 g protein, 2 g carbohydrates, 5 g total fat, 2 g saturated fat, 0 g fiber, 255 mg sodium

SUCCESS STORY
Maggie B. Lost 60 Pounds

In high school, my world was a magical place. If my hometown were a kingdom, I'd have been one of the glittering princesses. Dressed to the nines in evening gowns, hair coifed and makeup perfect, I competed in beauty pageants and even—well into my twenties—worked as a model. Beauty isn't everything—I think I knew that even back then—but it sure was nice seeing heads turn whenever I walked into a room.

But over the years, I turned in my tiaras for a sedentary job as a computer tech, and little by little that princess disappeared. Sitting in front of a computer all day—plus dealing with hormone problems and an addiction to carbs—I gained more than 100 pounds and weighed in at 235 by the time I turned 48. I had constant sacroiliac and sciatic nerve pain, terrible acid reflux, high blood pressure, and debilitating menopause symptoms. I was even on my way to full-blown diabetes.

In August 2011, I started reading *Wheat Belly,* and everything fell into place. Eliminating wheat products was easy. Less than a week later, my energy soared, my joints became more flexible, my skin rashes disappeared, and my tummy troubles subsided. After 3 more weeks, I lost 18 pounds. But the biggest surprise was losing fat in my belly, upper thighs, and even my back and arms!

Since May 2011, I've lost 60 pounds and regained my life. My acid reflux is completely gone, my skin is glowing, and my hair is long and silky again. The rosacea on my face, neck, and chest disappeared, and so have my allergies, menopause symptoms, and digestive problems. My joints don't hurt nearly as much, and I actually crave exercise now—there isn't a cookie, candy bar, or potato chip out there that feels as good as the pleasure I get from my workouts!

Best of all: I'm healthier than ever, and I can wear pretty clothes again. I'm wearing shorts for the first time in 20 years! I have a newfound confidence and enjoyment of life, something I haven't felt since my twenties. It feels great to turn heads again! I still have some weight to lose, but I'm excited about the new me and my new future. Bring it on!

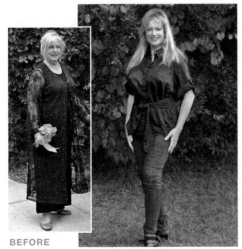

BEFORE

AFTER

THE WHEAT BELLY BAKERY

BASIC BREAD

PREP TIME: 15 MINUTES | TOTAL TIME: 1 HOUR 5 MINUTES

Makes 10 slices

This Basic Bread recipe is your starting place for many variations. As is, this bread can be toasted, can accompany dinner, or can be eaten simply spread with cream cheese, almond or peanut butter, or butter. If used for sandwiches, it may not hold up well with ingredients containing lots of moisture, so add ingredients like tomatoes just before consuming.

Easy variations include adding more cinnamon, another 3 tablespoons xylitol, and ½ to ¾ cup raisins for cinnamon raisin bread; adding garlic powder to the flour and grated Parmesan or Romano cheese sprinkled on top for a garlic bread; or adding orange peel, additional cinnamon, ground nutmeg, and cloves for a spicy orange bread.

A sweetener like xylitol is optional, though the xylitol does add a nice browning effect to the surface.

1¼ cups blanched almond flour

¼ cup + 2 tablespoons garbanzo bean (chickpea) flour

¼ cup ground golden flaxseeds

1½ teaspoons baking soda

1 teaspoon cinnamon (optional)

¼ teaspoon sea salt

5 eggs, separated

¼ cup butter, melted

1 tablespoon buttermilk

1 tablespoon xylitol or 4 drops liquid stevia or to desired sweetness

Preheat the oven to 350°F. Grease an 8½" × 4½" loaf pan.

In a food processor, combine the almond flour, garbanzo bean flour, flaxseeds, baking soda, cinnamon (if using), and salt. Pulse until well blended. Add the egg yolks, butter, buttermilk, and xylitol or stevia and pulse just until blended.

In a large bowl and using an electric mixer on high, beat the egg whites until soft peaks form. Pour into the flour mixture and pulse until the egg whites are evenly distributed, but do not run the machine at a constant speed. Spread into the pan and bake for 40 minutes, or until a wooden pick inserted in the center comes out clean.

Cool in the pan for 10 minutes. Remove and cool completely on a rack.

PER SLICE: 158 calories, 7 g protein, 7 g carbohydrates, 12 g total fat, 2 g saturated fat, 3 g fiber, 299 mg sodium

RYE BREAD

PREP TIME: 15 MINUTES | TOTAL TIME: 1 HOUR 15 MINUTES

Makes 14 slices (½" thick)

This recipe makes an incredible loaf of bread, rich with the unique flavor of caraway seeds. Use it as you would any other rye bread—for a ham and Swiss cheese sandwich, corned beef sandwich, or rye toast spread with butter.

If you're in the mood for the hearty richness of a pumpernickel rye, add 2½ teaspoons instant coffee granules and 2½ tablespoons unsweetened cocoa powder to the dry ingredients.

2½ cups almond meal/flour	1 tablespoon whole caraway seeds, divided
½ cup garbanzo bean (chickpea) flour	10 eggs, separated
½ cup ground golden flaxseeds	½ cup butter, melted
1 tablespoon baking soda	¼ cup buttermilk
½ teaspoon fine sea salt	1 tablespoon xylitol or 4 drops liquid stevia or to desired sweetness
1 tablespoon caraway seeds, finely ground in a spice grinder or coffee mill	

Preheat the oven to 350°F. Grease an 8½" × 4½" loaf pan.

In a food processor, combine the almond meal/flour, garbanzo bean flour, flaxseeds, baking soda, salt, and ground caraway seeds. Pulse on low speed until well mixed. Add 2 teaspoons of the whole caraway seeds, the egg yolks, butter, buttermilk, and xylitol or stevia and pulse just until blended.

In a large bowl and using an electric mixer on high, beat the egg whites until soft peaks form. Pour into the flour mixture and pulse just until the egg whites are evenly distributed, but do not run the food processor at a constant speed. Spread into the pan and sprinkle with the remaining 1 teaspoon caraway seeds. Bake for 50 to 60 minutes, or until a wooden pick inserted in the center comes out clean.

Cool in the pan on a rack for 10 minutes. Remove and cool completely on the rack.

PER SLICE: 233 calories, 11 g protein, 9 g carbohydrates, 19 g total fat, 4 g saturated fat, 4 g fiber, 412 mg sodium

WHEAT BELLY TORTILLAS

PREP TIME: 5 MINUTES   I   **TOTAL TIME:** 10 MINUTES

Makes 4 tortillas

These simple tortillas provide the starting place for endless variations: Mexican tortillas filled with sautéed poblano chile peppers and bell peppers, Cheddar cheese, sour cream, and salsa; Asian wraps with chicken, scallions, shredded fresh ginger, and Hoisin Sauce (page 217) or Asian Dipping Sauce (page 214); and Mediterranean wraps filled with spinach, sliced olives and avocado, and feta cheese, drizzled with olive oil. Unlike the Flaxseed Wraps (page 231) prepared in the microwave, these tortillas are prepared in the oven, 4 at a time.

Tortillas and wraps are, of course, portable and are therefore useful to pack for lunches.

1   cup ground golden flaxseeds

4   tablespoons almond meal/flour

¼   teaspoon sea salt

2   eggs

Preheat the oven to 375°F. Line a large baking sheet with parchment paper.

In a medium bowl, whisk together the flaxseeds, almond meal/flour, and salt. Whisk in the eggs just until combined. Divide the dough into 4 equal balls.

Roll each ball between 2 pieces of parchment paper until 6" round. Place on the baking sheet.

Bake for 5 minutes, or until golden.

PER SERVING: 205 calories, 11 g protein, 10 g carbohydrates, 16 g total fat, 1 g saturated fat, 9 g fiber, 136 mg sodium

BASIC FOCACCIA

PREP TIME: 15 MINUTES | TOTAL TIME: 35 MINUTES

Makes 12 servings

Flat focaccia breads are a natural fit for a wheat-free lifestyle since we don't need the "rise" as much as with loaf-style breads. I love this Basic Focaccia, as well as the Herbed Focaccia (page 230), because they hold up well when stuffed with meats and vegetables, as in the Reuben Sandwich (page 120).

FLAVORED OIL

3 tablespoons olive oil

½ teaspoon fine sea salt

2 large cloves garlic, minced

1–2 tablespoons minced fresh herbs (such as basil or rosemary)

DOUGH

2 cups almond meal/flour

1 cup garbanzo bean (chickpea) flour

½ cup ground golden flaxseeds

2 teaspoons baking powder

½ teaspoon fine sea salt

1 cup buttermilk

1 teaspoon instant (rapid rise) yeast (optional)

4 egg whites

To make the oil: In a small saucepan over low heat, combine the oil, salt, and garlic and simmer for 10 minutes. Remove from the heat. If using a delicate herb, such as basil, add it to the oil after you remove the oil from the heat. If using a hardier herb, such as rosemary, allow it to simmer for the full 10 minutes. Set aside. (Alternatively, you can skip this step and brush the focaccia with plain olive oil, then sprinkle your favorite seasonings on top.)

Preheat the oven to 400°F. Grease a 13" × 9" baking sheet with half of the oil, line it with parchment paper, and then liberally brush the paper with the reserved oil.

To make the dough: In a large bowl, combine the almond meal/flour, garbanzo bean flour, flaxseeds, baking powder, and salt. Stir or whisk to combine and break up the flour.

In a small bowl or glass measure, whisk the buttermilk and yeast, if using, until the yeast dissolves. Set aside. In a separate bowl, whip the egg whites with an electric mixer until stiff peaks form.

Add the yeast mixture to the flour mixture and stir until a rough dough ball forms. Gently fold in the egg whites until they're fairly well incorporated. The dough will not become completely smooth, and the whites will still be somewhat frothy.

Spread the dough in the pan with a spatula or spoon. Lightly coat your fingertips with cooking spray or dip them into the reserved oil and dimple the top of the dough. Pour the remaining oil mixture over the top of the dough, making sure it is entirely covered. (Oil will pool in the dimples.)

Bake for 20 minutes, or until golden and slightly spongy in the center. With a pizza cutter or knife, cut into the desired size and number of flatbreads. Serve warm.

PER SERVING: 205 calories, 9 g protein, 12 g carbohydrates, 15 g total fat, 1 g saturated fat, 4 g fiber, 275 mg sodium

HERBED FOCACCIA

PREP TIME: 15 MINUTES | TOTAL TIME: 40 MINUTES

Makes 2 servings

Though I use a 13" × 19" baking sheet, you can form this dough into whatever shape suits your needs. I make 2 focaccias, each 3" by 6", to use as the 2 bread slices. However, this recipe yields such an incredibly filling bread that the 2 slices can be halved to yield 2 very satisfying sandwiches to serve 2 people.

¼ cup extra-virgin olive oil, divided

2 cups almond meal/flour

½ cup ground golden flaxseeds

1 teaspoon baking soda

1 teaspoon baking powder

½ teaspoon sea salt

1½ teaspoons dried rosemary

1½ teaspoons dried oregano

1 teaspoon onion powder

1 teaspoon garlic powder

½ cup black or kalamata olives, roughly chopped

¼ cup sun-dried tomatoes, finely sliced

½ cup milk

2 teaspoons white or apple cider vinegar

3 egg whites

Preheat the oven to 350°F. Grease a 13" × 19" baking sheet. Line the baking sheet with parchment paper, then brush with some of the olive oil.

In a medium bowl, combine the almond meal/flour, flaxseeds, baking soda, baking powder, salt, rosemary, oregano, onion powder, and garlic powder and stir until well blended. Add the olives and tomatoes and mix well. Set aside.

In a small bowl, combine the milk, 2 tablespoons of the oil, and the vinegar.

In a large bowl and using an electric mixer on high, beat the egg whites until stiff.

Stir the milk mixture into the flour mixture until well blended. Mix in the egg whites until evenly distributed.

Spread the dough in the baking sheet. Brush the top with 1 tablespoon of the oil and sprinkle with additional sea salt. Dimple the surface with your fingertips or the handle end of a wooden spoon. Bake for 20 minutes. Brush the remaining oil on top of the focaccia and bake for 5 minutes, or until golden and firm to the touch.

Cool in the pan on a rack for 5 minutes. Remove to a cutting board and cut the desired size with a pizza cutter or knife.

PER SERVING: 188 calories, 7 g protein, 7 g carbohydrates, 16 g total fat, 2 g saturated fat, 4 g fiber, 271 mg sodium

FLAXSEED WRAP

PREP TIME: 5 MINUTES I TOTAL TIME: 15 MINUTES

Makes 1 serving

The Flaxseed Wraps introduced in the first *Wheat Belly* book proved so popular and such a useful staple that the recipe is reproduced here. Preparation requires several minutes, so I like to make several ahead of time and store for use later in the week.

Wraps made with flaxseeds and egg are surprisingly tasty. Once you get the hang of it, you can whip up a wrap or two in just a few minutes. If you have 2 pie pans, you can make 2 wraps at a time and accelerate the process (though they will need to be microwaved one at a time). Flaxseed Wraps can be refrigerated and will keep for a few days. Healthy variations are possible simply by using various vegetable juices (such as spinach or carrot) in place of the water called for.

3 tablespoons ground golden flaxseeds

¼ teaspoon baking powder

¼ teaspoon onion powder

¼ teaspoon paprika

Pinch of fine sea salt or celery salt

1 tablespoon coconut oil, melted, plus more for greasing the pan

1 tablespoon water

1 egg

In a small bowl, mix together the flaxseeds, baking powder, onion powder, paprika, and salt. Stir in the 1 tablespoon coconut oil. Beat in the water and egg until blended.

Grease a microwaveable glass pie pan with coconut oil. Pour in the batter and spread evenly over the bottom. Microwave on high power for 2 to 3 minutes, or until cooked. Let cool for 5 minutes.

To remove, lift up an edge with a spatula. If it sticks, use a pancake turner to gently loosen from the pan. Turn the wrap over and top with desired ingredients.

PER SERVING: 328 calories, 11 g protein, 9 g carbohydrates, 29 g total fat, 14 g saturated fat, 7 g fiber, 413 mg sodium

PIZZA CRUST I

PREP TIME: 15 MINUTES | **TOTAL TIME:** 45 MINUTES

Makes 12 servings

Here's a recipe for pizza crust that you can actually hold in your hands.

That may sound like nothing special, but when we eliminate wheat from our lives, we also eliminate the unique viscoelastic properties of wheat gluten, the quality that provides wheat foods' portability and the unique sturdiness that allows you to stuff a pita full of ingredients or hold a sandwich between your hands. In this recipe, we re-create these properties by using a plentiful quantity of cheese mixed with nonwheat flours. This confers sufficient strength to the dough to allow you to confidently eat a slice of pizza with your hands without a lapful of tomato sauce!

For a classic pizza, remove the baked crust from the oven and layer with pizza sauce, mozzarella cheese, Parmesan cheese, and your favorite toppings. Bake for an additional 10 minutes or until the cheese melts.

1½ cups shredded mozzarella cheese	½ teaspoon garlic powder
1½ cups ground almonds	½ teaspoon sea salt
¼ cup garbanzo bean (chickpea) flour	2 eggs
¼ cup ground golden flaxseeds	¼ cup extra-virgin olive oil
1 teaspoon onion powder	½ cup water

Preheat the oven to 350°F.

In a food processor, pulse the mozzarella until it becomes granular in size.

In a large bowl, combine the mozzarella, almonds, garbanzo bean flour, flaxseeds, onion powder, garlic powder, and salt. Stir in the eggs, oil, and water and mix thoroughly.

Spread a large sheet of parchment paper over a baking sheet. Place the dough on the parchment paper and lay a second sheet of parchment paper on top of the dough. Flatten with a rolling pin into a 14" round.

Carefully remove the top layer of parchment paper. Use a spoon or your hands to form a crust edge. Bake for 20 minutes.

PER SERVING: 185 calories, 9 g protein, 5 g carbohydrates, 16 g total fat, 3 g saturated fat, 2 g fiber, 153 mg sodium

PIZZA CRUST II

PREP TIME: 1 HOUR 15 MINUTES | TOTAL TIME: 1 HOUR 45 MINUTES

Makes 4 servings

Here's an alternative recipe for pizza crust minus the cheese for binding, but with yeast to provide the yeasty flavor some people miss. Without the cheese, this pizza crust may not be as sturdy but can usually still be eaten the old-fashioned way—with your hands rather than a fork.

For a classic pizza, remove the baked crust from the oven and layer with pizza sauce, mozzarella cheese, Parmesan cheese, and your favorite toppings. Bake for an additional 10 minutes or until the cheese melts.

¾ cup water (100–110°F)

1¼ teaspoons active dry yeast

1 cup garbanzo bean (chickpea) flour

1 cup almond meal/flour

½ cup ground golden flaxseeds

1 teaspoon sea salt

2 tablespoons olive oil

In a small bowl or glass measuring cup, whisk the water and yeast until the yeast dissolves. Let stand for 10 minutes.

In a medium bowl, combine the garbanzo bean flour, almond meal/flour, flaxseeds, and salt and mix well. Add the oil and stir. Add the yeast mixture and stir for 5 minutes, or until all the ingredients are evenly distributed and a loose ball of dough forms. Cover the bowl with plastic wrap and let stand for 1 hour.

Preheat the oven to 350°F.

Line a baking sheet with parchment paper. Place the dough on the parchment paper and lay a second sheet of parchment paper on top of the dough. Flatten with a rolling pin into a circle that is about 10" in diameter and ⅜" to ½" thick. Carefully remove the top layer of parchment paper. Use a spoon or your hands to form a crust edge. Alternatively, for a Sicilian-style pie, press the dough, using wet fingertips, into a 12½" × 9½" rimmed baking sheet.

Bake for 20 minutes.

PER SERVING: 377 calories, 15 g protein, 24 g carbohydrates, 27 g total fat, 2 g saturated fat, 10 g fiber, 347 mg sodium

SOFT PRETZELS

PREP TIME: 45 MINUTES | TOTAL TIME: 1 HOUR 10 MINUTES + COOLING TIME

Makes 12 pretzels

Two ingredients—yeast and baking soda—give these pretzels their traditional taste. The only thing that's missing is the stone-ground mustard.

These pretzels are best enjoyed warm from the oven. Alternatively, microwave for 10 seconds prior to serving.

1½ cups water (100–110°F)

1 package (¼ ounce) instant (rapid rise) yeast

2 cups garbanzo bean (chickpea) flour

2 cups almond meal/flour

1 cup ground golden flaxseeds

2 teaspoons kosher salt

4 tablespoons butter, melted

1 egg

1 tablespoon water

½ teaspoon baking soda

Coarse sea salt to taste

In a small bowl or glass measuring cup, whisk the water and yeast until the yeast dissolves. Let stand for 10 minutes.

In a large bowl or in the bowl of a stand mixer fitted with the dough hook, combine the garbanzo bean flour, almond meal/flour, flaxseeds, and kosher salt. Add the butter and stir or mix to combine. Add the yeast mixture and stir for 10 minutes or mix for 5 minutes, or until all the ingredients are evenly distributed and a loose ball of dough forms. If using a stand mixer, be sure to scrape down the sides and along the bottom of the mixing bowl. Cover the bowl with plastic wrap and let stand in a warm place for about 1 hour, or until the dough increases in size (it will not double like traditional gluten-containing dough).

Preheat the oven to 350°F. Set oven racks in the upper third and lower third of the oven. Line 2 baking sheets with parchment paper. In a small bowl, lightly beat the egg, water, and baking soda.

Lightly coat a work surface with oil or cooking spray (and lightly coat your hands, if necessary). Turn out the dough onto the work surface and knead a few times to bring the dough together. Divide into 12 pieces, and roll each piece into a ball. Cover the balls with plastic wrap while forming the pretzels.

Roll each dough ball into a 10" rope and then shape into a traditional pretzel or any shape you like. Transfer to the baking sheets and reshape if necessary. (If the dough cracks or breaks, simply pinch it back together.) Brush the pretzels with the egg wash and sprinkle with the coarse sea salt.

Bake for 25 minutes, or until the pretzels are golden and slightly firm to the touch.

PER SERVING: 265 calories, 11 g protein, 19 g carbohydrates, 18 g total fat, 3 g saturated fat, 8 g fiber, 359 mg sodium

BREADSTICKS

PREP TIME: 45 MINUTES | **TOTAL TIME:** 1 HOUR 10 MINUTES + COOLING TIME

Makes 16

Even though there's no gluten or sugar here, the yeast in this recipe does cause a bit of a rise in this dough. Flavor your breadsticks with seeds and spices, such as poppy seeds, garlic powder, or rosemary, to complement whatever you've having for dinner, such as Fettuccine Alfredo (page 191) or Eggplant Parmesan (page 192).

These breadsticks are best enjoyed warm from the oven. To reheat, microwave for 10 seconds prior to serving.

1½ cups water (100–110°F)	4 tablespoons butter, melted
1 package (¼ ounce) instant (rapid rise) yeast	1 egg
2 cups garbanzo bean (chickpea) flour	1 tablespoon water
2 cups almond meal/flour	Fine sea salt to taste
1 cup ground golden flaxseeds	Assorted seeds and spices (sesame seeds, poppy seeds, fennel seeds, cracked pepper, rosemary, garlic powder, etc.) to taste
2 teaspoons kosher salt	

In a small bowl or glass measuring cup, whisk the water and yeast until the yeast dissolves. Let stand for 10 minutes.

In a large bowl or in the bowl of a stand mixer fitted with the dough hook, combine the garbanzo bean flour, almond meal/flour, flaxseeds, and kosher salt. Add the butter and stir or mix to combine. Add the yeast mixture and stir for 10 minutes or mix with the mixer for 5 minutes, or until all the ingredients are evenly distributed and a loose ball of dough forms. If using a stand mixer, be sure to scrape down the sides and along the bottom of the mixing bowl. Cover the bowl with plastic wrap and let stand in a warm place for 1 hour, or until the dough increases in size (it won't double like traditional gluten-containing dough).

Preheat the oven to 350°F. Line a baking sheet with parchment paper. In a small bowl, lightly beat the egg and water.

Lightly coat a work surface with oil or cooking spray (and lightly coat your hands, if necessary). Turn out the dough onto the work surface and knead a few times to bring the dough together. Divide into 8 pieces, and roll each piece into a ball. Cover the balls with plastic wrap while forming the breadsticks.

Roll each dough ball into a breadstick 6 inches long. If the dough cracks or breaks, simply pinch it back together or reshape the ball tighter and try again. Transfer to the baking sheet. (They can be somewhat close together, though they will puff up slightly.) Brush the breadsticks with the egg wash and sprinkle with the sea salt and any desired seeds and spices.

Bake for 25 minutes, or until the breadsticks are golden and slightly firm to the touch.

PER BREADSTICK: 199 calories, 8 g protein, 14 g carbohydrates, 14 g total fat, 2 g saturated fat, 6 g fiber, 230 mg sodium

CARROT MUFFINS

PREP TIME: 20 MINUTES | TOTAL TIME: 1 HOUR

Makes 12

If you need a secret weapon to persuade that person in your household who doesn't believe that life without wheat is still worth living, then pull out some of these delicious carrot muffins.

While wheat-free, low-carb bread recipes can occasionally be a bit temperamental, muffins tend to be more forgiving due to their smaller size and less variation in internal cooking (a hurdle with wheat-free baking).

The carrots provide beta-carotene, the flaxseeds provide a near-zero carbohydrate source of fiber to keep your family wheat free and regular, the pecans provide crunch, and the spices and orange peel provide the zing. The optional raisins can add carbohydrates, so use them only when a higher-carbohydrate exposure is desired, such as to please kids or a fussy husband.

If no raisins are used, each muffin will yield approximately 4 grams of "net" carbs (total carbohydrates minus fiber), while adding raisins will increase carb exposure to 10 grams per muffin. (Compare this with typical wheat-based muffins that usually provide an incredible 36 to 52 grams of "net" carbohydrates per muffin.)

1½ cups almond meal/flour

1 cup chopped pecans

½ cup ground golden flaxseeds

2 teaspoons ground cinnamon

1½ teaspoons baking powder

1 teaspoon baking soda

1 teaspoon ground nutmeg

½ teaspoon ground cloves

½ teaspoon sea salt

1 cup shredded carrots

2 tablespoons orange peel

½ cup raisins (optional)

2 eggs, separated

½ cup xylitol or ¼ teaspoon liquid stevia or to desired sweetness

½ cup sour cream or coconut milk

¼ cup coconut oil, extra-light olive oil, or butter, melted

½ cup applesauce

¼ teaspoon cream of tartar

Preheat the oven to 350°F. Place paper liners in a 12-cup muffin pan or grease the cups.

In a large bowl, stir together the almond meal/flour, pecans, flaxseeds, cinnamon, baking powder, baking soda, nutmeg, cloves, and salt. Stir in the carrots, orange peel, and raisins (if using).

In a medium bowl, whisk together the egg yolks, xylitol or stevia, sour cream or coconut milk, oil or butter, and applesauce.

In a large bowl, with an electric mixer on high speed, beat the egg whites and cream of tartar until stiff peaks form. Gently fold the beaten whites into the egg yolk mixture until combined. Fold egg mixture into the flour mixture until well combined.

Divide the batter among the muffin cups, filling each about half full. Bake for 40 minutes, or until a wooden pick inserted in the center of a muffin comes out clean. Cool in the pan on a rack for 5 minutes. Remove from the pan and cool completely on the rack.

PER MUFFIN: 248 calories, 6 g protein, 9 g carbohydrates, 22 g total fat, 6 g saturated fat, 5 g fiber, 255 mg sodium

PEANUTS GONE WILD MUFFINS

PREP TIME: 15 MINUTES | TOTAL TIME: 1 HOUR 5 MINUTES

Makes 8

These triple-peanut muffins are intended for only the most hard-core of peanut lovers. This recipe throws peanuts at you in every form, from every direction. You'll beg for mercy.

If you cannot find preground peanut flour, you can easily grind it yourself in a food processor, coffee grinder, or food chopper.

1 cup almond meal/flour	2 eggs
½ cup peanut flour (28% fat)	½ cup buttermilk
3 tablespoons ground golden flaxseeds	3½ tablespoons extra-light olive oil
1 teaspoon baking soda	½ cup natural peanut butter, softened
1 teaspoon cinnamon (optional)	1 tablespoon vanilla extract
¼ teaspoon fine sea salt	½ cup chopped dry roasted, unsalted peanuts
½ cup xylitol (see note)	

Preheat the oven to 350°F. Place paper liners in 8 cups of a 12-cup muffin pan or grease the cups.

In a large bowl, sift together the almond meal/flour, peanut flour, flaxseeds, baking soda, cinnamon (if using), salt, and xylitol.

In a separate bowl, whisk the eggs. Add the buttermilk, oil, peanut butter, and vanilla and whisk to combine. Add the egg mixture to the flour mixture and whisk to combine. Fold in the peanuts.

Divide the batter among the muffin cups, filling each about ⅔ full. Bake for 20 minutes, or until a wooden pick inserted in the center of a muffin comes out clean. Remove from the pan and cool on a rack for 30 minutes.

Note: To prepare with stevia, omit the xylitol and add ¼ teaspoon liquid stevia, increase the baking soda to 1½ teaspoons, add 1 egg to the eggs, and add ½ cup unsweetened applesauce to the wet ingredients.

PER MUFFIN: 300 calories, 10 g protein, 19 g carbohydrates, 23 g total fat, 3 g saturated fat, 4 g fiber, 238 mg sodium

FLAXSEED CRACKERS

PREP TIME: 15 MINUTES | TOTAL TIME: 40 MINUTES + COOLING TIME

Makes approximately 40 crackers

The few flaxseed cracker brands on the market can be quite costly. Here's a recipe that will cut your costs by half or more yet easily match or improve on the taste. Dip Flaxseed Crackers in salsa, hummus, or onion or other sour cream–based dips.

This recipe yields a quantity of cracker dough that will require 2 baking sheets (approximately 18" × 13"). If you have only 1 baking sheet, divide the cracker dough in half and bake in 2 batches.

2 **cups ground golden flaxseeds**	1 **large egg**
3 **tablespoons whole flaxseeds or sesame seeds**	2 **tablespoons extra-light olive oil or coconut oil, melted**
½ **cup grated Parmesan cheese**	½ **cup water**
1 **teaspoon onion powder**	1 **teaspoon coarse sea salt or mix of spices (such as garlic, cumin, and chili)**
½ **teaspoon sea salt**	

Preheat the oven to 325°F.

In a large bowl, combine the ground flaxseeds, whole flaxseeds or sesame seeds, Parmesan, onion powder, and ½ teaspoon sea salt.

In a medium bowl, whisk together the egg, oil, and water. Pour into the flaxseed mixture and mix thoroughly.

Cover 2 baking sheets with parchment paper. Spoon half of the mixture onto each parchment, shape each into a loose ball, and cover each with another sheet of parchment paper. Using a rolling pin, flatten to ⅛" thickness.

Remove the top layer of parchment paper, sprinkle with coarse sea salt or desired spices, and bake for 25 minutes, or until the center is firm. Cool for at least 30 minutes. Break by hand or cut with a pizza cutter into crackers of desired size.

PER SERVING: 42 calories, 2 g protein, 2 g carbohydrates, 3 g total fat, 0 g saturated fat, 2 g fiber, 47 mg sodium

DATE-NUT QUICK BREAD

PREP TIME: 15 MINUTES | TOTAL TIME: 55 MINUTES

Makes 14 slices (½")

Some people lament the loss of their bagels or English muffins for breakfast in their new wheat-free lifestyle. Instead, try this Date-Nut Quick Bread toasted or as is and spread with cream cheese, butter, or your choice of nut butter.

If less carbohydrates are desired, reduce the quantity of dates, and make up for the difference with your sweetener of choice. For a more kid-friendly version, where carbohydrates do not have to be so limited, add ½ cup of raisins to the flour mixture.

1⅓ cups almond meal/flour	¾ cup pitted dates, chopped
⅓ cup ground golden flaxseeds	½ cup chopped pecans
1 teaspoon baking powder	2 eggs
½ teaspoon baking soda	1 egg white
1 teaspoon ground cinnamon	¼ cup butter, coconut oil, or extra-light olive oil, melted and cooled
¼ teaspoon ground nutmeg	
¼ teaspoon ground cloves	½ cup buttermilk
½ teaspoon sea salt	

Preheat the oven to 350°F. Grease an 8½" × 4½" loaf pan.

In a large bowl, sift together the almond meal/flour, flaxseeds, baking powder, baking soda, cinnamon, nutmeg, cloves, and salt. Add the dates and pecans and stir to combine.

In a small bowl, combine the eggs, egg white, butter or oil, and buttermilk and beat lightly to break up the yolks.

Pour the egg mixture into the flour mixture and mix thoroughly with a wooden spoon, just until moistened. Spoon the batter into the loaf pan and bake for 40 minutes, or until a wooden pick inserted in the center comes out clean and the bread is firm yet springy to the touch.

PER SERVING: 171 calories, 5 g protein, 11 g carbohydrates, 13 g total fat, 3 g saturated fat, 3 g fiber, 180 mg sodium

WALNUT RAISIN BREAD

PREP TIME: 15 MINUTES | **TOTAL TIME:** 55 MINUTES

Makes 10 slices (½")

This Walnut Raisin Bread serves as the bread for finger sandwiches, such as in the Goat Cheese Apricot Finger Sandwiches recipe on page 127.

1⅓ cups almond meal/flour

⅓ cup ground golden flaxseeds

1 teaspoon baking powder

½ teaspoon baking soda

2 teaspoons ground cinnamon

½ teaspoon sea salt

¾ cup raisins

½ cup chopped walnuts

2 eggs

1 egg white

¼ cup butter, coconut oil, or extra-light olive oil, melted and cooled

½ cup buttermilk

Preheat the oven to 350°F. Grease an 8½" × 4½" loaf pan.

In a large bowl, sift together the almond meal/flour, flaxseeds, baking powder, baking soda, cinnamon, and salt. Add the raisins and walnuts and stir to combine.

In a small bowl, combine the eggs, egg white, butter or oil, and buttermilk and beat lightly to break up the yolks.

Pour the egg mixture into the flour mixture and mix thoroughly with a wooden spoon, just until moistened. Spoon the batter into the loaf pan and bake for 40 minutes, or until a wooden pick inserted in the center comes out clean and the bread is firm yet springy to the touch.

PER SERVING: 169 calories, 5 g protein, 11 g carbohydrates, 13 g total fat, 3 g saturated fat, 3 g fiber, 220 mg sodium

PB & J BREAD

PREP TIME: 15 MINUTES | **TOTAL TIME:** 1 HOUR 15 MINUTES

Makes 14 slices (½")

As its name suggests, this bread tastes like good old-fashioned peanut butter and jelly. In my experience, kids of all sizes love this bread, even the Big Kid you're married to! I love this bread spread thickly with cream cheese.

If you cannot purchase peanut flour preground, you can easily grind it yourself in a food processor, coffee grinder, or food chopper.

1 cup almond meal/flour	½ cup natural peanut butter, at room temperature
½ cup peanut flour (28% fat)	
3 tablespoons ground golden flaxseeds	½ cup buttermilk
	3½ tablespoons extra-light olive oil
1 teaspoon baking powder	1 tablespoon vanilla extract
1 teaspoon baking soda	¼ teaspoon liquid stevia or to desired sweetness
½ teaspoon fine sea salt	
½ teaspoon allspice	¼ cup unsweetened spreadable fruit
2 eggs	

Preheat the oven to 350°F. Grease an 8½" × 4½" loaf pan.

In a medium bowl, sift together the almond meal/flour, peanut flour, flaxseeds, baking powder, baking soda, salt, and allspice.

In a separate bowl, combine the eggs, peanut butter, buttermilk, oil, vanilla, and stevia and stir until smooth.

Pour the egg mixture into the flour mixture and blend until just moistened. Pour into the pan and bake for 45 minutes.

In a small saucepan over medium-low heat, heat the spreadable fruit until it liquefies. When the bread is done, remove it from the oven and poke holes all over the top with a wooden pick. Spread the hot fruit over the top and return to the oven. Bake for 5 minutes. Allow to cool for 10 minutes on a rack to let the jam set. Remove to a rack to cool completely.

PER SERVING: 178 calories, 6 g protein, 9 g carbohydrates, 14 g total fat, 2 g saturated fat, 2 g fiber, 270 mg sodium

BASIC BISCUITS

Makes 8

Sometimes uncomplicated is best! These simple and wonderfully wheat-free biscuits will do the trick when you have an appetite for sausages with (healthy wheat-free) gravy and biscuits or require something to accompany a turkey dinner.

Easy variations include adding ¼ cup grated cheese, Italian seasonings, or cinnamon with your choice of sweetener.

1 cup almond meal/flour

1 cup ground golden flaxseeds

4 teaspoons baking powder

4 tablespoons cold butter, cut into cubes

4 egg whites

Preheat the oven to 350°F. Line a baking sheet with parchment paper.

In a large bowl, mix together the almond meal/flour, flaxseeds, and baking powder. Cut in the butter until combined.

In a medium bowl, beat the egg whites on high until soft peaks form. Gently fold the egg whites into the flour ingredients until well blended.

Spoon the dough into 8 rounds on the baking sheet. Flatten to approximately ¾" thickness. Bake for 15 minutes, or until golden brown.

PER SERVING: 209 calories, 8 g protein, 9 g carbohydrates, 18 g total fat, 4 g saturated fat, 6 g fiber, 348 mg sodium

CHEDDAR CHEESE BISCUITS

PREP TIME: 10 MINUTES | **TOTAL TIME:** 20 MINUTES

Makes 8

These simple biscuits, rich with the flavor of Cheddar cheese and butter, can accompany chili, be used as a hamburger bun, or make a quick sausage biscuit.

1 cup almond meal/flour

1 cup ground golden flaxseeds

4 teaspoons baking powder

½ teaspoon onion powder

4 tablespoons cold butter, cut into cubes

½ cup shredded sharp Cheddar cheese

4 egg whites

Preheat the oven to 350°F. Line a baking sheet with parchment paper.

In a bowl, mix together the almond meal/flour, flaxseeds, baking powder, and onion powder. Cut in the butter until combined. Stir in the Cheddar.

In a small bowl, beat the egg whites with a hand mixer until soft peaks form. Gently fold the egg whites into the dry ingredients until combined.

Spoon the dough into 8 rounds on the baking sheet. Flatten to approximately ¾" thickness.

Bake for 15 minutes, or until golden brown.

PER SERVING: 237 calories, 10 g protein, 9 g carbohydrates, 19 g total fat, 5 g saturated fat, 6 g fiber, 447 mg sodium

ROSEMARY–ROMANO CHEESE BISCUITS

PREP TIME: 15 MINUTES | **TOTAL TIME:** 35 MINUTES

Makes 8

These mouthwateringly delicious biscuits feature Italian herbs, Romano cheese, and the seductive taste of sun-dried tomatoes topped off with some more Romano cheese. Dip them into extra-virgin olive oil while they're still warm and you will knock your spouse out of the way to get another!

To make the recipe as written, you will need both shredded and grated Romano cheese. If preparing from an intact piece of Romano cheese, you can just shred and grate the specified amounts.

1 cup almond meal/flour

1 cup ground golden flaxseeds

4 teaspoons baking powder

¼ cup shredded Romano cheese

1 teaspoon dried rosemary

½ teaspoon dried oregano

2 tablespoons sun-dried tomatoes (soaked in oil), finely chopped

4 tablespoons cold butter, cut into cubes

4 egg whites

2 tablespoons grated Romano cheese

Preheat the oven to 350°F. Line a baking sheet with parchment paper.

In a large bowl, mix together the almond meal/flour, flaxseeds, baking powder, shredded Romano, rosemary, and oregano. Stir in the tomatoes. Cut in the butter until combined.

In a large bowl, beat the egg whites with a mixer on high speed until soft peaks form. Gently fold the egg whites into the flour mixture until combined.

Divide the dough into 8 rounds on the baking sheet. Flatten to approximately ¾" thickness. Sprinkle with the grated Romano.

Bake for 15 minutes, or until golden brown.

PER SERVING: 234 calories, 10 g protein, 9 g carbohydrates, 19 g total fat, 5 g saturated fat, 6 g fiber, 447 mg sodium

CLASSIC SCONES

PREP TIME: 10 MINUTES | **TOTAL TIME:** 30 MINUTES

Makes 8

A little secret: Because they contain no wheat, these Classic Scones are not *really* classic. However, they re-create all the simple pleasures of having a traditional scone with tea, coffee, or fried eggs, but with none of the wheat hassles.

Use this recipe as the basic starting place for fruit scones with currants, blueberries, cherries, or other berries; cheese scones with grated Parmesan, Romano, or any other variety of cheese; and herb scones with rosemary, oregano, garlic, or onion. At the holidays, pumpkin scones spiced up with ground cinnamon, nutmeg, and cloves are perfect served steaming hot, broken open, and topped with butter.

Fashion your scones into any desired shape: round, triangular, or with a depression in the middle to puddle your no-sugar-added fruit jam.

1 cup ground golden flaxseeds	2 tablespoons xylitol or 8–12 drops liquid stevia or to desired sweetness
¾ cup almond meal/flour	5 tablespoons cold butter
¼ cup coconut flour	¼ cup heavy cream
1½ teaspoons baking powder	2 eggs
¼ teaspoon fine sea salt	1 teaspoon vanilla extract

Preheat the oven to 350°F. Line a baking sheet with parchment paper.

In a medium bowl, combine the flaxseeds, almond meal/flour, coconut flour, baking powder, salt, and xylitol, if using. Cut the butter into the flour mixture until it's combined.

In another bowl, whisk together the stevia (if using), cream, eggs, and vanilla. Stir into the flour mixture until well blended.

Evenly divide the dough into 8 pieces and place on the baking sheet. Flatten to approximately ¾" thickness.

Bake for 18 minutes, or until golden brown.

PER SERVING: 258 calories, 8 g protein, 13 g carbohydrates, 22 g total fat, 7 g saturated fat, 7 g fiber, 228 mg sodium

CRANBERRY CINNAMON SCONES

PREP TIME: 10 MINUTES | TOTAL TIME: 30 MINUTES

Makes 8

Scones are wonderfully easy to whip up and carry to work, have for a quick and easy breakfast, or enjoy as a snack. Because these scones are, like their original wheat-based counterparts, essentially nonsweet, enjoy them with a dab of preserves or jam on top.

1 cup ground golden flaxseeds

¾ cup almond meal/flour

¼ cup coconut flour

1 tablespoon ground cinnamon

1½ teaspoons baking powder

¼ teaspoon fine sea salt

2 tablespoons xylitol or 8–12 drops liquid stevia or to desired sweetness

5 tablespoons cold butter, cut into cubes

¼ cup heavy cream (see note)

2 eggs

1 teaspoon vanilla extract

½ cup dried unsweetened cranberries, currants, or other dried unsweetened berries

Preheat the oven to 350°F. Line a baking sheet with parchment paper.

In a medium bowl, mix the flaxseeds, almond meal/flour, coconut flour, cinnamon, baking powder, salt, and xylitol, if using. Cut the butter into the flour mixture until it's the size of peas.

In another bowl, whisk together the stevia (if using), cream, eggs, and vanilla until combined. Stir into the dry ingredients until well blended. Add the dried fruit, and stir until evenly distributed.

Evenly divide the dough into 8 pieces and place on the baking sheet. Flatten to approximately ¾" thickness.

Bake for 18 minutes, or until golden brown.

Note: If using stevia, use an additional 1 tablespoon heavy cream.

PER SERVING: 268 calories, 8 g protein, 16 g carbohydrates, 22 g total fat, 7 g saturated fat, 8 g fiber, 252 mg sodium

GINGER APRICOT SCONES

PREP TIME: 15 MINUTES | TOTAL TIME: 35 MINUTES

Makes 8

The combination of ginger and apricots is magical! The scones provide a rich mix of tastes and go great with coffee, serve as the finish to lunch or dinner, or even serve as a meal themselves.

1 cup ground golden flaxseeds

¾ cup almond meal/flour

¼ cup coconut flour

1½ teaspoons baking powder

½ teaspoon ground ginger

¼ teaspoon fine sea salt

2 tablespoons xylitol or 8–12 drops liquid stevia or to desired sweetness

5 tablespoons cold butter, cut into cubes

¼ cup heavy cream

2 eggs

1 teaspoon vanilla extract

½ cup dried unsweetened apricots, finely chopped

1 tablespoon finely grated fresh ginger (from a 2" piece of ginger)

Preheat the oven to 350°F. Line a baking sheet with parchment paper.

In a medium bowl, mix the flaxseeds, almond meal/flour, coconut flour, baking powder, ground ginger, salt, and xylitol, if using. Cut the butter into the flour mixture until it's the size of peas.

In another bowl, whisk together the stevia (if using), cream, eggs, and vanilla until combined. Stir into the flour mixture until well blended. Add the apricots and fresh ginger, and stir until they are evenly distributed.

Evenly divide the dough into 8 pieces and place on the baking sheet. Flatten to approximately ¾" thickness.

Bake for 18 minutes, or until golden brown.

PER SERVING: 259 calories, 8 g protein, 13 g carbohydrates, 22 g total fat, 7 g saturated fat, 7 g fiber, 252 mg sodium

STRAWBERRY SHORTCAKES

PREP TIME: 15 MINUTES | TOTAL TIME: 20 MINUTES

Makes 8 servings

Thought you'd never experience the rich taste of strawberry shortcake again? Well, here you go, every bit as delicious as anything conjured up out of wheat flour!

3 cups strawberries, hulled and thinly sliced

⅓ cup xylitol or ¼ teaspoon liquid stevia or to desired sweetness

¾ cup whipping cream

¾ teaspoon vanilla extract

8 Basic Biscuits (page 245), halved horizontally

In a bowl, combine the strawberries and xylitol or stevia. Using a large spoon or potato masher, bruise the strawberries lightly. Stir well. Set aside.

In a medium bowl, and using an electric mixer on high, beat the cream and vanilla until soft peaks form.

Place the bottom halves of the shortcakes on 8 plates. Reserve ¼ cup of the strawberries. Divide the whipped cream and the remaining strawberries on top of the biscuits. Cover with the biscuit tops and top with the remaining berries.

PER SERVING: 324 calories, 9 g protein, 22 g carbohydrates, 38 g total fat, 14 g saturated fat, 6 g fiber, 568 mg sodium

MINI MOCHA CAKES

PREP TIME: 20 MINUTES | **TOTAL TIME:** 45 MINUTES

Makes 12

Living a wheat-free life does not mean eating foods that are tasteless or boring. I've had these mocha cakes for breakfast many times, and they're filling and delicious.

Because there's no flour, they "soufflé up" during baking and then fall as they cool, leaving a perfect little indentation to fill with whipped cream. If you're looking for a special presentation dessert, this recipe easily converts into an 8" cake (see note).

8 ounces bittersweet (85% cacao) chocolate, coarsely chopped

12 tablespoons butter

½ cup xylitol (see note)

2 teaspoons instant espresso powder

5 eggs

2 teaspoons vanilla extract

½ cup heavy whipping cream or ready-made whipped cream (unsweetened; no high-fructose corn syrup)

Unsweetened cocoa powder or dark chocolate shavings, for garnish (optional)

Preheat the oven to 350°F. Place paper liners in a 12-cup muffin pan or grease the cups.

In a large glass bowl, microwave the chocolate and butter on high power for 1 minute, stirring once. If not completely melted, microwave, stirring every 20 seconds, until melted. Stir in the xylitol and espresso powder until completely melted.

Add the eggs, one at a time, blending well after each egg. Stir in the vanilla.

Divide the batter among the muffin cups, filling each about three-quarters full.

Bake for 20 minutes, or until firm to the touch and a wooden pick inserted in the center of a cake comes out with moist crumbs. Cool in the pan on a rack for 5 minutes. Remove to the rack to cool completely.

If using whipping cream, just before serving, in a medium bowl and using an electric mixer on high, beat the whipping cream until stiff peaks form. Dollop or pipe whipped cream onto the cakes. Sprinkle with the cocoa or chocolate shavings, if desired.

Note: To prepare with stevia, omit the xylitol and add ¼ teaspoon liquid stevia and ⅓ cup plain Greek yogurt to the chocolate mixture, after adding the last egg.

To make this recipe as a 12-serving cake, coat an 8" springform pan with oil or cooking spray and line it with parchment paper. Coat the paper with oil or cooking spray. Pour the batter into the pan and bake for 45 minutes, or until a wooden pick inserted in the center comes out with moist crumbs. Cool completely on a rack. Refrigerate for several hours or overnight before serving.

PER SERVING: 297 calories, 5 g protein, 16 g carbohydrates, 26 g total fat, 15 g saturated fat, 3 g fiber, 115 mg sodium

VANILLA CUPCAKES WITH CHOCOLATE FROSTING

PREP TIME: 25 MINUTES | TOTAL TIME: 50 MINUTES

Makes 10

Okay, so your 10-year-old (or 50-year-old) needs some cupcakes, but you don't want to sacrifice health and contribute to obesity, diabetes, or myriad other health problems. Can you ever serve cupcakes again?

Yes, you can! And they can be every bit as delicious as their wheat-based counterparts, just minus the appetite stimulation and other health problems.

CUPCAKES

- 2 cups almond meal/flour
- ¼ cup coconut flour
- ¼ cup ground golden flaxseeds
- 2 teaspoons baking powder
- ½ teaspoon baking soda
- ½ teaspoon fine sea salt
- 2 eggs, separated
- ¼ cup coconut oil or butter, melted

- ⅓ cup xylitol (see note)
- 2 tablespoons buttermilk
- 1 tablespoon vanilla extract

FROSTING

- 1 square (1 ounce) semisweet baking chocolate or 2 tablespoons semisweet chocolate chips
- 4 ounces cream cheese, softened
- ¼ teaspoon stevia powder

Preheat the oven to 350°F. Place 10 paper liners in a 12-cup muffin pan.

To make the cupcakes: In a medium bowl, whisk together the almond meal/flour, coconut flour, flaxseeds, baking powder, baking soda, and salt.

In a large bowl, whisk the egg yolks, oil or butter, xylitol, buttermilk, and vanilla until well blended. Set aside.

In a large bowl, with an electric mixer on high speed, beat the egg whites until stiff peaks form.

Gently fold the egg whites into the egg yolk mixture. Then fold the egg mixture into the flour mixture until well combined. Divide among the paper liners.

Bake for 20 minutes, or until the tops are golden and a wooden pick inserted in the center of a cupcake comes out clean. Allow to cool in the pan for 5 minutes. Remove to a rack to cool completely.

To make the frosting: In a small bowl, microwave the chocolate on high power for 15 seconds. Stir until smooth, microwaving again if necessary. In a medium bowl, with an electric mixer on low speed, beat the cheese until smooth. Add the chocolate and stevia and beat on low speed until smooth. Spread over the cooled cupcakes.

Note: To prepare the cupcakes with stevia, omit the coconut flour and xylitol. Add ¼ teaspoon liquid stevia and 1 additional egg, and increase the coconut oil to 6 tablespoons, the buttermilk to ½ cup, and the vanilla to 1½ tablespoons. Add ⅓ cup unsweetened applesauce to the egg yolk mixture.

PER SERVING: 290 calories, 8 g protein, 17 g carbohydrates, 24 g total fat, 9 g saturated fat, 5 g fiber, 353 mg sodium

RASPBERRY CHOCOLATE CHEESECAKE

PREP TIME: 20 MINUTES | TOTAL TIME: 3 HOURS + COOLING TIME

Makes 16 servings

This is the recipe for the cheesecake I made for my wife's birthday. She loved it!

I used a basic cheesecake recipe with a few modifications: I added ingredients to make a thin layer of dark chocolate that provided a nice added dimension to the raspberry cheesecake filling. This is a bit more complicated than my usual simple recipes, but it was worth watching my wife really enjoy the rich taste after she blew out the candles. If you're looking for even more chocolate, replace the crust in this recipe with the chocolate crust from the Chocolate Cream Pie (page 266).

CRUST

- 1½ cups ground pecans or walnuts
- 4 tablespoons butter or coconut oil, melted
- 2 teaspoons xylitol or 1 drop liquid stevia or to desired sweetness
- 2 teaspoons unsweetened cocoa powder

FILLING

- 16 ounces cream cheese, at room temperature
- ¾ cup sour cream
- 3 eggs
- 1 tablespoon vanilla extract
- ½ cup xylitol or ¼ teaspoon liquid stevia or to desired sweetness
- 1¼ cups fresh or frozen sugar-free raspberries, pureed and strained
- ¼ cup raspberries for garnish

CHOCOLATE GLAZE

- ¼ cup bittersweet (85% cacao) chocolate chips
- 2 tablespoons butter
- 1 teaspoon milk or half-and-half

Preheat the oven to 350°F.

To make the crust: In a large bowl, stir together the nuts, butter or oil, xylitol or stevia, and cocoa. Press onto the bottom of a 9" springform pan.

Bake for 10 minutes, or until browned around the edges. Set aside.

To make the filling: In a large bowl and using an electric mixer on medium speed, beat the cheese, sour cream, eggs, vanilla, and xylitol or stevia until smooth. Stir in the pureed raspberries.

Pour into the crust.

Bake for 40 minutes, or until a knife inserted in the center comes out clean. Cool completely on a rack. Refrigerate until ready to serve. Remove from the spring-form pan and place on a serving dish. Glaze.

To make the glaze: In a small microwaveable bowl, microwave the chocolate chips and butter on high power for 15 seconds. Stir until smooth, microwaving again if necessary until melted and smooth. Stir in the milk or half-and-half. Drizzle over the cooled cake. Refrigerate for 30 minutes, or until the glaze is set. Garnish with raspberries, if desired.

PER SERVING: 284 calories, 5 g protein, 12 g carbohydrates, 26 g total fat, 11 g saturated fat, 2 g fiber, 142 mg sodium

CHOCOLATE-FROSTED YELLOW CAKE

PREP TIME: 30 MINUTES | **TOTAL TIME:** 1 HOUR 15 MINUTES

Makes 12 servings

This basic Yellow Cake will serve you well as is or as the starting point for numerous variations. Try adding different base ingredients to the batter or adding unique toppings. For example, to really punch up the almond flavor, add ½ teaspoon almond extract. For a chocolate layer cake, add ¼ cup cocoa powder to the flour mixture. To make a lemon poppy seed cake, add the peel of 2 lemons and a 3-ounce bottle of poppy seeds.

As written, this recipe yields a single layer cake with enough icing to cover it. To make a double-layer cake, double all ingredients and separate the batter into 2 baking pans. For a change of pace, instead of frosting, drizzle the cooled cake with chocolate glaze: Melt ¼ cup bittersweet chocolate chips and 2 tablespoons butter in a small glass bowl and microwave on high power in 15-second increments, stirring in between, until melted.

Because most cakes work best with a lighter texture, use almond flour, not the meal ground from whole almonds, for this yellow cake.

2 cups almond flour

¼ cup coconut flour

¼ cup ground golden flaxseeds

2 teaspoons baking powder

½ teaspoon baking soda

½ teaspoon fine sea salt

3 eggs, separated

6 tablespoons butter, melted

⅓ cup xylitol (see note)

1 tablespoon vanilla extract

½ cup buttermilk

Chocolate Frosting (page 254), recipe doubled

Preheat the oven to 350°F. Grease an 8" round baking pan and line it with a circle of parchment paper. Grease the paper.

In a large bowl, sift together the almond flour, coconut flour, flaxseeds, baking powder, baking soda, and salt.

In a large bowl, with an electric mixer on high speed, beat the egg whites until stiff peaks form.

In a separate bowl, whisk the egg yolks until smooth. Add the butter, xylitol, vanilla, and buttermilk and mix until combined. Gently fold the egg whites into the yolk mixture. Then fold the egg mixture into the flour mixture until well combined. Pour into the cake pan.

Bake for 35 minutes, or until the top is golden and a wooden pick inserted in the center comes out clean. Allow to cool in the pan for 10 minutes, then invert onto a rack to cool completely. Frost with the chocolate frosting.

Note: To prepare with stevia, omit the coconut flour, replace the xylitol with ¼ teaspoon liquid stevia, and add ⅓ cup unsweetened applesauce to the wet ingredients.

PER SERVING: 309 calories, 8 g protein, 16 g carbohydrates, 26 g total fat, 10 g saturated fat, 4 g fiber, 380 mg sodium

LEMON CHEESECAKE CUPCAKES

PREP TIME: 25 MINUTES | TOTAL TIME: 1 HOUR

Makes 12

Does anyone *not* love cheesecake? And you thought that cheesecake was unhealthy!

This variation converts its sugary, fattening counterpart into healthy, bite-size treats that even kids will snatch up.

1 cup walnuts, ground	2 eggs
1 teaspoon ground cinnamon	½ cup sour cream or canned coconut milk
3 tablespoons butter or coconut oil, melted	2 teaspoons grated lemon peel
12 ounces cream cheese, softened	3 tablespoons lemon juice
½ cup xylitol or ¼ teaspoon liquid stevia or to desired sweetness	Strawberries, shaved dark chocolate, or mint leaves for garnish

Preheat the oven to 350°F. Place paper liners in a 12-cup muffin pan.

In a small bowl, mix together the walnuts and cinnamon. Stir in the butter or oil. Divide among the muffin cups and press down with a spoon or fingertips until evenly distributed. Bake for 10 minutes, or until firm to the touch. Cool on a rack.

In a large bowl, with an electric mixer on medium speed, beat the cheese and xylitol or stevia until creamy. Add the eggs, one at a time, and beat until well blended, scraping down the sides of the bowl after each addition. Add the sour cream or coconut milk, lemon peel, and lemon juice and beat until thoroughly mixed. Divide among the paper liners.

Bake for 30 minutes, or until a knife inserted in the center of a cupcake comes out almost clean. Cool in the pan for 5 minutes. Remove to a rack and cool completely.

Garnish each cupcake with a strawberry, chocolate shavings, or a mint leaf, if desired. Refrigerate until ready to serve.

PER SERVING: 237 calories, 4 g protein, 11 g carbohydrates, 22 g total fat, 9 g saturated fat, 1 g fiber, 130 mg sodium

BASIC PIE CRUST

PREP TIME: 1 HOUR 15 MINUTES + RESTING TIME | TOTAL TIME: 1 HOUR 40 MINUTES

Makes 8 servings (one 9" bottom pie crust)

Here's your starting place for beautiful custard, lemon meringue, chocolate cream, or other pies.

Use almond flour ground from blanched almonds for this recipe. Without the strength of gluten to hold the flours together, this crust is a bit delicate. If you decide to try making a top crust for a pie (double the recipe for top and bottom crusts) or pot pie, roll it according to the directions, then place—parchment paper and all—on a baking sheet and freeze for 20 minutes. That will give the crust enough strength to be transferred to the top of your pie.

1 cup walnuts	½ teaspoon sea salt
1 cup almond flour, divided	½ cup unsalted butter, cut into cubes
⅔ cup ground golden flaxseeds	1 egg
2 teaspoons baking powder	1 tablespoon vinegar
½ teaspoon guar gum	1 tablespoon water
½ teaspoon xanthan gum	

In a food processor, pulse the walnuts until chopped. Add ⅓ cup almond flour, the flaxseeds, baking powder, guar gum, xanthan gum, and salt. Pulse until well blended. Add the butter and pulse 10 times. Add the egg, vinegar, and water, and pulse until just combined. The dough will be wet.

Dust a work surface and your hands with some almond meal/flour. Place the dough on the work surface. Knead the remaining almond meal into the dough. Form into a disk. Wrap the dough with plastic wrap. Refrigerate for at least 1 hour.

To roll out, dust a piece of parchment paper with almond meal. Place the dough on the paper and dust with more almond meal. Top with a second piece of paper. With a rolling pin, roll to a 10" round. Peel off the top paper. Place a 9" pie plate upside down over the dough and turn the dough onto the pie plate. Gently peel off the parchment paper. Trim any overhang and crimp the edges. Chill until ready to use.

To prebake, preheat the oven to 350°F. Bake for 23 minutes, or until the crust is golden and no longer moist to the touch.

PER SERVING: 319 calories, 8 g protein, 9 g carbohydrates, 31 g total fat, 9 g saturated fat, 6 g fiber, 233 mg sodium

BASIC NUT CRUST

PREP TIME: 5 MINUTES | TOTAL TIME: 30 MINUTES

Makes 8 servings (one 9" bottom pie crust)

Contemplating a unique cheesecake or quiche? Here is the Basic Nut Crust to get you started.

Just about any ground nut will serve you well. Add ½ teaspoon unsweetened cocoa powder for a "darker" taste.

1⅓ **cups ground nuts (pecans, walnuts, almonds, macadamia nuts)**

⅔ **cup ground golden flaxseeds**

6 **tablespoons butter, melted and cooled**

In a large bowl, stir together the nuts, flaxseeds, and butter until well blended.

Press into a 9" pie plate.

To prebake, preheat the oven to 350°F. Cover the pie crust with foil. Bake for 15 minutes. Remove the foil, turn the pie plate, and bake for 10 minutes, or until the crust is golden and no longer moist to the touch.

PER SERVING: 257 calories, 4 g protein, 6 g carbohydrates, 26 g total fat, 7 g saturated fat, 5 g fiber, 61 mg sodium

KEY LIME PIE

Makes 8 servings

Surely this Key Lime Pie will convince any wheat-consuming holdouts that life is good without wheat!

This version adds a unique coconut-based crust. It may also be made with a prebaked Basic Nut Crust using macadamia nuts.

CRUST

- 3 tablespoons butter
- 1½ cups flaked unsweetened coconut

FILLING

- 1 cup heavy whipping cream
- 8 ounces cream cheese or Neufchâtel cheese, softened
- 3 tablespoons xylitol, finely ground, or 6 drops liquid stevia or to desired sweetness
- ½ cup bottled key lime juice
- 1 teaspoon lime peel (optional)

To make the crust: In a medium skillet over medium heat, melt the butter. Add the coconut and stir until coated. Cook for 5 minutes, stirring constantly, or until the coconut is lightly toasted. Press into a 9" pie plate.

To make the filling: In a large bowl, with an electric mixer on high speed, beat the cream until stiff peaks form.

In a large bowl, with the same beaters on medium speed, beat the cheese, xylitol or stevia, lime juice, and lime peel (if using) until well blended. Fold the whipped cream into the lime mixture. Pour into the pie crust.

Serve immediately or refrigerate until ready to serve.

PER SERVING: 370 calories, 3 g protein, 10 g carbohydrates, 36 g total fat, 25 g saturated fat, 2 g fiber, 153 mg sodium

PUMPKIN PIE

PREP TIME: 20 MINUTES | **TOTAL TIME:** 1 HOUR 20 MINUTES

Makes 8 servings

Pumpkin pie is one of those fixtures of Thanksgiving dinner that, when re-created without wheat, can be enjoyed without worry. No worries over weight gain, increased blood sugar, triglycerides, blood pressure. No leg edema, abdominal cramps, or diarrhea. No depression, moodiness, or crabbiness—except that aimed at your weird brother-in-law who keeps on licking his fingers after touching everything.

CRUST

- 1⅓ cups ground pecans
- ⅔ cup ground golden flaxseeds
- 6 tablespoons butter or coconut oil, melted

FILLING

- 8 ounces cream cheese, at room temperature
- ½ cup xylitol (see note)
- 2 eggs
- 1 can (15 ounces) pumpkin puree
- ½ cup canned coconut milk
- 1 teaspoon vanilla extract
- 1 teaspoon ground cinnamon
- ½ teaspoon ground nutmeg
- ½ teaspoon ground ginger
- ¼ teaspoon ground cloves
- Unsweetened whipped cream for garnish

Preheat the oven to 350°F.

To make the crust: In a medium bowl, stir together the pecans, flaxseeds, and butter or oil. Press into a 9" pie plate. Bake for 15 minutes, or until lightly browned.

To make the filling: In a large bowl, with an electric mixer on medium speed, beat the cheese and xylitol until smooth. Add the eggs, one at a time, scraping down the sides of the bowl after each addition. Add the pumpkin, coconut milk, vanilla, cinnamon, nutmeg, ginger, and cloves. Beat on low speed until well blended.

Pour into the pie crust. Place on a baking sheet. Bake for 45 minutes, or until a knife inserted in the center comes out clean. Place on a rack to cool completely. If desired, top with the whipped cream.

Note: To prepare with stevia, omit the xylitol and coconut milk. Use ¼ teaspoon liquid stevia and ⅔ cup heavy cream in the pumpkin mixture. Increase the vanilla to 1½ teaspoons.

PER SERVING: 452 calories, 8 g protein, 24 g carbohydrates, 40 g total fat, 15 g saturated fat, 7 g fiber, 175 mg sodium

CHOCOLATE CREAM PIE

PREP TIME: 15 MINUTES | TOTAL TIME: 40 MINUTES + COOLING TIME

Makes 8 servings

Pile the whipped cream high on this delicious and decadent Chocolate Cream Pie!

The filling for this pie is best paired with a darker crust, so a generous portion of cocoa powder is included in the crust mix.

The filling is easily halved and makes a wonderful mousse, parfait, or frozen dessert. For a mousse, simply serve in a dish with a dollop of whipped cream (sweetened with a sugar substitute to your liking). For a parfait, spoon some filling into a tall glass, add a layer of whipped cream, and then alternate layers of chocolate and cream until you reach the top of the glass, finishing with the cream and chocolate shavings. Or freeze your mousse for 1 to 2 hours for a refreshing summer treat.

CRUST

 1 cup almond meal/flour

 ½ cup ground golden flaxseeds

 ⅛ teaspoon liquid stevia or to desired sweetness

 ¼ cup unsweetened cocoa powder

 ¼ cup butter, melted

 2 tablespoons light canned coconut milk or almond milk

 1 tablespoon vanilla extract

FILLING

 ¼ teaspoon liquid stevia or to desired sweetness

 2 tablespoons coconut flour

 1 teaspoon instant espresso powder

 Pinch of sea salt

 2 cans (14 ounces each) coconut milk

 1 square (1 ounce) semisweet baking chocolate, finely chopped

 1 square (1 ounce) unsweetened baking chocolate, finely chopped

 2 tablespoons vanilla extract

 Unsweetened whipped cream (optional)

 Chocolate shavings for garnish (optional)

Preheat the oven to 325°F. Grease a 9" pie plate.

To make the crust: In a large bowl, whisk the almond meal/flour, flaxseeds, stevia, and cocoa until well blended. Add the butter, milk, and vanilla and stir until combined. The dough will be thick.

Press into the pie plate. Prick the bottom multiple times with a fork. Cover with foil. Bake for 20 minutes, or until firm to the touch.

To make the filling: In a medium saucepan, combine the stevia, coconut flour, espresso powder, and salt. Whisk in the coconut milk until smooth. Bring to a boil over medium heat, stirring constantly. Boil for 1 minute, or until thickened. Remove from the heat and whisk in the semisweet chocolate, unsweetened chocolate, and vanilla until smooth.

Pour the chocolate mixture into the cooled pie crust. Let cool for 5 minutes. Place a piece of plastic wrap directly on the chocolate filling. Refrigerate for at least 2 hours, or until set. Carefully remove the plastic wrap. Garnish with whipped cream and chocolate shavings, if desired.

PER SERVING: 428 calories, 8 g protein, 15 g carbohydrates, 40 g total fat, 26 g saturated fat, 7 g fiber, 60 mg sodium

PEANUT BUTTER PIE

PREP TIME: 25 MINUTES | TOTAL TIME: 45 MINUTES + COOLING TIME

Makes 8 servings

Here's a way to wallop the kids with healthy protein and fat, cleverly disguised as a Peanut Butter Pie!

CRUST

- 1 cup almond meal/flour
- ½ cup ground golden flaxseeds
- ⅛ teaspoon liquid stevia or to desired sweetness
- ¼ cup unsweetened cocoa powder
- ¼ cup butter, melted
- 2 tablespoons canned coconut milk or almond milk
- 1 tablespoon vanilla extract

FILLING

- 1 cup heavy cream
- 1 teaspoon vanilla extract
- 8 ounces cream cheese, softened
- 10 drops liquid stevia or to desired sweetness
- 1 cup creamy natural peanut butter
- 2 tablespoons canned coconut milk

  Melted chocolate for garnish

Grease a 9" pie plate.

To make the crust: In a large bowl, whisk together the almond meal/flour, flaxseeds, stevia, and cocoa. Stir in the butter, milk, and vanilla. Press into the pie plate. Prick the bottom with a fork. Cover with foil. Bake for 20 minutes, or until firm to the touch.

To make the filling: In a large bowl, with an electric mixer on high speed, beat the cream and vanilla until stiff peaks form. Set aside.

In a medium bowl, with the same beaters on medium speed, beat the cheese and stevia until well blended. Beat in the peanut butter and coconut milk. (If the mixture is too thick, add more coconut milk, 1 tablespoon at a time, to reach a smooth and slightly creamy consistency.) Fold the whipped cream into the peanut butter mixture until well blended.

Pour into the cooled pie crust. Refrigerate for at least 2 hours, or until set. Top with melted chocolate, if desired.

PER SERVING: 564 calories, 16 g protein, 16 g carbohydrates, 51 g total fat, 18 g saturated fat, 7 g fiber, 274 mg sodium

LEMON-BLUEBERRY TART

PREP TIME: 20 MINUTES | **TOTAL TIME:** 1 HOUR 30 MINUTES

Makes 10 servings

Despite looking like a beautiful and delicious dessert, this Lemon-Blueberry Tart is really just eggs, nuts, and the rich protein and fat of cream that nutritionally complement any meal with none of the problems of sugared-up or wheat flour–containing versions.

1 cup lemon juice

2 teaspoons lemon peel (optional)

4 eggs

2 egg yolks

1 teaspoon xanthan gum

¼ teaspoon liquid stevia

12 tablespoons unsalted butter, at room temperature, cut into small cubes

1 cup heavy whipping cream

1 prebaked Basic Pie Crust (page 261), baked in a 9" tart or pie pan

1 cup blueberries

In a medium saucepan over medium-high heat, bring the lemon juice and lemon peel, if using, to a boil. Remove from the heat.

Meanwhile, in a medium bowl, whisk together the eggs, egg yolks, xanthan gum, and stevia until well blended. Gradually whisk the hot lemon juice mixture into the egg mixture until blended.

Pour back into the saucepan. Cook over medium-low heat, whisking constantly, for 10 minutes, or until thick. Remove from the heat and whisk in the butter, a little at a time, until smooth and well blended.

Pour into a bowl and cover with plastic wrap. Refrigerate for at least 1 hour, or until completely cold.

Meanwhile, in a small bowl, with an electric mixer on high speed, beat the cream until stiff peaks form. Refrigerate until the lemon mixture is cold.

Fold the whipped cream into the cold lemon mixture. Pour into the tart shell. When ready to serve, pile the blueberries in the center of the tart.

Note: If you find the egg mixture lumpy, strain the hot lemon-egg mixture through a small sieve into a bowl before adding the butter.

PER SERVING: 516 calories, 10 g protein, 12 g carbohydrates, 50 g total fat, 22 g saturated fat, 5 g fiber, 228 mg sodium

MOCHA WALNUT BROWNIES

PREP TIME: 10 MINUTES | TOTAL TIME: 40 MINUTES

Makes 12

Richer than a cookie, heavier than a muffin, brownies are ordinarily an indulgence that leaves you ashamed of your lack of restraint. Have one . . . or two or three, and you will surely pack on a pound of belly fat.

Serve these brownies plain or topped with cream cheese or natural peanut or almond butter, or dip them in coffee.

8 ounces bittersweet (85% cacao) chocolate, chopped

¾ cup butter

2 teaspoons instant espresso powder

½ teaspoon liquid stevia

4 eggs

¼ cup canned coconut milk

2 teaspoons vanilla extract

½ cup chopped walnuts

2 tablespoons coconut flour

¼ cup ground golden flaxseeds

Preheat the oven to 350°F. Grease a 9" × 9" baking pan.

In a large glass bowl, combine the chocolate and butter. Microwave on high power for 1 minute, stirring once halfway through the cooking time. If not completely melted, microwave, stirring every 20 seconds, until melted. Stir in the espresso powder until completely melted.

Add the eggs, one at a time, blending well after each egg. Stir in the coconut milk and vanilla.

Stir in the walnuts, coconut flour, and flaxseeds until well blended.

Pour into the pan and bake for 25 minutes, or until a wooden pick inserted in the center comes out clean.

PER SERVING: 285 calories, 5 g protein, 13 g carbohydrates, 26 g total fat, 13 g saturated fat, 3 g fiber, 106 mg sodium

TRAIL MIX BARS

PREP TIME: 10 MINUTES | TOTAL TIME: 1 HOUR

Makes 8

These bars have many of the wonderful nuts and seeds and much of the crunch of a trail mix but without the sugar load. They pose only a modest carbohydrate exposure, with the dates providing 4 grams of sugar per date.

If you are a marathon runner, triathlete, or other long-duration exerciser and would like to use these bars as your carbohydrate source during exercise, they are easily modified to increase carbohydrate content to suit your needs. You can add 2 or 3 additional dates, for instance, or add raisins or apricots, ground in your food chopper or food processor in the first step. If you are *not* a long-duration athlete, leave these bars as is!

½ cup shredded unsweetened coconut

¼ cup raw pumpkin seeds

¼ cup raw sunflower seeds

4 whole pitted Deglet Noor dates

¼ cup coarsely chopped walnuts

¼ cup cacao nibs

2 teaspoons ground cinnamon

¼ cup coconut milk, at room temperature

2 tablespoons almond butter, at room temperature

Preheat the oven to 200°F. Grease a 9" × 5" loaf pan.

In a food processor, combine the coconut, pumpkin seeds, sunflower seeds, and dates. Chop or pulse until the mixture is the consistency of coarse coffee grounds. Pour into a large bowl.

With a spoon, stir in the walnuts, cacao nibs, and cinnamon. Stir in the coconut milk and almond butter until well blended. Press into the pan. Bake for 50 minutes, or until firm to the touch. Cool on a rack. Cut into 8 bars.

PER SERVING: 186 calories, 4 g protein, 9 g carbohydrates, 15 g total fat, 6 g saturated fat, 2 g fiber, 23 mg sodium

CHOCOLATE BARS

PREP TIME: 15 MINUTES | TOTAL TIME: 1 HOUR 5 MINUTES

Makes 12

These bars are wonderfully portable to eat as snacks. Because they are extra filling, they can even serve as a meal replacement. I make a batch or two every week to keep handy for times when I'm in a hurry and need something to go.

Use the darkest mini chocolate chips you can find to keep sugar exposure down. Cacao nibs are an especially healthy replacement for chocolate chips because they provide the taste of cocoa with virtually no sugar and provide extra crunch. (As always, if you are among the most gluten-sensitive, use gluten-free dark chocolate chips.)

5 tablespoons shredded unsweetened coconut

5 tablespoons raw sunflower seeds

4 tablespoons raw pumpkin seeds

4 Deglet Noor dates

1 cup almond meal/flour

½ cup coconut flour

½ cup extra-dark mini chocolate chips or cacao nibs

4 tablespoons coarsely chopped walnuts

2 tablespoons whey powder

2 teaspoons unsweetened cocoa powder

Sweetener equivalent to ½ cup sugar (optional)

½ cup canned coconut milk

¼ cup almond butter, at room temperature

Preheat the oven to 200° F. Line a 9" × 9" baking pan with parchment paper.

In a food processor, combine the coconut, sunflower seeds, pumpkin seeds, and dates. Pulse until the mixture is the consistency of coarse coffee grounds. Pour into a large bowl.

With a spoon, stir in the almond meal/flour, coconut flour, chocolate chips or cacao nibs, walnuts, whey powder, cocoa, and sweetener (if using).

Stir in the coconut milk and almond butter. Spread into the pan. Bake for 50 minutes, or until firm to the touch.

PER SERVING: 340 calories, 11 g protein, 19 g carbohydrates, 26 g total fat, 8 g saturated fat, 9 g fiber, 52 mg sodium

CHOCOLATE ALMOND BISCOTTI

PREP TIME: 15 MINUTES | TOTAL TIME: 1 HOUR 40 MINUTES

Makes 15

Biscotti are twice-baked biscuits or cookies. The twofold baking process confers sturdiness that makes these delicious wheat-free biscotti perfect for dipping into coffee, latte, or espresso.

These biscotti are rich with the naturally delicious combination of chocolate and almonds.

2 eggs

½ cup ricotta cheese or canned coconut milk, at room temperature

¼ cup butter or coconut oil, melted

¼ cup almond butter, at room temperature

¼ cup xylitol or ¼ teaspoon liquid stevia or to desired sweetness

¼ cup milk, unsweetened almond milk, or carton-variety coconut milk

1 teaspoon almond extract

3 cups almond meal/flour

2 tablespoons coconut flour

½ cup slivered almonds

¼ cup unsweetened cocoa powder

2½ ounces extra-dark chocolate, chopped

Preheat the oven to 350°F. Line a baking sheet with parchment paper.

In a large bowl, whisk together the eggs, ricotta or coconut milk, butter or coconut oil, almond butter, xylitol or stevia, milk, and almond extract.

Stir in the almond meal/flour, coconut flour, almonds, cocoa, and chocolate. Stir until well blended.

Place on the baking sheet and shape into a loaf approximately 12" long and 4" wide. Bake for 40 minutes.

Remove from the oven and reduce the heat to 300°F. Cool on the baking sheet on a rack for 15 minutes. Using a serrated knife, cut crosswise into ¾" slices and lay each slice on its side on the baking sheet. Bake for 30 minutes, turning the biscotti once halfway through the baking time, or until firm and dry.

Cool on the rack for 30 minutes, or until completely cooled.

PER SERVING: 264 calories, 9 g protein, 10 g carbohydrates, 23 g total fat, 6 g saturated fat, 5 g fiber, 67 mg sodium

GINGERBREAD COOKIES

PREP TIME: 20 MINUTES | **TOTAL TIME:** 35 MINUTES + CHILLING TIME

Makes 2 dozen

Here's a recipe for wheat-free, sugar-free Gingerbread Cookies. They're rich with the spices that smell like the holidays: ginger, nutmeg, cloves, and cinnamon. They're great plain, spread with cream cheese (pumpkin cream cheese, in particular), or dipped in coffee. (See note for a quick and yummy decorator icing.)

This dough does roll out, so you can also make gingerbread people!

3 cups almond meal/flour

¼ cup coconut flour

¼ cup ground golden flaxseeds

2 teaspoons ground ginger

1½ teaspoons ground cinnamon

1 teaspoon baking soda

1 teaspoon unsweetened cocoa powder

1 teaspoon ground nutmeg

½ teaspoon ground cloves

¼ teaspoon fine sea salt

¾ cup gluten-free, sugar-free maple syrup

¼ cup coconut oil or butter, melted

1 egg

2 teaspoons vanilla extract

Preheat the oven to 350°F. Line 2 baking sheets with parchment paper.

In a large bowl, whisk together the almond meal/flour, coconut flour, flaxseeds, ginger, cinnamon, baking soda, cocoa, nutmeg, cloves, and salt.

In a small bowl, combine the maple syrup, coconut oil or butter, egg, and vanilla. Whisk until smooth. Stir into the flour mixture until well blended.

Shape into 1" balls and place on the baking sheets. Flatten to ¾" thickness. Bake for 15 minutes, or until the cookies are golden around the edges.

Cool on a rack for 2 minutes. Remove the cookies and place on the racks to cool completely.

Note: To make gingerbread people, divide the dough into 2 disks and wrap each in plastic wrap. Refrigerate for 1 hour. Place 1 disk on a sheet of parchment paper on a work surface. Top with another sheet of parchment and roll to ½" thickness. Remove the top sheet of parchment. Place a shallow bowl of water on the work surface. Dip each cookie cutter into the water and cut into the dough. Place the cookies on the baking sheets. Gently knead the scraps of dough and reroll as needed. Bake for 12 minutes, or until lightly browned. Cool on a rack for 2 minutes. Remove the cookies to racks to cool completely. Repeat with the remaining dough.

If you prefer iced cookies, in a small bowl, combine 1 tablespoon softened cream cheese, 2 teaspoons heavy cream, and 1 teaspoon gluten-free, sugar-free maple syrup. Stir until smooth and creamy. Transfer to a small sandwich bag. With a scissors, snip off a small corner of the bag. Pipe designs on the completely cooled cookies and allow to set before storing between layers of parchment paper or waxed paper in an airtight container.

PER SERVING: 143 calories, 4 g protein, 7 g carbohydrates, 12 g total fat, 3 g saturated fat, 3 g fiber, 103 mg sodium

CHOCOLATE CHIP COOKIES

PREP TIME: 10 MINUTES | TOTAL TIME: 35 MINUTES

Makes 30

These Chocolate Chip Cookies are like the kind you buy at the bakery: rich and moist, with that just-baked taste you can't get in store-bought cookies. They are a bit of an indulgence, however, since they're rich in sugar-containing chocolate chips.

Try to use the darkest chocolate chips you can find to minimize sugar exposure. Using Hershey's Special Dark chocolate chips, each cookie will contain about 5 grams of carbohydrates, which can add up after a few cookies. By using the darkest chocolate chips you can find—or by making your own dark chocolate chunks by chopping dark chocolate (85% or greater cacao) into bite-size pieces—you can reduce carbohydrate exposure to about 2 to 3 grams per cookie.

4 cups almond meal/flour

1 teaspoon baking soda

½ teaspoon sea salt

4 eggs

½ cup butter or coconut oil, melted

¼ cup sour cream or coconut milk

2 teaspoons vanilla extract

½ teaspoon liquid stevia

10 ounces bittersweet or dark chocolate chips

Preheat the oven to 350°F. Line a baking sheet with parchment paper.

In a large bowl, whisk together the almond meal/flour, baking soda, and salt.

In a small bowl, whisk together the eggs, butter or coconut oil, sour cream or coconut milk, vanilla, and stevia. Stir into the flour mixture just until combined. Stir in the chips.

Drop by heaping tablespoons onto the baking sheet. Using a spoon or glass, press each cookie to ½" thickness.

Bake for 25 minutes, or until the edges are lightly browned. Remove to a rack to cool completely.

PER SERVING: 176 calories, 5 g protein, 8 g carbohydrates, 15 g total fat, 5 g saturated fat, 2 g fiber, 80 mg sodium

PEANUT BUTTER CHOCOLATE CHIP COOKIES

PREP TIME: 20 MINUTES | TOTAL TIME: 35 MINUTES

Makes 20

Tell the kids that these cookies are peanut butter cups disguised as cookies!

Cookies like these, rich in the healthy fats of peanuts and coconut, are surprisingly filling. They may go further than you think!

1½ cups almond meal/flour	1 cup milk
½ cup peanut flour	1 egg
1 teaspoon baking powder	2 teaspoons vanilla extract
½ teaspoon sea salt	½ teaspoon liquid stevia
1 cup natural, unsweetened peanut butter, at room temperature	1 cup bittersweet chocolate chips

Preheat the oven to 350°F. Line a baking sheet with parchment paper.

In a large bowl, whisk together the almond meal/flour, peanut flour, baking powder, and salt.

In a medium bowl, whisk together the peanut butter, milk, egg, vanilla, and stevia until smooth. Stir into the flour mixture just until combined. Stir in the chips.

Drop by heaping tablespoons onto the baking sheet. Using a spoon or glass, press each cookie to ½" thickness.

Bake for 15 minutes, or until the edges are lightly browned. Remove to a rack to cool completely.

Note: To prepare with stevia, omit the coconut flour and xylitol. Add ½ teaspoon liquid stevia and increase the milk to 1 cup.

PER SERVING: 203 calories, 7 g protein, 11 g carbohydrates, 16 g total fat, 4 g saturated fat, 3 g fiber, 146 mg sodium

ORANGE CREAM COOKIES

PREP TIME: 20 MINUTES | TOTAL TIME: 40 MINUTES

Makes 20

Remember the delightful combination of orange and cream you tasted in an ice cream pop as a kid? Well, these cookies will be reminiscent of that flavor, with the orange from orange peel and the creamy vanilla combination of vanilla extract and cream.

2 cups almond meal/flour

¾ cup xylitol or ¼ teaspoon liquid stevia or to desired sweetness

½ cup finely chopped pecans

¼ cup golden raisins

3 tablespoons shredded unsweetened coconut

1 tablespoon grated orange peel

1 teaspoon baking soda

¼ teaspoon sea salt

½ cup whipping cream or canned coconut milk

1 egg

2 tablespoons coconut oil, melted

1 tablespoon vanilla extract

Preheat the oven to 350°F. Line a baking sheet with parchment paper.

In a large bowl, combine the almond meal/flour, xylitol or stevia, pecans, raisins, coconut, orange peel, baking soda, and salt.

In a small bowl, whisk together the cream or coconut milk, egg, coconut oil, and vanilla. Stir into the flour mixture just until combined.

Drop by heaping tablespoons onto the baking sheet. Using a spoon or glass, press each cookie to ½" thickness. Bake for 18 minutes, or until golden. (Bake cookies prepared with stevia for 12 minutes.)

Remove to a rack to cool completely.

PER SERVING: 149 calories, 3 g protein, 12 g carbohydrates, 12 g total fat, 3 g saturated fat, 2 g fiber, 89 mg sodium

CHOCOLATE COCONUT ICE MILK

PREP TIME: 35 MINUTES | TOTAL TIME: 35 MINUTES + FREEZING TIME

Makes 7 servings (3½ cups)

This is a wheat- and dairy-free variation on an old favorite: chocolate chip ice cream.

1 **can (13.6 ounces) coconut milk**

⅓ **cup bittersweet chocolate chips, melted**

2 **tablespoons unsweetened cocoa powder**

1 **teaspoon natural vanilla liquor or vanilla extract**

⅛ **teaspoon liquid stevia**

In a large bowl, whisk together the coconut milk, melted chocolate, cocoa, vanilla, and stevia.

Pour into an ice cream maker and freeze according to the manufacturer's directions.

Serve immediately for soft-serve consistency or freeze for 2 hours for a firmer ice cream consistency.

PER SERVING (½ CUP): 168 calories, 2 g protein, 9 g carbohydrates, 15 g total fat, 13 g saturated fat, 2 g fiber, 8 mg sodium

PEACH ALMOND FROZEN YOGURT

PREP TIME: 25 MINUTES | **TOTAL TIME:** 50 MINUTES + CHILLING AND FREEZING TIME

Makes 8 servings (4 cups)

Roasting the peaches intensifies their flavor, making this dessert the quintessential summer treat.

2 medium peaches, pitted, peeled, and sliced into quarters

1 quart plain Greek yogurt

¼ teaspoon liquid stevia or ½ cup xylitol or to desired sweetness

2 teaspoons vanilla extract

½ teaspoon almond extract

½ cup sliced almonds, toasted, for garnish

Preheat the oven to 350°F.

In a glass baking dish, place the peaches. Roast for 20 minutes. Set aside to cool briefly. In a food processor or blender, puree until smooth. Refrigerate for 1 hour, or until completely cold.

In a large bowl, combine the yogurt, stevia or xylitol, vanilla, and almond extract and stir well. Pour into an ice cream maker and follow the manufacturer's directions. Toward the last few minutes of turning, pour in the peaches.

Remove and store in the freezer for at least 2 hours. Before serving, allow to soften for 10 minutes. Sprinkle with toasted almonds, if desired.

PER SERVING (½ CUP): 168 calories, 8 g protein, 7 g carbohydrates, 12 g total fat, 9 g saturated fat, 1 g fiber, 33 mg sodium

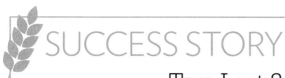

Tara Lost 8 Pounds

Me? I'm a gym rat. You'd think I'd be the world's fittest person. If there's a class, I take it—from yoga to water aerobics to cardio-training boot camps. I work out with a trainer, run about 50 kilometers a week, and hit the trails every chance I get.

But even though I was getting stronger, my belly was getting fatter. I kept taking more and more things out of my diet, and replacing "bad" foods with "healthy" ones like Bran Buds, Wasa crackers, and whole wheat bread.

So why was I so fat? I'd been steadily gaining weight since my thirties, going from a healthy 125 pounds all the way up to 155 this past Christmas—and I'm only 4 foot 11. When I started having terrible belly pains, I went to a surgeon to see if I had a hernia. The diagnosis, though, was a lot different: a torn pelvic-floor muscle due to overtraining at boot camp. The good news was that the doctor took the time to listen to me. When she heard that for years I'd been taking laxatives for chronic painful constipation, a red flag went up, and she insisted that I quit them cold turkey. Instead, she suggested, I should increase my fiber to 30 grams a day.

So I added more bran and whole grains, and 2 months later my regularity had improved, but my belly hurt from my ribs to my pelvis, and I was exhausted and filled with pain. So back to the surgeon I went. She was the first doctor—and I've been to lots of doctors—to suggest that I have a gluten sensitivity.

I started cutting back on all bread and pasta, but I thought that as long as it was brown, it was healthy. Was I wrong! Luckily, though, a friend told me about *Wheat Belly,* and I decided to give it a shot.

Since giving up wheat on my 45th birthday in March 2012, I've lost 8 pounds and 3 inches around my belly. My roly-poly back has smoothed out, and my jeans are loose. Best of all, I'm running like I'm 30 again, with energy to burn after my workout. And I go to sleep easily and wake up totally refreshed. I'm working hard at removing wheat from my home and getting my husband and kids off wheat, too.

I used to think that being gluten free was just another hippie health kick, but now I know better. For the first time in my life, I've found the key to good health.

APPENDIX A

Wheat, Wheat Everywhere

THE MOST CONFIDENT way to minimize your exposure to the Evil Grain is to focus on single-ingredient, natural foods. This includes vegetables such as spinach, kale, radicchio, and green peppers. It also includes fruits, poultry, beef, pork, fish, nuts, seeds, and dairy (preferably organic, unsweetened, unflavored). Single-ingredient natural foods have nothing to do with wheat or gluten unless, of course, somebody added it.

When you venture outside of single-ingredient natural foods, or eat in social situations, go to restaurants, or purchase prepared meals, then there is always going to be potential for inadvertent wheat and gluten exposure.

Inadvertent wheat and gluten exposure has real-world implications. Someone with celiac disease, for instance, may have to endure days to weeks of abdominal cramping, diarrhea, even intestinal bleeding from an inadvertent encounter with some wheat gluten on an unwashed knife used to cut her pork tenderloin. Even after the nasty rash of dermatitis herpetiformis heals, it can flare with just a dash of wheat-containing soy sauce. Or someone who experiences inflammatory neurological symptoms can experience abrupt decline in coordination

for weeks because the gluten-free beer really wasn't. For many others who don't have celiac disease or gluten sensitivity, accidental exposure to wheat can bring on ravenous hunger, diarrhea, asthma, mental "fog," joint pains or swelling, leg edema, emotional outbursts, the "high" of bipolar illness, or the paranoia of schizophrenia.

Many people therefore have to be vigilant about exposure to wheat. Those with celiac disease and its equivalents, including dermatitis herpetiformis, cerebellar ataxia, and peripheral neuropathy attributable to gluten exposure, as well as those with gluten sensitivity, also need to avoid other gluten-containing grains: rye, barley, spelt, triticale, kamut, bulgur, and oats. In addition, they need to be aware of the potential for cross-contamination, that is, potential gluten contamination from utensils, airborne particles, or liquids. If a food is labeled "gluten free," then it should have been prepared in a facility where cross-contamination should not have occurred. Cross-contamination is especially tricky when you order at restaurants; very few establishments have the ability to avoid cross-contamination, though this is just beginning to become available in some progressive restaurants.

In the list that follows, you will see that

wheat and gluten come in an incredible variety of forms, often hidden away in the form of some additive, thickener, or coating. Couscous, matzo, orzo, graham, and bran are all wheat. So are faro, panko, and rusk. Names and package appearances can be misleading. For instance, the majority of breakfast cereals contain wheat flour, wheat-derived ingredients, or gluten, despite names such as Corn Flakes or Rice Krispies.

Oats remain a topic of controversy, since oat products contain a glutenlike protein called avenin to which only a minority of people with celiac react (a phenomenon that is not currently testable outside research settings). Oat products are also often processed on the same equipment or in the same facility as wheat products, providing potential for cross-contamination. Most celiac sufferers therefore avoid oats as well. (Note that the absence of intestinal symptoms after consuming a food such as oats is *not* a reliable method of assessing safety; intestinal damage and other effects may not be perceived.) Anyway, oat products make your blood sugar skyrocket and, in my view, are awful for health. Heart healthy they are *not*.

To qualify as gluten free by FDA criteria, manufactured products (not restaurant-produced products) must be both free of gluten and produced in a gluten-free facility to prevent cross-contamination. The FDA's proposed cutoff for qualifying as "gluten free" is no more than 20 parts per million (ppm), the threshold for detection and the standard used in many other countries.

This means that, for the seriously sensitive, even an ingredient label that does not list wheat or any buzzwords for wheat such as "modified food starch" can *still* contain some measure of gluten. If in doubt, a call or e-mail to the customer service department may be necessary to inquire whether a gluten-free facility was used. Also, more manufacturers are starting to specify whether products are gluten free or not gluten free on their Web sites.

Note that wheat free does *not* equate with gluten free in food labeling. Wheat free can mean, for instance, that barley malt or rye is used in place of wheat, but both also contain gluten. It's important that those who are very gluten-sensitive, such as those with celiac, do not assume that wheat free is necessarily gluten free.

You already know that wheat and gluten can be found in abundance in obvious foods such as breads, pastas, and pastries. But there are some not-so-obvious foods that can contain wheat, as listed here.

Baguette

Barley

Beignet

Bran

Brioche

Bulgur

Burrito

Couscous

Crepe

Croutons

Durum

Einkorn

Emmer

Farina

Farro

Focaccia

Fu (gluten in Asian foods)

Gnocchi

Graham flour

Gravy

Hydrolyzed vegetable protein

Hydrolyzed wheat starch

Kamut

Matzo

Modified food starch

Orzo

Panko (bread crumbs used in Japanese cooking)

Ramen

Roux (wheat-based sauce or thickener)

Rusk

Rye

Seitan (nearly pure gluten used in place of meat)

Semolina

Soba (mostly buckwheat, but usually also includes wheat)

Spelt

Strudel

Tabbouleh

Tart

Textured vegetable protein

Triticale

Triticum

Udon

Vital wheat gluten

Wheat bran

Wheat germ

Wraps

Wheat-Containing Products

Wheat reflects the inventiveness of the human species, as we've transformed this grain into an incredible multitude of shapes and forms. Beyond the many configurations that wheat can take listed above, there is an even greater variety of foods that contain some measure of wheat or gluten. These are listed beginning on the next page.

Please keep in mind that, due to the extraordinary number and variety of products on the market, this list cannot include every possible wheat- and gluten-containing item. The key is to remain vigilant and ask—or walk away—whenever in doubt.

Many foods listed below also come in gluten-free versions. Some gluten-free versions are both tasty and healthy, such as vin-aigrette salad dressing without hydrolyzed vegetable protein. But bear in mind that the growing world of gluten-free breads, breakfast cereals, and flours, which are typically made with rice starch, cornstarch, potato starch, or tapioca starch, does *not* offer healthy substitutes. Nothing that generates diabetic-range blood sugar responses should be labeled "healthy," gluten free or otherwise. These products serve best as an occasional indulgence, not staples, if they are consumed *at all*. Note that nearly every food that can be created with the usual destructive junk carbohydrates of gluten-free ingredients can also be created with healthy ingredients, such as those used in the recipes in this cookbook.

There is also an entire world of stealth

sources of wheat and gluten that cannot be deciphered from the label. It's not uncommon for even manufacturers not to know if gluten is present, since they may purchase ingredients with uncertain gluten cross-contamination status. If the listed ingredients include nonspecific terms such as "starch," "emulsifiers," or "leavening agents," then the food contains gluten until proven otherwise.

There is also doubt surrounding the gluten content of some foods and ingredients, such as caramel coloring. Caramel coloring is the caramelized product of heated sugars that is nearly always made from corn syrup, but an occasional manufacturer makes it from a wheat-derived source. Such uncertainties are noted on the list below with a question mark beside the listing.

Not everybody needs to be extra vigilant about the minutest exposure to gluten. The listings that follow are simply meant to raise your awareness of just how ubiquitous wheat and gluten are, and provide a starting place for people who really *do* need to be extremely vigilant about their gluten exposure.

Here's a list of unexpected sources of wheat and gluten.

Beverages (also see Assembling Your Wheat Belly Kitchen on page 58)

Ales, beers, lagers
There are increasing numbers of gluten-free beers, such as Bard's, Green's, and Redbridge. Anheuser Buschs' Bud Lite is not gluten free, but is made from rice with only minor traces of barley gluten; it is therefore safe for anyone without celiac or gluten sensitivity who wishes to avoid the appetite-stimulating effect of wheat gliadin.

Bloody Mary mixes

Coffees, flavored

Herbal teas made with wheat, barley, or malt

Malt liquor

Teas, flavored

Vodkas distilled from wheat (Absolut, Grey Goose, Ketel One, SKYY, Stolichnaya) or other gluten-containing grains (Belvedere, Finlandia, Van Gogh)

Wine coolers (containing barley malt)

Whiskey distilled from wheat or barley (Jack Daniels, Bushmills, Jameson)

Breakfast cereals

Sometimes it's obvious: Shredded Wheat, Wheaties, Mini Wheats. However, there are many that do not feature wheat prominently yet still contain the Evil Grain. A simple rule: Avoid breakfast cereals altogether, even if free of wheat, as they are high in sugar and other junk carbohydrates like corn, puffed rice, and oats. The *only* safe breakfast cereals I know of are the ones you make yourself, such as the granola recipe provided in this cookbook.

Bran cereals (All Bran, Bran Buds, Raisin Bran)

Corn flakes (Corn Flakes, Crunchy Corn Bran, Frosted Flakes)

Cream of Wheat

Farina

Granola cereals

"Healthy" cereals (Grape-Nuts, Smart Start, Special K, Trail Mix Crunch)

Malt-O-Meal

Muesli, Mueslix

Oat bran

Oat cereals (Cheerios, Cracklin' Oat Bran, Honey Bunches of Oats)

Oatmeal

Popped corn cereals (Corn Pops)

Puffed rice cereals (Rice Krispies)

Cheese

Most cheeses are completely safe, but because cultures to ferment some cheeses, especially blue cheese and Roquefort, are grown on breads such as rye, they may not be strictly gluten free and can potentially present a gluten exposure risk.

Blue cheese

Cottage cheese (some)

Gorgonzola cheese

Roquefort

Coloring/fillers/texturizers/thickeners

These hidden sources can be among the most problematic, since they are often buried deep in the ingredient list or bear misleading names that suggest they have nothing to do with wheat or gluten. Unfortunately, there is often no way to tell from the label, nor will the manufacturer be able to tell you, since these ingredients are often produced by a supplier. A useful rule of thumb: Whenever possible, avoid processed foods that are likely to contain such ingredients.

Artificial colors

Artificial flavors

Caramel coloring

Caramel flavoring

Dextrimaltose

Emulsifiers

Hydrolyzed vegetable protein

Hydrolyzed wheat starch

Maltodextrin

Modified food starch

Stabilizers

Textured vegetable protein

Energy, protein, and meal replacement bars

With few exceptions, energy bars are essentially candy with a few healthy ingredients or health claims added. The list below cites bars that contain wheat/gluten. (See the bar recipes in this cookbook to understand how to make truly healthy energy bars.)

Clif Bars

Gatorade Pre-Game Fuel Nutrition bars

GNC Pro Performance bars

Kashi GoLean bars

Power Bars

Slim-Fast meal bars

Fast food

At many fast-food restaurants, the oil used to fry bread crumb–coated chicken patties may be the same oil used to fry french fries. Likewise, cooking surfaces may be shared. Foods you wouldn't ordinarily regard as containing wheat often do, such as scrambled eggs cooked on the same grill as pancakes or Taco Bell nacho chips and potato bites. Fast-food sauces, sausages, and burritos typically contain wheat or wheat-derived ingredients.

Foods that don't contain wheat or gluten are the rare exception at fast-food restaurants. It is therefore difficult, some say near impossible, to confidently obtain wheat- and gluten-free foods at these places. However, some chains, such as Subway, Arby's, Wendy's, and Chipotle Mexican Grill, confidently claim that many of their products are gluten free and/or offer a gluten-free menu. A word to the wise: Avoid fast-food restaurants whenever possible and don't chance it, especially if you have celiac disease or gluten sensitivity.

Meats, poultry, and fish

Meats, poultry, and fish, of course, are perfectly safe, whether or not the animal they came from was wheat free. However, manufacturers often add wheat-containing ingredients, usually to stretch out the quantity or modify texture or taste. Look for meats with the fewest ingredients, ideally only the meat itself. Note that deli meats sliced at the grocery or butcher shop are typically cross-contaminated by the equipment used to slice wheat-containing meats.

Breaded meats, poultry, fish

Canned meats

Chicken, self-basting

Deli meats (lunchmeats, salami)

Ham

Hamburger (if bread crumbs are added)

Hot dogs

Imitation bacon

Imitation crabmeat

Meatballs (if bread crumbs are added)

Pepperoni

Sausage

Turkey, self-basting

Miscellaneous

This can be a real problem area, since identifiable wheat- or gluten-containing ingredients may not be listed on product labels. A call to the manufacturer may be necessary.

Envelopes (glue)

Lip glosses and balms

Lipstick

Nutritional supplements
Many manufacturers will specify "gluten free" on the label.

Play-Doh

Prescription and over-the-counter medications
A useful online resource can be found at www.glutenfreedrugs.com, a listing maintained by a pharmacist.

Stamps (glue)

Sauces, salad dressings, condiments

Gravies thickened with wheat flour

Ketchup

Malt syrup

Malt vinegar

Marinades

Miso

Mustards containing wheat
(Simple mustards made with mustard seeds, vinegar, and salt are generally safe. Occasionally, a manufacturer will add a gluten-containing ingredient, such as wheat flour, beer, or malt vinegar, and these mustards should be avoided.)

Salad dressings

Soy sauce

Teriyaki sauce

Seasonings

Most herbs and seasonings have little potential for wheat/gluten exposure, except for these occasional exceptions:

Bacon bits, imitation

Curry powder

Seasoning mixes

Taco seasoning

Snacks and desserts

Cookies, crackers, and pretzels are obvious wheat-containing snacks. But there are plenty of not-so-obvious items.

Cake frosting

Candy bars

Chewing gum (powdered coating)

Chex mixes

Corn chips

Dried fruit (lightly coated with flour)

Dry roasted peanuts

Fruit fillings with thickeners

Granola bars

Ice cream (cookies and cream, Oreo Cookie, cookie dough, cheesecake, chocolate malt)

Ice cream cones

Jelly beans (not including Jelly Belly and Starburst)

Licorice

Nut bars

Pies

Potato chips (including Pringles)

Roasted nuts

Tiramisu

Tortilla chips, flavored

Trail mixes

Soups

Bisques

Broths, bouillon

Canned soups

Soup mixes

Soup stocks and bases

Soy and vegetarian products

Vegetarian "chicken" strips

Vegetarian chili

Vegetarian hot dogs and sausages

Vegetarian "scallops"

Vegetarian "steaks"

Veggie burgers (Boca Burgers, Gardenburgers, Morningstar Farms)

Sweeteners

Barley malt, barley extract

Dextrin and maltodextrin

Malt, malt flavoring, malt syrup

Wheat- and Gluten-Safe and *Healthy* Foods

Remember: Just because a food is free of wheat or gluten does *not* necessarily make it healthy. Table sugar and gumdrops are free of wheat and gluten, as is gluten-free multigrain bread made with tapioca, rice, and potato starch—but they are terribly unhealthy.

Gluten-free books and cookbooks lavish you with all the gluten-free flours and baked foods that you can make by replacing wheat with gluten-free baking mixes, or some combination of tapioca starch, rice starch, potato starch, or cornstarch. *This is a big mistake.* Yes, you lose the gluten, but you replace wheat and gluten with starches that are extravagant triggers of blood sugar, grow visceral fat, and contribute to diabetes, cataracts, and arthritis. So let me be absolutely clear on this: **Avoid gluten-free flours and foods made with junk carbohydrates like the plague!**

So here's a starting place for foods that won't expose you to the Evil Grain but also will fit into a healthy lifestyle, one that won't make you fat and diabetic (because I hate when that happens!). I don't list all the vegetables and fruits that are naturally free of wheat and gluten, as this should be fairly obvious.

Dairy Products

Few dairy products have added wheat or gluten. The notable exceptions are some cheeses, such as some cottage cheeses and Gorgonzola and blue cheeses, and yogurts flavored with granola, cookie fragments, nuts coated in wheat flour, or other added ingredients.

Buttermilk

Cream

Cream cheese

Greek yogurt, unsweetened, unflavored

Kefir, unsweetened, unflavored

Milk

Yogurt, unsweetened, unflavored

Fish and Shellfish

As with meats, when shopping for fish and shellfish, look for those without added ingredients, just plain fish and shellfish. You can be confident any saltwater or freshwater fish is free of wheat and gluten, provided no human has added it.

Catfish	**Oysters**
Clams	**Perch**
Cod	**Red snapper**
Crab	**Salmon**
Halibut	**Shrimp**
Lobster	**Squid**
Mahi mahi	**Trout**
Mussels	**Walleye**
Octopus	

Grains

It pains me to list *any* grains, but I have to admit that they are occasionally useful, despite the bad rap their mutated cousin, wheat, has brought to them. These non-wheat, nongluten grains may be useful, for instance, for people who are not carbohydrate intolerant (uncommon) or kids' dishes, since kids tolerate carbohydrates better than adults do.

Also, note that, while I list corn and rice, these grains are increasingly likely to be genetically modified and should be consumed cautiously, if at all.

Amaranth

Buckwheat

Corn

Millet

Quinoa

Rice, white and brown

Sorghum

Teff

Wild rice

Herbs and Spices

Single-ingredient fresh and dried herbs and spices are free of wheat and gluten.

Allspice	**Cardamom**
Anise	**Celery seed**
Basil	**Cilantro**
Bay leaf	**Cinnamon**
Caraway	**Clove**

Coriander	**Pepper, black, red, white**
Dill	
Fennel	**Rosemary**
Fenugreek	**Saffron**
Garlic	**Sage**
Marjoram	**Salt, sea salt**
Mint	**Star anise**
Mustard	**Tarragon**
Oregano	**Thyme**
Paprika	**Turmeric**
Parsley	**Wasabi**

Legumes

As with vegetables, fruits, and nuts, legumes will contain wheat or gluten only if someone put it there. Legumes are naturally free of wheat and gluten, but the baked beans in sauce may contain added wheat flour, as well as high-fructose corn syrup and sugar.

Black beans

Black-eyed peas

Carob

Chickpeas (also known as garbanzo beans)

Kidney beans

Lentils

Mesquite

Peanuts

Peas

Pinto beans

Red beans

Soybeans

Spanish beans

Vanilla, vanilla beans

Meats, Poultry, and Eggs

Meats without additives are your safest bet.

Beef

Buffalo

Chicken

Duck

Eggs, any variety

Elk

Lamb

Ostrich

Pheasant

Pork

Quail

Turkey

Nuts and Seeds

Raw nuts and seeds are free of wheat and gluten, as are dry roasted if nothing is added. Nuts and seeds with added ingredients, such as wheat flour and various starches, typical of mixed nuts, "party" mixes, and flavored nuts, should be avoided.

Almonds	**Pecans**
Brazil nuts	**Pistachios**
Cashews	**Pumpkin seeds**
Chia seeds	
Filberts	**Sesame seeds**
Flaxseeds	**Sunflower seeds**
Hazelnuts	
Peanuts	**Walnuts**

APPENDIX B

Wheat-Free Resources

THERE ARE PLENTY of resources available for people with celiac disease or gluten sensitivity. They are primarily useful to help identify hidden sources of gluten, locate restaurants and stores that sell gluten-free foods, and identify physicians familiar with the special needs of people who have celiac disease. Sources for such information are listed below.

Because *Wheat Belly* and the *Wheat Belly Cookbook* introduce the concept that wheat elimination is not just for people with celiac disease or gluten sensitivity, but is for *everyone*, the list of resources that target this larger audience is still limited, though it will undoubtedly grow rapidly as this concept catches on.

In the meantime, some resources for products, additional wheat-free recipes, and more information are listed below.

Nuts, Seeds, Nut Meals, and Flours

Sources for nuts, seeds, nut meals, and flours may be as close as your supermarket. However, it really pays to shop around, as prices vary widely (as much as sixfold—600 percent!). The most economical method is usually to grind nut meals and flours yourself in a food chopper, food processor, or coffee grinder. However, most major supermarkets and health food stores carry preground nut meals and flours. Seed meals are rarely sold preground but are very easy to grind from whole sesame, sunflower, chia, or pumpkin seeds.

Bob's Red Mill is a nationally distributed brand and an excellent source of high-quality (often organic) almond flour, coconut flour, garbanzo bean (chickpea) flour, and xanthan gum.

Trader Joe's is a very affordable source for nearly all the whole nuts and seeds you need. They also have ground almond meal for a great price. Whole Foods Market is another, though high-cost, source for most nuts, seeds, meals, and flours.

The online retailers below have extensive choices of nuts, seeds, and nut and seed flours and meals, including almond meal, almond flour, and chia.

www.nuts.com
www.ohnuts.com

Sweeteners

Start with your grocery store or health food store for liquid stevia, powdered stevia (pure stevia or made with inulin), or Truvía. Health food stores, in particular, typically have several choices of stevia, since it has been available for several years as a nutritional supplement.

Erythritol and xylitol are not always available in grocery stores. Check health food stores, but you may need to order online. Nuts.com carries xylitol, and Amazon carries several brands of xylitol and erythritol, including NOW, KAL, and Emerald Forest.

Shirataki Noodles

Bigger and better-stocked grocery stores will often carry shirataki noodles, though look for them in the refrigerated section, not on the pasta shelf. If not available in your grocery store, these noodles can be purchased online. Miracle and House Foods are two good brands.

Celiac Disease Resources

Here are additional resources for individuals with celiac disease or gluten sensitivity. They are useful for helping identify foods containing gluten, and some of these organizations maintain lists of restaurants that accommodate safe gluten-free eating. The Gluten Intolerance Group, for instance, maintains a list of gluten-free restaurants searchable by state or zip code. The Celiac Disease Foundation Web site also provides links to the Web sites of the various gluten-free food manufacturers. The Celiac Sprue Association provides a wealth of resources, including a phone-in hotline for members ($50 for a 2-year membership).

These organizations also provide support to restaurants and food manufacturers needing guidance on creating a gluten-free food preparation environment. The National Foundation for Celiac Awareness, for instance, offers a food service training program.

These organizations are supported by donations and product sales. However, buyer beware: Much of the revenue that supports these organizations comes from manufacturers of gluten-free foods. It means that they tend to steer you toward these products, which are best avoided entirely. Nonetheless, these organizations can serve as a useful starting place for more information relevant to celiac disease and gluten sensitivity.

Celiac Disease Foundation
www.celiac.org

Celiac Sprue Association
www.csaceliacs.info

Gluten Intolerance Group
www.gluten.net

National Foundation for Celiac Awareness
www.celiaccentral.org

Gluten-Free Prescription Drugs and Nutritional Supplements

This Web site, maintained by PhD pharmacist Steve Plogsted, is a good starting place to investigate the gluten content of prescription drugs.

With nutritional supplements, always check the label. Nutritional supplements are often labeled "gluten-free," as well as listing the absence of other potential undesirable components, such as lactose.

www.glutenfreedrugs.com

Additional Recipes

Cookbooks in the low-carbohydrate and "paleo" diets overlap to a great extent with the sorts of foods advocated in this cookbook. Their recipes are wheat free and focus on real food ingredients.

Just be careful: Some of the recipes in these cookbooks tend to use unhealthy sweeteners such as maple syrup, honey, and agave, or occasionally rely too heavily on "safe" starches like sweet potatoes or yams and rice. These carbohydrate sources are indeed safer than wheat and sugar, but they are not entirely healthy when consumed in larger quantities, such as more than a ½-cup serving.

Likewise, be careful with gluten-free cookbooks, as they often use unhealthy gluten-free replacements, such as rice starch, cornstarch, potato starch, tapioca starch, or premixed gluten-free flours. My advice: Never use these starches. Avoid the recipes that call for them, and select only the ones that do not use these gluten-free flours.

Web Sites

Stay-at-home mom turned wheat/gluten-free, low-carb recipe writer Carolyn Ket-chum provides great recipes accompanied by excellent photography.

www.alldayidreamaboutfood.com

Elana Amsterdam's beautiful and creative mostly almond flour–based recipes are featured on her Web site/blog, as well as in her cookbook listed in the next section.

www.elanaspantry.com

Formally trained in culinary arts, blogger Michelle provides great recipes that are free of wheat/gluten and corn.

www.glutenfreefix.com

Nutritionist Maria Emmerich is a wheat-free, limited-carbohydrate champion! She is among the few nutritionists who truly understand these important health concepts. The photography on her Web site is also stunningly beautiful. Maria's excellent cookbook is listed below.

www.mariahealth.blogspot.com

Books

The Art of Eating Healthy—Sweets: Grain Free Low Carb Reinvented, by Maria Emmerich (CreateSpace, 2011)

Everyday Paleo, by Sarah Fragoso (Victory Belt Publishing, 2011)

The G-Free Diet: A Gluten-Free Survival Guide, by Elisabeth Hasselbeck (Center Street, 2011)

The Gluten-Free Almond Flour Cookbook, by Elana Amsterdam (Celestial Arts, 2009)

The Gluten-Free Asian Kitchen: Recipes for Noodles, Dumplings, Sauces, and More, by Laura B. Russell (Celestial Arts, 2011)

The Gluten-Free Bible: The Thoroughly Indispensable Guide to Negotiating Life without Wheat, by Jax Peters Lowell (Holt Paperbacks, 2005)

The Gluten-Free Edge: Get Skinny the Gluten-Free Way! by Gini Warner and Chef Ross Harris (Adams Media, 2011)

Grain-Free Gourmet, by Jodi Bager and Jenny Lass (Whitecap Books Ltd., 2010)

The Healthy Gluten-Free Life: 200 Delicious Gluten-Free, Dairy-Free, Soy-Free and Egg-Free Recipes, by Tammy Credicott (Victory Belt Publishing, 2012)

Make It Paleo, by Bill Staley and Hayley Mason (Victory Belt Publishing, 2011)

1001 Low-Carb Recipes, by Dana Carpender (Fair Winds Press, 2010)

Paleo Comfort Foods, by Julie and Charles Mayfield (Victory Belt Publishing, 2011)

The Primal Blueprint Cookbook: Primal, Low Carb, Paleo, Grain-Free, Dairy-Free and Gluten-Free, by Mark Sisson (Primal Nutrition, 2010)

More *Wheat Belly* Resources

Wheat Belly: Lose the Wheat, Lose the Weight, and Find Your Path Back to Health (Rodale, 2011)

This is the original book, released in August 2011, that details all the reasons why humans have no business eating modern wheat.

The Wheat Belly Blog provides ongoing discussions about many issues relevant to wheat and living wheat free, as well as real stories of people who have discovered this lifestyle. I also post new recipes here.

Many articles, podcasts, and TV interviews are archived on the blog.

www.wheatbellyblog.com

Wheat-Free Research and Education Foundation

This is the organization I've helped establish that will, in the future, fund research, provide education, and help inform the public about the need to recognize the dangers of wheat consumption and the health benefits of ridding your life of it.

www.wheatfreeref.org

REFERENCES

Introduction

Duffey KJ, Popkin BM. Energy density, portion size, and eating occasions: Contributions to increased energy intake in the United States, 1977–2006. *PLoS Medicine* 2011 June;8(6):1001050.

Popkin BM, Duffey KJ. Does hunger and satiety drive eating anymore? Increasing eating occasions and decreasing time between eating occasions in the United States. *Am J Clin Nutr* 2010 May;91(5):1342–7.

Frankengrain

Alaedini A, Okamoto H, Briani C et al. Immune cross-reactivity in celiac disease: anti-gliadin antibodies bind to neuronal synapsin I. *J Immunol* 2007 May 15;178(10):6590–5.

Bardella MT, Fredella C, Prampolini L et al. Body composition and dietary intakes in adult celiac disease patients consuming a strict gluten-free diet. *Am J Clin Nutr* 2000 Oct;72(4):937–9.

Barera G, Mora S, Brambill P et al. Body composition in children with celiac disease and the effects of a gluten-free diet: a prospective case-control study. *Am J Clin Nutr* 2000 Jul;72(1):72–5.

Branum A, Lukacs S. Food allergy among U.S. children: Trends in prevalence and hospitalizations. *National Center for Health Statistics Data Brief.* 2008. Retrieved from http://www.cdc.gov/nchs/data/databriefs/db10.htm.

Bray GA. Medical consequences of obesity. *J Clin Endocrinol Metab* 2004 Jun;89(6):2583–9.

Castro-Antunes MM, Crovella S, Brandão LA et al. Frequency distribution of HLA DQ2 and DQ8 in celiac patients and first-degree relatives in Recife, northeastern Brazil. *Clinics* (Sao Paulo) 2011;66(2):227–31.

Centers for Disease Control, National Center for Health Statistics at http://www.cdc.gov/diabetes/statistics/incidence/fig1.htm.

Cheng J, Brar PS, Lee AR, Green PH. Body mass index in celiac disease: beneficial effect of a gluten-free diet. *J Clin Gastroenterol* 2010 April;44(4):267–71.

Cohen MR, Cohen RM, Pickar D, Murphy DL. Naloxone reduces food intake in humans. *Psychosomatic Med* 1985 March/April;47(2):132–8.

Cordain L. Cereal grains: Humanity's double-edged sword, in Simopoulous AP (ed), Evolutionary aspects of nutrition and health. *World Rev Nutr Diet* 1999;84:19–73.

Cordain L, Toohey L, Smith MJ, Hickey MS. Modulation of immune function by dietary lectins in rheumatoid arthritis. *Br J Nutr* 2000;83:207–17.

Dickey W, Kearney N. Overweight in celiac disease: prevalence, clinical characteristics, and effect of a gluten-free diet. *Am J Gastroenterol* 2006 Oct;101(10):2356–9.

Drewnowski A, Krahn DD, Demitrack MA et al. Naloxone, an opiate blocker, reduces the consumption of sweet high-fat foods in obese and lean female binge eaters. *Am J Clin Nutr* 1995;61:1206–12.

Dubcovsky J, Dvorak J. Genome plasticity a key factor in the success of polyploidy wheat under domestication. *Science* 2007 June 29;316:1862–6.

Duffey KJ, Popkin BM. Energy density, portion size, and eating occasions: contributions to increased energy intake in the United States, 1977–2006. *PLoS Med* 2011 June;8(6):e1001050.

Espinosa JF, Asensio JL, Garcia JL et al. NMR investigations of protein-carbohydrate interactions: Binding studies and refined three-dimensional solution structure of the complex between the B domain of wheat germ agglutinin and N,N',N''-triacetylchitotriose. *Eur J Biochem* 2000;267:3965–78.

Gao X, Liu SW, Sun Q, Xia GM. High frequency of HMW-GS sequence variation through somatic hybridization between *agropyron elongatum* and common wheat. *Planta* 2010 Jan;23(2):245–50.

Gosnell BA, Levine AS. Reward systems and food intake: role of opioids. *Int J Obes (Lond)* 2009 Jun;33 Suppl 2:S54–8.

Greene WC, Goldman CK, Marshall ST et al. Stimulation of immunoglobulin biosynthesis in human B cells by wheat germ agglutinin. 1. Evidence that WGA can produce both a positive and negative signal for activation of human lymphocytes. *J Immunol* 1981 Aug;127(2):799–804.

Greenway FL, Fujioka K, Plodkowski RA et al. Effect of naltrexone plus bupropion on weight loss in overweight and obese adults (COR-I): a multicentre, randomised, double-blind, placebo-controlled, phase 3 trial. *Lancet* 2010 Aug 21;376(9741):595–605.

Grün F, Blumberg B. Minireview: the case for obesogens. *Mol Endocrinol* 2009 Aug;23(8): 1127–34.

Krupicková S, Tucková L, Flegelová Z et al. Identification of common epitopes on gliadin, enterocytes, and calreticulin recognised by antigliadin antibodies of patients with coeliac disease. *Gut* 1999 Feb;44(2):168–73.

Larré C, Lupi R, Gombaud G et al. Assessment of allergenicity of diploid and hexaploid wheat genotypes: Identification of allergens in the albumin/globulin fraction. *J Proteomics* 2011 Aug 12;74(8):1279–89.

Livingston JN, Purvis BJ. The effects of wheat germ agglutinin on the adipocyte insulin receptor. *Biochim Biophys Acta* 1981 Dec;678(2):194–201.

Lorenzsonn V, Olsen WA. In vivo responses of rat intestinal epithelium to intraluminal dietary lectins. *Gastroenterol* 982;82: 838–48.

Magaña-Gómez JA, Calderón de la Barca AM. Risk assessment of genetically modified crops for nutrition and health. *Nutr Rev* 2009;67(1):1–16.

Marriott BP, Cole N, Lee E. National estimates of dietary fructose intake increased from 1977 to 2004 in the United States. *J Nutr* 2009 Jun;139(6):1228S–35S.

Molberg Ø, Uhlen AK, Jensen T et al. Mapping of gluten T-cell epitopes in the bread wheat ancestors: implications for celiac disease. *Gastroenterol* 2005;128:393–401.

Murray JA, Watson T, Clearman B, Mitros F. Effect of a gluten-free diet on gastrointestinal symptoms in celiac disease. *Am J Clin Nutr* 2004 Apr;79(4):669–73.

Nachbar MS, Oppenheim JD. Lectins in the United States diet: a survey of lectins in commonly consumed foods and a review of the literature. *Am J Clin Nutr* 1980 Nov;33:2338–45.

Pastorello EA, Farioli L, Conti A et al. Wheat IgE-mediated food allergy in European patients: alpha-amylase inhibitors, lipid transfer proteins and low-molecular-weight glutenins. Allergenic molecules recognized by double-blind, placebo-controlled food challenge. *Int Arch Allergy Immunol* 2007;144(1):10–22.

Pearce S, Saville R, Vaughan S et al. Molecular characterization of *Rht-1* dwarfing genes in hexaploid wheat. *Plant Physiol* 2011 Dec;157:1820–31.

Peumans WJ, Stinissen HM, Carlier AR. A genetic basis for the origin of six different isolectins in hexaploid wheat. *Planta* 1982;154(6):562–7.

Pusztai A, Ewen SW, Grant G et al. Antinutritive effects of wheat-germ agglutinin and other N-acetylglucosamine-specific lectins. *Br J Nutr* 1993 Jul;70(1):313–21.

Rice RH. Wheat germ agglutinin. Evidence for a genetic basis of multiple forms. *Biochim Biophys Acta* 1976 Aug 24;444(1):175–80.

Rojas E, Llinas P, Rodriguez-Romero A et al. Hevein, an allergenic lectin from rubber latex, activates human neutrophils' oxidative burst. *Glyconj J* 2001 Apr;18(4):339–45.

Rubio-Tapia A, Kyle RA, Kaplan E et al. Increased prevalence and mortality in undiagnosed celiac disease. *Gastroenterol* 2009 July;137(1):88–93.

Sabelli P, Shewry PM. Characterization and organization of gene families at the *Gli-1* loci of bread and durum wheat by restriction fragment analysis. *Theor Appl Genet* 1991;83:209–16.

Sapone A, Lammers KM, Casolaro V et al. Divergence of gut permeability and mucosal immune gene expression in two gluten-associated conditions: celiac disease and gluten sensitivity. *BMC Med* 2011 Mar 9;9:23.

Sestili F, Janni M, Doherty A et al. Increasing the amylose content of durum wheat through silencing of the SBEIIa genes. *BMC Plant Biol* 2010 Jul 14;10:144.

Shan L, Molberg Ø, Parrot I et al. Structural basis for gluten intolerance in celiac sprue. *Science* 2002 Sep 27;297(5590):2275–9.

Shewry PR. Wheat. *J Exp Bot* 2009;60(6):1537–53.

Shewry PR, Halford NG, Belton PS, Tatham AS. The structure and properties of gluten: an elastic protein from wheat grain. *Phil Trans Roy Soc London* 2002;357:133–42.

Sibbitt LD. The quality of some semidwarf and conventional height hard red spring wheat varieties. *N Dak Farm Res* 1971 Jan/Feb;28(3):8–13.

Sjolander A, Magnusson KE, Latkovic S. Morphological changes of rat small intestine after short-time exposure to concanavalin A or wheat germ agglutinin. *Cell Struct Func* 1986;11:285–93.

Slattery CJ, Kavakli IH, Okita TW. Engineering starch for increased quantity and quality. *Trends in Plant Science* 2000;5:291–8.

Smecuol E, Gonzalez D, Mautalen C et al. Longitudinal study on the effect of treatment on body composition and anthropometry of celiac disease patients. *Am J Gastroenterol* 1997 April;92(4):639–43.

Sollid LM, Kolberg J, Scott H et al. Antibodies to wheat germ agglutinin in coeliac disease. *Clin Exp Immunol* 1986;63:95–100.

Song X, Ni Z, Yao Y et al. Identification of differentially expressed proteins between hybrid and parents in wheat (*Triticum aestivum L.*) seedling leaves. *Theor Appl Genet* 2009 Jan;118(2):213–25.

Stanhope KL. Role of fructose-containing sugars in the epidemics of obesity and metabolic syndrome. *Annu Rev Med* 2012;63:329–43.

Tchernychev B, Wilchek M. Natural human antibodies to dietary lectins. *FEBS Lett* 1996 Nov 18;397(2–3):139–42.

Tjon JM, van Bergen J, Koning F. Celiac disease: how complicated can it get? *Immunogenetics* 2010 Oct;62(10):641–51.

Van den Broeck HC, de Jong HC, Salentijn EMJ et al. Presence of celiac disease epitopes in modern and old hexaploid wheat varieties: wheat breeding may have contributed to increased prevalence of celiac disease. *Theor Appl Genet* 2010;121:1527–39.

Vasil V, Srivastava V, Castillo AM et al. Rapid production of transgenic wheat plants by direct bombardment of cultured immature embryos. *Biotechnology* 1993;11:1553–8.

Venkatasubramani N, Telega G, Werlin SL. Obesity in pediatric celiac disease. *J Pediat Gastroenterol Nutr* 2010 Sep;51(3):295–7.

Wadden TA, Foreyt JP, Foster GD et al. Weight loss with naltrexone SR/bupropion SR combination therapy as an adjunct to behavior modification: the COR-BMOD trial. *Obesity* (Silver Spring) 2011 Jan;19(1):110–20.

Wang JR, Wei YM, Yan ZH, Zheng YL: Detection of single nucleotide polymorphisms in the 24 kDa dimeric α-amylase inhibitors from cultivated wheat and its diploid putative progenitors. *Biochem Biophys Acta* 2005;1723(1–3):309–20.

Wright CS, Raikhel N. Sequence variability in three wheat germ agglutinin isolectins: products of multiple genes in polyploidy wheat. *J Mol Evol* 1989 Apr;28(4):327–36.

Zhao XL, Xia XC, He ZH et al. Characterization of three low-molecular-weight Glu-D3 subunit genes in common wheat. *Theor Appl Genet* 2006 Nov;113(7):1247–59.

Zioudrou C, Streaty RA, Klee WA. Opioid peptides derived from food proteins. The exorphins. *J Biol Chem* 1979 Apr 10;254(7):2446–9.

Why Does My Stomach Hurt?

Behall KM, Scholfield DJ, Hallfrisch J. The effect of particle size of whole-grain flour on plasma glucose, insulin, glucagon and thyroid-stimulating hormone in humans. *J Am Coll Nutr* December 1999;18(6):591–7.

Biesiekierski JR, Newnham ED, Irving PM et al. Gluten causes gastrointestinal symptoms in subjects without celiac disease: a double-blind randomized placebo-controlled trial. *Am J Gastroenterol* 2011 Mar;106(3):508–14.

Briani C, Samaroo D, Alaedini A. Celiac disease: from gluten to autoimmunity. *Autoimmun Rev* 2008 Sep;7(8):644–50.

Centers for Disease Control, 2011 National Diabetes Fact Sheet at http://www.cdc.gov/diabetes/pubs/references11.htm.

Cermak SA, Curtin C, Bandini LG. Food selectivity and sensory sensitivity in children with autism spectrum disorders. *J Am Diet Assoc* 2010 Feb;110(2):238–46.

Chiu CJ, Liu S, Willett WC et al. Informing food choices and health outcomes by use of the dietary glycemic index. *Nutr Rev* 2011 Apr;69(4):231–42.

DeNarci VG, Johnson MS, Whaley-Connell AT, Sowers JR. Cytokine abnormalities in the etiology of the cardiometabolic syndrome. *Curr Hypertens Rep* 2010 Apr;12(2):93–8.

Dickerson F, Stallings C, Origoni A et al. Markers of gluten sensitivity in acute mania: A longitudinal study. *Psychiatry Res* 2012 Mar 2 [Epub ahead of print].

Dohan FC. Coeliac disease and schizophrenia. *Brit Med J* 1973 July 7;51–2.

Duffey KJ, Popkin BM. Energy density, portion size, and eating occasions: contributions to increased energy intake in the United States, 1977–2006. *PLoS Med* 2011 June;8(6):e1001050.

Eisenmann A, Murr C, Fuchs D et al. Gliadin IgG antibodies and circulating immune complexes. *Scand J Gastroenterol* 2009;44(2):168–71.

Fasano A, Berti I, Gerarduzzi T et al. Prevalence of celiac disease in at-risk and not-at-risk groups in the United States: a large multicenter study. *Arch Intern Med* 2003 Feb 10;163(3):286–92.

Flegal KM, Carroll MD, Ogden CL, Curtin LR. Prevalence and trends in obesity among US adults, 1999–2008. *JAMA* 2010;303(3):235–41.

Garrote JA, Gómez-González E, Bernardo D et al. Celiac disease pathogenesis: the proinflammatory cytokine network. *J Pediatr Gastroenterol Nutr* 2008 Aug;47 Suppl 1:S27–32.

Green PH. The many faces of celiac disease: clinical presentation of celiac disease in the adult population. *Gastroenterol* 2005 Apr;128(4 Suppl 1):S74–8.

Hadjivassiliou M, Grunewald R, Davies-Jones G. Gluten sensitivity as a neurological illness. *J Neurol Neurosurg Psychiatry* 2002 May;72(5):560–3.

Hadjivassiliou M, Sanders DS, Grünewald RA et al. Gluten sensitivity: from gut to brain. *Lancet* 2010 March;9:318–30.

Harpoer E, Moses H, Lagrange A. Occult celiac disease presenting as epilepsy and MRI changes that responded to gluten-free diet. *Neurology* 2007;68:533.

Hu WT, Murray JA, Greenaway MC et al. Cognitive impairment and celiac disease. *Arch Neurol* 2006 Oct;63(10):1440–6.

Humbert P, Pelletier F, Dreno B et al. Gluten intolerance and skin diseases. *Eur J Dermatol* 2006 Jan–Feb;16(1):4–11.

Jönsson T, Olsson S, Ahrén B et al. Agrarian diet and diseases of affluence—do evolutionary novel dietary lectins cause leptin resistance? *BMC Endocr Disord* 2005 Dec 10;5:10.

Knivsberg AM, Reichelt KL, Hoien T, Nodland M. A randomized, controlled study of dietary intervention in autistic syndromes. *Nutr Neurosci* 2002;5:251–61.

Lamarche B, Lemieux I, Després JP. The small, dense LDL phenotype and the risk of coronary heart disease: epidemiology, patho-physiology and therapeutic aspects. *Diabetes Metab* 1999 Sept;25(3):199–211.

Lee Y, Pratley RE. Abdominal obesity and cardiovascular disease risk: the emerging role of the adipocyte. *J Cardiopulm Rehab Prev* 2007;27:2–10.

Lohi S, Mustalahti K, Kaukinen K et al. Increasing prevalence of celiac disease over time. *Aliment Pharmacol Ther* 2007;26:1217–25.

Ludvigsson JF, Montgomery SM, Ekbom A et al. Small-intestinal histopathology and mortality risk in celiac disease. *JAMA* 2009 Sep 16;302(11):1171–8.

Mavroudi A, Karatza E, Papastravrou T et al. Successful treatment of epilepsy and celiac disease with a gluten-free diet. *Pediatr Neurol* 2005;33:292–5.

Niederhofer H, Pittschieler K. A preliminary investigation of ADHD symptoms in persons with celiac disease. *J Atten Disord* 2006 Nov;10(2):200–4.

Rubio-Tapia A, Kyle RA, Kaplan E et al. Increased prevalence and mortality in undiagnosed celiac disease. *Gastroenterol* 2009 July;137(1):88–93.

Ruuskanan A, Luostarinen L, Collin P et al. Persistently positive gliadin antibodies without transglutaminase antibodies in the elderly: gluten intolerance beyond coeliac disease. *Dig Liver Dis* 2011 Oct;43(10):772–8.

Stalenhoef AF, de Graaf JH. Association of fasting and nonfasting serum triglycerides with cardiovascular disease and the role of remnant-like lipoproteins and small dense LDL. *Curr Opin Lipidol* 2008;19:355–61.

Sturm R. Increases in clinically severe obesity in the United States, 1986–2000. *Arch Intern Med* 2003 Oct 13;163(18):2146–8.

Vlissides DN, Venulet A, Jenner FA. A double-blind gluten-free/gluten-load controlled trial in a secure ward population. *Br J Psych* 1986;148:447–52.

Volta U, Tovoli F, Cicola R et al. Serological tests in gluten sensitivity (nonceliac gluten intolerance). *J Clin Gastroenterol* 2011 Dec 5 [Epub ahead of print].

Yeomans MR, Gray RW. Opioid peptides and the control of human ingestive behaviour. *Neurosci Biobehav Rev* 2002 Oct;26(6):713–28.

Zarkadas M, Cranney A, Case S et al. The impact of a gluten-free diet on adults with coeliac disease: results of a national survey. *J Hum Nutr Diet* 2006 Feb;19(1):41–9.

Zioudrou C, Streaty RA, Klee WA. Opioid peptides derived from food proteins. The exorphins. *J Biol Chem* 1979 Apr 10;254(7):2446–9.

Welcome to the Wonderful State of Wheatlessness

Allan K, Devereux G. Diet and asthma: nutrition implications from prevention to treatment. *J Am Diet Assoc* 2011 Feb;111(2):258–68.

Barera G, Bonfanti R, Viscardi M et al. Occurrence of celiac disease after onset of type 1 diabetes: a 6-year prospective longitudinal study. *Pediatrics* 20021;109:833–8.

Boyle JP, Thompson TJ, Gregg EW et al. Projection of the year 2050 burden of diabetes in the US adult population: dynamic modeling of incidence, mortality, and prediabetes prevalence. *Population Health Metrics* 2010;8:29, doi:10.1186/1478-7954-8-29.

Buschard K. What causes type 1 diabetes? Lessons from animal models. *APMIS Suppl* 2011 Jul;132:1–19. doi:10.1111/j.1600-0463.2011.02765.x.

Cermak SA, Curtin C, Bandini LG. Food selectivity and sensory sensitivity in children with autism spectrum disorders. *J Am Diet Assoc* 2010 Feb;110(2):238–46.

Cooke W, Smith W. Neurological disorders associated with adult coeliac disease. *Brain* 1966;89:683–722.

Corazza GR, Andreani ML, Venturo N et al. Celiac disease and alopecia areata: report of a new association. *Gastroenterol* 1995 Oct;109(4):1333–7.

Cordain L, Lindeberg S, Hurtado M et al. Acne vulgaris: A disease of Western Civilization. *Arch Dermatol* 2002 Dec;138:1584–90.

Dickerson F, Stallings C, Origoni A et al. Markers of gluten sensitivity and celiac disease in bipolar disorder. *Bipolar Disord* 2011 Feb;13(1):52–8. doi: 10.1111/j.1399-5618.2011.00894.x.

Dohan FC. Coeliac disease and schizophrenia. *Brit Med J* 1973 July 7;51–2.

Hadjivassiliou M, Davies-Jones G, Sanders DS, Grünewald RA. Dietary treatment of gluten ataxia. *J Neurol Neurosurg Psychiatry* 2003;74:1221–4.

Hadjivassiliou M, Sanders DS, Grünewald RA et al. Gluten sensitivity: from gut to brain. *Lancet* 2010 March;9:318–30.

Hafström I, Ringertz B, Spångberg A et al. A vegan diet free of gluten improves the signs and symptoms of rheumatoid arthritis: the effects on arthritis correlate with a reduction in antibodies to food antigens. *Rheumatol* 2001;1175–9.

Hansen AK, Ling F, Kaas A et al. Diabetes preventive gluten-free diet decreases the number of caecal bacteria in non-obese diabetic mice. *Diabetes Metab Res Rev* 2006;22:220–5.

Hansen D, Bennedbaek FN, Hansen LK et al. High prevalence of celiac disease in Danish children with type 1 diabetes mellitus. *Acta Paediatr* 2001 Nov;90(11):1238–43.

Hiraiwa H, Sakai T, Mitsuyama H et al. Inflammatory effect of advanced glycation end products on human meniscal cells from osteoarthritic knees. *Inflamm Res* 2011 Nov;60(11):1039–48.

Hu WT, Murray JA, Greenway MC et al. Cognitive impairment and celiac disease. *Arch Neurol* 2006;63:1440–6.

Knivsberg AM, Reichelt KL, Hoien T, Nodland M. A randomized, controlled study of dietary intervention in autistic syndromes. *Nutr Neurosci* 2002;5:251–61.

Mavroudi A, Karatza E, Papastravrou T et al. Successful treatment of epilepsy and celiac disease with a gluten-free diet. *Pediatr Neurol* 2005;33:292–5.

Millward C, Ferriter M, Calver S et al. Gluten- and casein-free diets for autistic spectrum disorder. *Cochrane Database Syst Rev* 2008 Apr 16;(2):CD003498.

Niederhofer H, Pittschieler K. A preliminary investigation of ADHD symptoms in persons with celiac disease. *J Atten Disord* 2006 Nov;10(2):200–4.

Nousia-Arvanitakis S, Fotoulaki M, Tendzidou K et al. Subclinical exocrine pancreatic dysfunction resulting from decreased cholecystokinin secretion in the presence of intestinal villous atrophy. *J Pediatr Gastroenterol Nutr* 2006 Sep;43(3):307–12.

Peltola M, Kaukinen K, Dastidar P et al. Hippocampal sclerosis in refractory temporal lobe epilepsy is associated with gluten sensitivity. *J Neurol Neurosurg Psychiatry* 2009 Jun;80(6):626–30.

Sanz Y, Santacruz A, Gauffin P. Gut microbiota in obesity and metabolic disorders. *Proc Nutr Soc* 2010 Aug;69(3):434–41.

Smith RN, Mann NJ, Braue A et al. A low-glycemic–load diet improves symptoms in acne vulgaris patients: a randomized controlled trial. *Am J Clin Nutr* 2007 Jul;86(1):107–15.

Tjellström B, Stenhammar L, Högberg L et al. Gut microflora associated characteristics in children with celiac disease. *Am J Gastroenterol* 2005 Dec;100(12):2784–8.

Toda Y, Toda T, Takemura S et al. Change in body fat, but not body weight or metabolic correlates of obesity, is related to symptomatic relief of obese patients with knee osteoarthritis after a weight control program. *J Rheumatol* 1998 Nov;25(11):2181–6.

Westman EC, Yancy WS Jr, Mavropoulos JC et al. The effect of a low-carbohydrate, ketogenic diet versus a low-glycemic index diet on glycemic control in type 2 diabetes mellitus. *Nutr Metab (London)* 2008 Dec 19;5:36.

Whiteley P, Haracopos D, Knivsberg AM et al. The ScanBrit randomised, controlled, single-blind study of a gluten- and casein-free dietary intervention for children with autism spectrum disorders. *Nutr Neurosci* 2010 Apr;13(2):87–100.

Assembling Your Wheat Belly Kitchen

Abou-Donia MB, El-Masry EM, Abdel-Rahman AA et al. Splenda alters gut microflora and increases intestinal p-glycoprotein and cytochrome p-450 in male rats. *J Toxicol Environ Health A* 2008;71(21):1415–29.

Allayee H, Roth N, Hodis HN. Polyunsaturated fatty acids and cardiovascular disease: implications for nutrigenetics. *J Nutrigenet Nutrigenomics* 2009;2(3):140–8.

Astrup A, Dyerberg J, Elwood P et al. The role of reducing intakes of saturated fat in the prevention of cardiovascular disease: where does the evidence stand in 2010? *Am J Clin Nutr* 2011 Apr;93(4):684–8.

Cattaneo A, Ballabio C, Bertelli AA et al. Evaluation of residual immunoreactivity in red and white wines clarified with gluten or gluten derivatives. *Int J Tissue React* 2003;25(2):57–64.

Knekt P, Järvinen R, Dich J et al. Risk of colorectal and other gastro-intestinal cancers after exposure to nitrate, nitrite and N-nitroso compounds: a follow-up study. *Int J Cancer* 1999 Mar 15;80(6):852–6.

Lang IA, Galloway TS, Scarlett A et al. Association of urinary bisphenol A concentration with medical disorders and laboratory abnormalities in adults. *JAMA* 2008;300(11):1303–10.

Marchioli R, Barzi F, Bomba E et al. Early protection against sudden death by n-3 polyunsaturated fatty acids after myocardial infarction: time-course analysis of the results of the Gruppo Italiano per lo Studio della Sopravvivenza nell'Infarto Miocardico (GISSI)-Prevenzione. *Circulation* 2002 Apr 23;105(16):1897–903.

Mozaffarian D, Aro A, Willett WC. Health effects of trans-fatty acids: experimental and observational evidence. *Eur J Clin Nutr* 2009 May;63 Suppl 2:S5–21.

Natah SS, Hussien KR, Tuominen JA et al. Metabolic response to lactitol and xylitol in healthy men. *Am J Clin Nutr* 1997 Apr;65(4):947–50.

Nilsson M, Stenberg M, Frid AH et al. Glycemia and insulinemia in healthy subjects after lactose-equivalent meals of milk and other food proteins: the role of plasma amino acids and incretins. *Am J Clin Nutr* 2004 Nov;80(5):1246–53.

Paik DC, Saborio DV, Oropeza R, Freeman HP. The epidemiological enigma of gastric cancer rates in the US: was grandmother's sausage the cause? *Int J Epidemiol* 2001 Feb;30(1):181–2.

Siener R, Ehrhardt C, Bitterlich N et al. Effect of a fat spread enriched with medium-chain triacylglycerols and a special fatty acid-micronutrient combination on cardiometabolic risk factors in overweight patients with diabetes. *Nutr Metab (Lond)* 2011 Apr 8;8:21.

Simonato B, Mainente F, Tolin S et al. Immunochemical and mass spectrometry detection of residual proteins in gluten fined red wine. *J Agric Food Chem* 2011 Apr 13;59(7):3101–10.

Siri-Tarino PW, Sun Q, Hu FB et al. Saturated fat, carbohydrate, and cardiovascular disease. *Am J Clin Nutr* 2010 Mar;91(3):502–9.

Stanhope KL, Schwarz JM, Keim NL et al. Consuming fructose-sweetened, not glucose-sweetened, beverages increases visceral adiposity and lipids and decreases insulin sensitivity in overweight/obese humans. *J Clin Invest* 2009 May;119(5):1322–34. doi:10.1172/JCI37385.

Uribarri J, Woodruff S, Goodman S et al. Advanced glycation end products in foods and a practical guide to their reduction in the diet. *J Am Diet Assoc* 2010 Jun;110(6):911–16.

Urpi-Sarda M, Casas R, Chiva-Blanch G et al. Virgin olive oil and nuts as key foods of the Mediterranean diet effects on inflammatory biomarkers related to atherosclerosis. *Pharmacol Res* 2012 Mar 18 [Epub ahead of print].

ACKNOWLEDGMENTS

THE RELEASE OF the original *Wheat Belly* created a huge and largely unmet need for practical solutions and, yes, recipes to successfully follow this new path for health. The clamoring for better wheat-free food ideas and recipes therefore led to this cookbook. In fact, the demand was so great that we completed this project in record time. I am therefore deeply grateful to all the people who came together to create this project.

No one person could have accomplished what is contained herein without plenty of help. My editor at Rodale, Anne Egan, took this cookbook project head-on, acting as coach and quarterback, helping me organize the considerable effort required to create, modify, and test all these unique recipes. Anne brought her extensive experience of having helped to create dozens of cookbooks and thousands of recipes over her career, offering suggestions to better craft these unique creations sans wheat. This finished cookbook project is largely due to Anne's skillful guidance. Thank you, Anne!

I could not have completed this cookbook project on such an ambitious timeline without the tireless assistance of the wonderful professionals in the Rodale Test Kitchen. My grateful thanks therefore go to Annie De Walt, Jennifer Kushnier, and Test Kitchen Director JoAnn Brader, who tested and retested these recipes until we got them right. This was no small matter! As readers can readily see, we've re-created familiar dishes by removing unhealthy ingredients and putting new ingredients to work, disrupting many of the basic rules of cooking and baking that food professionals are accustomed to following. Because these changes modify the performance of the overall recipe—more or less liquid, gain some new ingredients, lose some old, novel techniques required to generate "rise" and viscoelasticity in breads, changes in cooking time, etc.—all of them had to be tested to ensure proper recipe performance. Nonetheless, we tackled this cookbook project and accomplished it faster than I thought possible. I could never have gotten this project done in such an ambitiously short time without their help. Thank you!

My agent and friend, Rick Broadhead, has seen me through the entire *Wheat Belly* effort. Rick has proven to be a valuable ally with his unfailing support and incredible eye for detail. Rick is a professional in every sense, bringing his deep experience as author as well as agent. My gratitude for Rick's support and guidance is boundless.

Besides owing her many thanks for bearing all the home and family burdens that I neglected during this project, I owe my wife, Dawn, an additional thank-you for allowing me to bring a tsunami of cooking activity into our kitchen while she continued to prepare our everyday meals. And her discerning palate helped me refine many of these recipes, as she, better than anyone else I know, is one of those people who can identify all the individual flavors amidst the clamor of tastes and scents in a dish. And thanks, too, for helping me eat both my successes and my failures!

All the followers of Wheat Belly social media and online discussions at the Wheat Belly Blog (www.wheatbellyblog.com) and elsewhere deserve a big thank-you, because they provided the stories and discussions that revealed the tremendous demand for recipes consistent with the Wheat Belly approach. These discussions reflect how the Wheat Belly message is being received and put to work worldwide. These are the people showing us how to accomplish wheatlessness in unique and faraway places, as well as in neighborhoods throughout North America. They are also the people who remind me every day just how far-reaching and important this message is to the health of billions of people. This project would never have gotten its start without the wonderful support of readers and viewers worldwide.

INDEX

Underscored page references indicate boxed text and tables. An asterisk (*) indicates that photographs appear in the color insert pages.

Coronary heart disease, cause of, 26
Cough, chronic, wheat-free diet relieving, 51
Crackers
    Flaxseed Crackers, 241
Cramps, 14, 31, 32, 47, 50, 51. *See also*
        Gastrointestinal problems
Cranberries
    Cranberry Cinnamon Scones, 249
Cravings, food, wheat-free diet eliminating, 27,
        152, 169, 210
Cream
    Orange Cream Cookies, 278
Cream of tartar, 79
Crepes
    Crepes with Ricotta and Strawberries, 100
Crohn's disease, 31, 35, 47–48
Cross-contamination
    avoiding, 62, 64, 77
    in restaurant food preparation, 61, 65, 282
Croutons
    avoiding, in restaurants, 61
    Caesar Salad with Wheat-Free Croutons, 135
Cucumbers
    Panzanella, 138
    Wasabi Cucumbers, 148
Cupcakes
    Lemon Cheesecake Cupcakes, 260
    Vanilla Cupcakes with Chocolate Frosting,
        254–55
Curry
    Indian Chicken Curry, 184
    Thai Chicken Curry Soup, 160

D

Dairy intolerance, replacement foods for, 93
Dairy products
    fat in, 71
    organic, 81, 83
    wheat- and gluten-safe, 289
Dandruff, viii, 22, 36
Dates
    Date-Nut Quick Bread, 242
    Goat Cheese and Olive Stuffed Dates, 148
Deli meats, avoiding, 60, 83
Dementia, 22, 34
Depression, 22
    weight gain from, 91
    wheat-free diet relieving, 39, 194
Dermatitis herpetiformis, 22, 37, 52, 64–65, 282

Desserts. *See* Bars; Brownies; Cakes; Cookies;
        Frozen treats; Pies
Diabetes. *See also* Prediabetes
    bowel flora and, 50
    causes of, 19, 26, 29–31
    as epidemic, x
    nonwheat carbohydrates and, 44, 45
    reversing, 43, 46, 57
    type 1, 43
Diabetes medications, precautions about, 46,
        48–49
Diarrhea
    from gluten sensitivity and celiac disease, 31, 32
    with irritable bowel syndrome, 47, 51
    from wheat allergy, 14
    from wheat withdrawal, 41
Dietary sensitivities, replacement foods for, 93
Digestive problems. *See* Gastrointestinal
        problems
Dijon mustard
    Mustard Sauce, 212
Dinkel wheat, 5, 6, 7
Dips
    Almond Red Pepper Dip, 144
    Artichoke and Spinach Dip, 143
Dressing
    Cauliflower Mushroom Dressing, 197
Dried fruit, 79
Dumplings
    Chicken and Dumplings,* 161

E

Eating away from home, precautions when, 61,
        65, 282
Eczema, 14
Eggplant
    Eggplant Parmesan, 192
    Olive Oil and Balsamic Roasted Vegetables, 198
Eggs
    Breakfast Egg Biscuits,* 112
    Broccoli and Mushroom Frittata, 103
    Cheddar Egg Muffins, 111
    Cheese and Egg Quesadillas,* 101
    Good-Morning Soufflé, 104–5
    Greek Frittata, 108
    Green Chile and Chorizo Strata, 107
    Grilled Cheese Breakfast Bake, 102
    Italian Sausage Frittata, 109
    organic, 79–80

Frozen treats
    Chocolate Coconut Ice Milk, 279
    Peach Almond Frozen Yogurt, 280
Fructose, as problem sweetener, 73, 83–84. *See
    also* High-fructose corn syrup
Fruit juice, 84–85
Fruits. *See also specific fruits*
    dried, 79

G

Garbanzo bean flour, 68, 72
Gastrointestinal problems
    from wheat, 31–34
    after wheat elimination, 50–51
    wheat-free diet relieving, 46–48, 115, 194,
        223
Genetically modified organisms (GMOs), 19
Genetics of wheat, ix, xiv, 1, 2–3, 4–13, 14–15, 17,
        18, 20, 22–23, 24, 56
Ginger
    Ginger Apricot Scones, 250
    Gingerbread Cookies, 274–75
    Ginger Chicken Lettuce Cups, 130
Glia-α9 sequence, 8, 9, 11, 38
Gliadin antibody test, 55
Gliadin protein
    addictive quality of, x, 9, 26–27, 31, 38, 40, 53,
        60
    appetite stimulation from, ix, x, 9, 10–11, 19,
        26–27, 28, 31, 38, 42, 43, 73
    characteristics of, 8–9
    foods lacking, 44
    health effects from, x, 25, 34–35, 36, 53
Gluten. *See also* Wheat/gluten
    celiac disease and gluten sensitivity from,
        9–10, 31
    characteristics of, 9
    foods lacking, 44
    genetic manipulation of, 9, 10–12
    in wines, 88–89
Gluten-free cookbooks, cautions about, xiii, 294
Gluten-free ingredients, in recipes, 92, 294
Gluten-free products
    cost of, 77
    FDA criteria for, 283
    guidelines for selecting, 62
    health problems from, xiii, 63, 289
    unhealthy ingredients in, xii, 284, 289
Gluten-free snacks, 210

Gluten-sensitive individuals. *See also* Celiac
        disease sufferers
    cross-contamination concerns for, 61, 62, 64,
        65, 77
    fast-food restaurant avoidance by, 61, 65
    gluten-free products for, 62
    kitchen cleanup guidelines for, 59, 81
    precautions for, 64–65, 77
    reading food labels, 60
    resources for, 292, 293
Gluten sensitivity, 22. *See also* Celiac disease
    gluten and, 9–10
    gluten-free ingredients with, 92
    medical doubts about, 32–33
    patient story about, 281
    symptoms of, 31, 32
    testing for, 55
Glycemic index
    of common foods, 25–26
    diabetes and, 30
    of nonwheat grains, 44
GMOs, 19
Gout, dietary precautions and, 93
Grains
    wheat- and gluten-safe, 290
    whole (*see* Whole grains)
Granola
    Grainless Granola, 114
Gravy
    thickening, 67–68
    Wheat-Free Turkey Gravy, 213
Green beans
    Green Bean Casserole,* 199
    Mock Potato and Snap Bean Salad, 139
Ground golden flaxseed, 66, 68, 72
Guar gum, 80

H

Hair loss, 37, 52
Ham
    Wasabi Ham and Swiss Sandwiches, 121
Hazelnut meal, 68, 80
Healthy eating guidelines, general, 83–85
Heart attack, cause of, 26
Heartburn
    from gluten sensitivity and celiac disease, 31
    wheat-free diet relieving, 40
Heart disease, 19, 22, 26
Heart-healthy food claims, ignoring, 60

Herbs, 80
    Herbed Chicken, 182
    Herbed Focaccia, 230
    wheat- and gluten-safe, 290
High blood pressure, wheat-free diet lowering, 169
High-fructose corn syrup
    as problem sweetener, 18–19, 73, 83–84
    removing food sources of, 59
High-temperature cooking, avoiding, 85
Honey, as problem sweetener, 73, 84
Horseradish sauce
    Grilled Salmon with Horseradish Sauce, 187
Hunger
    from eating whole grains, 27
    lack of, on wheat-free diet, 40, 115, 152
Hydrogenated oils, avoiding, 85
Hypoglycemia, in diabetics eliminating wheat, 46, 48–49

I

Ice cream maker, 82
Ice milk
    Chocolate Coconut Ice Milk, 279
Indian-style dish
    Indian Chicken Curry, 184
Inflammation
    causes of, 19, 22, 26, 33, 35–36, 63
    wheat-free diet reducing, 43
Inflammatory arthritis, 54–55
Inflammatory bowel disease. See Crohn's disease;
    Ulcerative colitis
Insulin, factors increasing, 19, 26, 71, 73
Insulin resistance, 19, 26, 30, 43
Inulin, in stevia, 74, 75, 80
Irritable bowel syndrome, 22, 31, 40, 47, 51
Italian sausage
    Italian Sausage Frittata, 109

J

Joint pain, wheat-free diet relieving, 40, 54–55, 91, 169, 194, 210, 223

K

Kalamata olives
    Goat Cheese and Olive Stuffed Dates, 148
    Greek Frittata, 108
    Panzanella, 138
KAL stevia, 74

Kamut, 5–6, 7, 21, 282
Kid-friendly dishes
    appetizers
        Buffalo Chicken with Blue Cheese Sauce, 146
        Cheese Fondue, 145
        Mozzarella Sticks, 150
        Teriyaki Meatballs, 147
    breads
        Basic Bread,* 225
        Basic Focaccia,* 228–29
        Breadsticks, 236–37
        Carrot Muffins, 238–39
        Cheddar Cheese Biscuits, 246
        Date-Nut Quick Bread, 242
        Flaxseed Wrap, 231
        PB & J Bread, 244
        Peanuts Gone Wild Muffins, 240
        Walnut Raisin Bread, 243
        Wheat Belly Tortillas, 227
    breakfast
        Breakfast Egg Biscuits,* 112
        Cheddar Egg Muffins, 111
        Cheese and Egg Quesadillas,* 101
        French Toast,* 95
        Grainless Granola, 114
        Grilled Cheese Breakfast Bake, 102
        Homemade Turkey Sausage Patties, 110
        Italian Sausage Frittata, 109
        Wheat-Free Pancakes, 96–97
    desserts
        Chocolate Bars, 272
        Chocolate Chip Cookies,* 276
        Chocolate Coconut Ice Milk, 279
        Chocolate Cream Pie, 266–67
        Chocolate-Frosted Yellow Cake,* 258–59
        Gingerbread Cookies, 274–75
        Lemon Cheesecake Cupcakes, 260
        Mini Mocha Cakes, 252–53
        Mocha Walnut Brownies, 270
        Orange Cream Cookies, 278
        Peach Almond Frozen Yogurt, 280
        Peanut Butter Chocolate Chip Cookies,* 277
        Peanut Butter Pie,* 268
        Pumpkin Pie, 264–65
        Strawberry Shortcakes, 251
        Trail Mix Bars, 271
        Vanilla Cupcakes with Chocolate Frosting, 254–55

homegrown, <u>87</u>
Olive Oil and Balsamic Roasted Vegetables, 198
organic, 84
Steak and Veggie Fajita, 128
Vegetarian main dishes
Eggplant Parmesan, 192
Fettuccine Alfredo,* 191
No-Macaroni 'n Cheese, 193
Vegetarian products, wheat- or gluten-containing, 288
Vinegars, 80
balsamic
Balsamic Glazed Pork Tenderloin, 176
Olive Oil and Balsamic Roasted Vegetables, 198
Visceral fat
causes of, 19, 22, 26, 28, 63
health problems from, 19, 30
inflammation from, 36
wheat-free diet for losing, 42, 43
Vodka, 86, 89–90

W

Waffle maker, 82
Waist circumference, wheat-free diet reducing, 42, 43
Walnut meal, 66, 69, 80
Walnut oil, 71
Walnuts
Mocha Walnut Brownies, 270
Walnut Raisin Bread, 243
Wasabi
Wasabi Cream Sauce, 219
Wasabi Cucumbers, 148
Wasabi Ham and Swiss Sandwiches, 121
Water, as recommended beverage, 85
Weight gain. *See also* Overweight and obesity
diabetes and prediabetes from, 30
nonnutritive sweeteners and, 73
from wheat consumption, x, 28–29
Weight loss
from calorie reduction, 27
nonwheat carbohydrates stalling, <u>44</u>
success stories about (*see* Success stories)
from wheat elimination, xi, <u>10</u>, 30, 38, 42–43
Wheat. *See also* Wheat/gluten
addiction to, x, 26–27, 37, 40–41
allergies to, 13–15, 18, 22

Frankengrain analogy about, xiv, <u>16–17</u>
genetic alteration of, ix, xiv, 1, 2–3, 4–13, <u>14–15</u>, <u>17</u>, 18, <u>20</u>, 24, 56
future of, 22–23
health problems from, viii, 1, 19, 22, 24, 25, 55, 56
blood sugar abnormalities, 25–26
diabetes, 29–31
gastrointestinal illnesses, 31–34
inevitability of, 37, 55, 56
inflammation, 33, 35–36
neurological impairment, 22, 34–35, 282
obesity, <u>10–11</u>
skin conditions, 22, 36–37
weight gain, x, 28–29
old forms of, 5, 7, 20
Wheat- and gluten-safe foods, 289–91
shopping for, 60
Wheat belly, as visceral fat. *See* Visceral fat
Wheat Belly Bakery. *See* Baked goods
Wheat Belly Blog, 93
Wheat Belly: Lose the Wheat, Lose the Weight, and Find Your Path Back to Health, viii, ix, x
Wheat-free cookbooks, cautions about, 294
Wheat-free diet
calorie reduction from, <u>11</u>, 27, <u>86</u>
enjoyment of food in, xii–xiii
health benefits from, xi–xii, 1, 39, 41–42, 56
diabetes prevention or reversal, 30, 31, 43, 46
gastrointestinal health, 46–48, <u>115</u>, <u>194</u>, <u>223</u>
joint pain relief, 40, 54–55, <u>91</u>, <u>169</u>, <u>194</u>, <u>210</u>, <u>223</u>
nervous system health, 53–54
respiratory health, 49–51
skin improvements, 52–53, <u>91</u>, <u>141</u>, <u>194</u>, <u>223</u>
sleep improvement, 40, <u>281</u>
weight loss, xi, <u>10</u>, 38, 42–43
social media on benefits of, x–xi
subjective effects of, 39–40
success stories about (*see* Success stories)
Wheat-free foods
cost of, 77
vs. gluten-free foods, 283
scarcity of, 62–63
Wheat-free lifestyle, newness of, 93
Wheat-free resources, 292–95